AF133655

Old and New Actors and Phenomena in the Three-M Processes of Life and Society: Medicalization, Moralization and Misinformation

Old and New Actors and Phenomena in the Three-M Processes of Life and Society: Medicalization, Moralization and Misinformation

Editors

Violeta Alarcão
Sónia Cardoso Pintassilgo

MDPI • Basel • Beijing • Wuhan • Barcelona • Belgrade • Manchester • Tokyo • Cluj • Tianjin

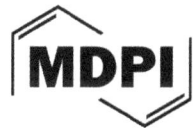

Editors
Violeta Alarcão
Iscte—Instituto Universitário de Lisboa
Portugal

Sónia Cardoso Pintassilgo
Iscte—Instituto Universitário de Lisboa
Portugal

Editorial Office
MDPI
St. Alban-Anlage 66
4052 Basel, Switzerland

This is a reprint of articles from the Special Issue published online in the open access journal *Societies* (ISSN 2075-4698) (available at: https://www.mdpi.com/journal/societies/special_issues/Life_Society).

For citation purposes, cite each article independently as indicated on the article page online and as indicated below:

LastName, A.A.; LastName, B.B.; LastName, C.C. Article Title. *Journal Name* **Year**, *Volume Number*, Page Range.

ISBN 978-3-0365-6477-7 (Hbk)
ISBN 978-3-0365-6478-4 (PDF)

© 2023 by the authors. Articles in this book are Open Access and distributed under the Creative Commons Attribution (CC BY) license, which allows users to download, copy and build upon published articles, as long as the author and publisher are properly credited, which ensures maximum dissemination and a wider impact of our publications.

The book as a whole is distributed by MDPI under the terms and conditions of the Creative Commons license CC BY-NC-ND.

Contents

About the Editors vii

Violeta Alarcão and Sónia Pintassilgo
Old and New Actors and Phenomena in the Three-M Processes of Life and Society:
Medicalization, Moralization and Misinformation
Reprinted from: *Societies* **2023**, *13*, 17, doi:10.3390/soc13010017 1

Brígida Riso
"Not Storing the Samples It's Certainly Not a Good Service for Patients": Constructing the
Biobank as a Health Place
Reprinted from: *Societies* **2022**, *12*, 113, doi:10.3390/soc12040113 5

Catarina Barata
"Mix of Races, Bad Uterus": Obstetric Violence in the Experiences of Afro-Brazilian Migrants
in Portugal
Reprinted from: *Societies* **2022**, *12*, 78, doi:10.3390/soc12030078 21

Luís Gouveia and Catarina Delaunay
'Focusing and Unfocusing'—Cognitive, Evaluative, and Emotional Dynamics in the
Relationship with Human Embryos among ART Beneficiaries
Reprinted from: *Societies* **2022**, *12*, 7, doi:10.3390/soc12010007 37

Chiara Pussetti
Because You're Worth It! The Medicalization and Moralization of Aesthetics in Aging Women
Reprinted from: *Societies* **2021**, *11*, 97, doi:10.3390/soc11030097 57

Violeta Alarcão and Bilyana Zdravkova
Attitudes and Practices towards HPV Vaccination and Its Social Processes in Europe:
An Equity-Focused Scoping Review
Reprinted from: *Societies* **2022**, *12*, 131, doi:10.3390/soc12050131 73

Alain Giami
Medicalization of Sexuality and Trans Situations: Evolutions and Transformations
Reprinted from: *Societies* **2023**, *13*, 3, doi:10.3390/soc13010003 95

Diogo Silva da Cunha and Hélder Raposo
A New Time of Reckoning, a Time for New Reckoning: Views on Health and Society, Tensions
between Medicine and the Social Sciences, and the Process of Medicalization
Reprinted from: *Societies* **2022**, *12*, 119, doi:10.3390/soc12040119 109

About the Editors

Violeta Alarcão

Violeta Alarcão, Ph.D., has extensive experience as a medical sociologist and in clinical and epidemiological research. She was a researcher at the Institute of Preventive Medicine and Public Health (IMP&SP), Faculty of Medicine of the University of Lisbon (FMUL) from 2004 to 2019, having participated in and coordinated several research projects. Currently, she is a Researcher at the Centre for Research and Studies in Sociology (CIES-Iscte) of the University Institute of Lisbon and collaborates as a researcher at the Institute of Environmental Health (ISAMB-FMUL). Her research interests are multiple and interdisciplinary, having come increasingly to include topics such as sexuality, gender, and ethnicity, from a transdisciplinary perspective.

Sónia Cardoso Pintassilgo

Sónia Cardoso Pintassilgo, Ph.D., is an Assistant Professor at the Department of Social Research Methods and Researcher at CIES-Iscte in the Family, Generations and Health reserach line. She is the co-coordinator of Laboratório de Estudos Sociais sobre o Nascimento—nascer. She is a sub-director of School of Sociology and Public Policies at Iscte—Instituto Universitário de Lisboa (ESPP-Iscte), responsible for the advisory service to students of ESPP-Iscte and has been, in recent years, President of the Jury of the M23 of the same school. She is a member of the Plenary of the Scientific Council of Iscte and of the Scientific Committee of the Department of Social Research Methods. Since 2019, she has been part of the Scientific Committee of the special competitions for access to Iscte, in the context of which, she has been contributing to the design of training responses and the monitoring of an increasingly diverse student body, aimed at improving not only access but also the academic and social experience of students. She has conducted research regarding the Demography, Population Sociology and Sociology of Birth and Motherhood.

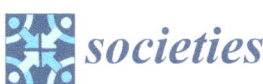

Editorial

Old and New Actors and Phenomena in the Three-M Processes of Life and Society: Medicalization, Moralization and Misinformation

Violeta Alarcão [1,2,*] and Sónia Pintassilgo [1]

[1] Centro de Investigação e Estudos de Sociologia, Instituto Universitário de Lisboa (Iscte), Avenida das Forças Armadas, 1649-026 Lisboa, Portugal
[2] Instituto de Saúde Ambiental, Faculdade de Medicina, Universidade de Lisboa, 1649-028 Lisboa, Portugal
* Correspondence: violeta_sabina_alarcao@iscte-iul.pt

Medicalization has been a key concept in the field of the sociology of health and illness over the past 50 years, capturing the expanding social control of everyday life by medical experts [1–4]. Sociologists and other social scientists have used this concept most generally to refer to a negative development of abusive medical authority in Western societies, although medical doctors are not the only agents in the medicalization process, and the relationship between the highly technoscientific biomedical and lay perspectives is multidirectional, multi-sited, and of increasing complexity in the context of pluralist and global perspectives [5–8].

In this debate, women have been typically presented as a group who are particularly vulnerable to the medicalization of their life events, health, and bodies, with pre-menstrual syndrome, menstruation, pregnancy, childbirth, and menopause being defined and treated as diseases, despite the extent to which they have actively participated in medicalization because of their own gendered, aged, classed, and race-based needs and motives [9–12]. New conditions, including many that are specific to men's experiences such as erectile dysfunction and andropause, have become subject to medicalization processes, and have been critically addressed in new studies of the medicalization of men's bodies and lives [13–16], highlighting the need for a better understanding of the multiple and intricate intersections between medicine, health, bodies, and gender. Processes of medicalization are not only part of new forms of political and economic power, but also illustrative of the redefinition of social, cultural, and moral practices.

In this Special Issue of *Societies*, a total of seven excellent articles presenting different perspectives on the medicalization of life and society are included, which contribute to the field by analyzing how people's lives, health, and illness are defined and influenced throughout life and across levels of influence by different processes of medicalization. Four of the contributions are research articles, two are concept papers, and one is a review. These articles represent the various forms of the medicalization of society, such as biobanks and biomedical research, the medicalization of pregnancy and childbirth, the medicalization and moralization of beauty and aging, the social construction of vaccination, the processes of medicalization and demedicalization, the depathologization and pharmacologization of sexuality, and the movement of medicalization critique, providing an insightful consideration of the range of complex aspects of medicalization processes and their implications for health and society. Below, we summarize the articles in order of appearance.

Riso [17] explores the construction of a biobank as a place of health, through ethnographic research and interviews of the biobank technicians, nurses, and medical doctors. Her description of the effort of the biobank staff to "humanize" the samples and to respect them as representing a person is a very interesting and innovative approach that also serves to give voice to the different emergent new professionals in the health field she interviewed. In Riso's words: "In shaping the biological samples as things in human objects, the biobank

Citation: Alarcão, V.; Pintassilgo, S. Old and New Actors and Phenomena in the Three-M Processes of Life and Society: Medicalization, Moralization and Misinformation. *Societies* **2023**, *13*, 17. https://doi.org/10.3390/soc13010017

Received: 9 January 2023
Accepted: 10 January 2023
Published: 12 January 2023

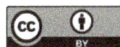

Copyright: © 2023 by the authors. Licensee MDPI, Basel, Switzerland. This article is an open access article distributed under the terms and conditions of the Creative Commons Attribution (CC BY) license (https://creativecommons.org/licenses/by/4.0/).

staff allow themselves to portray the biobank as a healthcare space and intrinsically entangled in healthcare system provision." This research represents a unique contribution to tracing the map of Portuguese biobanks, which are in their early stages.

Barata [18], in her very beautifully written and very interesting manuscript, addresses the issues of obstetric violence and racism in the Portuguese setting of obstetric care. Her research used qualitative methods and interviews with three Afro-Brazilian migrants about their perinatal experiences of obstetric care in the Portuguese public sector, between 2013 and 2019. This work contributes to revealing how multiple discriminations intertwine in reproductive healthcare and how, so often, these forms of violence operate in subtle and veiled ways. As Barata illustrates, the intersection between gender and race/coloniality is at the origin of the prejudice against Brazilian women, who seem to share the stigma of hypersexuality and the suffering of sexual violence.

Gouveia and Delaunay's [19] work represents a useful and original approach to the complexity of dealing with the varied and fluid ways in which doctors, embryologists, and beneficiaries of assisted reproductive technology (ART) think about and engage with embryos, eggs, and treatment processes. The data presented are the results from 69 interviews, both with individual users and with heterosexual and homosexual couples at different stages of their therapeutic trajectory, providing information to stimulate reflection and guide intervention to improve management, counseling, and support throughout decision-making processes involving lab-grown embryos.

Pussetti [20] presents a very interesting and thought-provoking study about gender, aging, and the perceptions of beauty. By employing in-depth ethnography and self-ethnography, the author describes the experience of the medicalization and moralization of beauty in Portuguese women aged 45–65 years, and highlights how they create personal variants of the hegemonic normative discourses on beauty and successful aging. However, as Pussetti puts it, "beauty, like youth, has an effective social value. Extending the privileges associated with beauty and youth means preserving one's own body capital to ensure social capital (social integration, the power of sexual attraction), symbolic capital (status and prestige) and economic capital (better salaries, professional mobility). Both are, however, ephemeral privileges and involve hard work, maintenance, and much economic investment, as well as suffering. At the same time, cosmetic procedures and choices are informed by cultural, economic and political structures and material inequalities."

Alarcão and Bilyana [21] present a comprehensive scoping review investigating the attitudes and practices related to HPV vaccination in Europe, with a particular focus on identifying social differences and understanding the social determinants of HPV vaccination. The authors found 28 studies discussing facilitators and barriers to immunization that took place in Europe and conclude that health-equity-focused programming is essential in promoting universal vaccination from the top down. The authors suggest that action plans to address specific perceptions and barriers towards HPV vaccination should be co-designed with the populations identified to be most at-risk, such as LGBT people, migrant and ethnic minorities, and several other populations.

Giami [22], in his concept paper, provides a very interesting analysis of the various forms of the medicalization of sexuality and gender, and demonstrates that medicalization is a very complex process, making a valuable addition to the literature. This article explores the evolution of the definition and the process of medicalization of sexuality during the second half of the 20th century, arguing that each of the different approaches studied (responses to the HIV-AIDS epidemic, conceptions of homosexuality, treatments for "sexual disorders", and gender-affirmative pathways for transgender and gender-diverse individuals) represents a particular form of medicalization, that is, a form of medicalized representation of sexuality or gender identity issues, which has social, political, economic, medical, and subjective implications. As Giami says, "while medicalization initially consisted of the medical appropriation of a field of human activity, more recent developments show how health has progressively become the foundation and justification of individual and collective moral values".

Cunha and Raposo [23], in their concept paper "A New Time of Reckoning, a Time for New Reckoning: Views on Health and Society, Tensions between Medicine and the Social Sciences, and the Process of Medicalization", provide an extensive and deep reflection with an enlarged knowledge-based orientation for standardizing the relationships between the health–illness–medicine complex and society. Their discussion of the concept of medicalization is a very useful illustration of its use in various fields, with new structures and new agents, and medicalization-related concepts, such as those of biomedicalization, camization, pharmaceuticalization, or therapeuticalization, this being indicative of the multiple contributions, the adaptative nature of the medicalization processes, and the elasticity of this concept itself.

This Special Issue has opened new directions and challenges in research and policy-making in the transforming healthcare landscape, such as the need to explore the emergence of new voices and actors in the field of biomedical research, analyzing their action possibilities, their interaction with other professionals, and the production of medical-scientific knowledge, and the need to further investigate the ethical dilemmas of the technoscientification of medicine and health care.

Author Contributions: V.A. wrote the first draft of the editorial, and S.P. provided comments and recommended amendments. All authors have read and agreed to the published version of the manuscript.

Funding: This research received no external funding.

Institutional Review Board Statement: Not applicable.

Informed Consent Statement: Not applicable.

Data Availability Statement: Not applicable.

Acknowledgments: We sincerely thank all the authors and reviewers who have participated in this Special Issue, and all the professional collaborations provided by the Editorial Office of *Societies* journal.

Conflicts of Interest: The authors declare no conflict of interest.

References

1. Zola, I.K. Medicine as an Institution of Social Control. *Sociol. Rev.* **1972**, *20*, 487–504. [CrossRef] [PubMed]
2. Conrad, P. Medicalization and Social Control. *Annu. Rev. Sociol.* **1992**, *18*, 209–232. [CrossRef]
3. Crawford, R. Healthism and the Medicalization of Everyday Life. *Int. J. Health Serv.* **1980**, *10*, 365–388. [CrossRef] [PubMed]
4. Busfield, J. The concept of medicalisation reassessed. *Sociol. Health Illn.* **2017**, *39*, 759–774. [CrossRef] [PubMed]
5. Conrad, P. The Shifting Engines of Medicalization. *J. Health Soc. Behav.* **2005**, *46*, 3–14. [CrossRef] [PubMed]
6. Clarke, A.E.; Shim, J.K.; Mamo, L.; Fosket, J.R.; Fishman, J.R. Biomedicalization: Technoscientific Transformations of Health, Illness, and U.S. Biomedicine. *Am. Sociol. Rev.* **2003**, *68*, 161–194. [CrossRef]
7. Correia, T. Revisiting Medicalization: A Critique of the Assumptions of What Counts As Medical Knowledge. *Front. Sociol.* **2017**, *2*, 14. [CrossRef]
8. Williams, S.J.; Coveney, C.; Gabe, J. The concept of medicalisation reassessed: A response to Joan Busfield. *Sociol. Health Illn.* **2017**, *39*, 775–780. [CrossRef]
9. Gabe, J.; Calnan, M. The limits of medicine: Women's perception of medical technology. *Soc. Sci. Med.* **1989**, *28*, 223–231. [CrossRef]
10. Riessman, C.K. Women and medicalization: A new perspective. *Soc. Policy* **1983**, *14*, 3–18.
11. Brubaker, S.J.; Dillaway, H.E. Medicalization, Natural Childbirth and Birthing Experiences. *Sociol. Compass.* **2009**, *3*, 31–48. [CrossRef]
12. Pintassilgo, S.; Carvalho, H. Trends and consequences of the technocratic paradigm of childbirth in Portugal: A population-based analysis of birth conditions and social characteristics of parents. *Sex. Reprod. Healthc.* **2017**, *13*, 58–67. [CrossRef] [PubMed]
13. Loe, M. *The Rise of Viagra: How the Little Blue Pill Changed Sex in America*; New York University Press: New York, NY, USA, 2004.
14. Marshall, B.L.; Katz, S. Forever Functional: Sexual Fitness and the Ageing Male Body. *Body Soc.* **2002**, *8*, 43–70. [CrossRef]
15. Wentzell, E. Aging respectably by rejecting medicalization: Mexican men's reasons for not using erectile dysfunction drugs. *Med. Anthropol. Q.* **2013**, *27*, 3–22. [CrossRef]
16. Alarcão, V.; Roxo, L.; Virgolino, A.; Machado, F.L. The Intimate World of Men's Sexual Problems: Portuguese Men's and Women's Narratives Explicated Through a Mixed Methods Approach. *Sex. Cult.* **2015**, *19*, 543–560. [CrossRef]

17. Riso, B. "Not Storing the Samples It's Certainly Not a Good Service for Patients": Constructing the Biobank as a Health Place. *Societies* **2022**, *12*, 113. [CrossRef]
18. Barata, C. "Mix of Races, Bad Uterus": Obstetric Violence in the Experiences of Afro-Brazilian Migrants in Portugal. *Societies* **2022**, *12*, 78. [CrossRef]
19. Gouveia, L.; Delaunay, C. "Focusing and Unfocusing"—Cognitive, Evaluative, and Emotional Dynamics in the Relationship with Human Embryos among ART Beneficiaries. *Societies* **2022**, *12*, 7. [CrossRef]
20. Pussetti, C. Because You're Worth It! The Medicalization and Moralization of Aesthetics in Aging Women. *Societies* **2021**, *11*, 97. [CrossRef]
21. Alarcão, V.; Zdravkova, B. Attitudes and Practices towards HPV Vaccination and Its Social Processes in Europe: An Equity-Focused Scoping Review. *Societies* **2022**, *12*, 131. [CrossRef]
22. Giami, A. Medicalization of Sexuality and Trans Situations: Evolutions and Transformations. *Societies* **2023**, *13*, 3. [CrossRef]
23. da Cunha, D.S.; Raposo, H. A New Time of Reckoning, a Time for New Reckoning: Views on Health and Society, Tensions between Medicine and the Social Sciences, and the Process of Medicalization. *Societies* **2022**, *12*, 119. [CrossRef]

Disclaimer/Publisher's Note: The statements, opinions and data contained in all publications are solely those of the individual author(s) and contributor(s) and not of MDPI and/or the editor(s). MDPI and/or the editor(s) disclaim responsibility for any injury to people or property resulting from any ideas, methods, instructions or products referred to in the content.

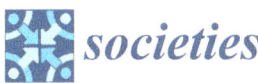

Article

"Not Storing the Samples It's Certainly Not a Good Service for Patients": Constructing the Biobank as a Health Place

Brígida Riso [1,2,3]

[1] Faculdade de Medicina, Universidade de Lisboa, Avenida Professor Egas Moniz, 1649-028 Lisboa, Portugal; brigida.riso@medicina.ulisboa.pt
[2] Instituto de Saúde Ambiental, Faculdade de Medicina, Universidade de Lisboa, 1649-028 Lisboa, Portugal
[3] Iscte—Instituto Universitário de Lisboa, CIES-Iscte, 1649-026 Lisboa, Portugal

Abstract: Biobanks have been established from the beginning of the millennium as relevant infrastructures to support biomedical research. These repositories have also transformed the paradigm of collecting and storing samples and associated clinical data, moving these practices from the healthcare services and research laboratories to dedicated services. In Portugal, the establishment of biobanks is happening in the absence of a specific legal framework, turning it difficult to fully understand the scope of their action. This ethnographic research explored how establishing a biobank challenges the dynamics between healthcare and biomedical research. The ethnography intended to follow the path of biological samples from the hospital, where they were collected, to the biobank in a research institute, where they were stored. Findings suggest that although the nature of the biobank's technical work seemed to inscribe it as a research-oriented setting, the biobank's daily work was performed through symbolic action in the logic of care. Biobank staff constantly recalled the human nature of the samples, and they built complex illness narratives of each sample, promoting a connection with the absent donor. These practices were crucial to constructing the biobank as a health place, one that was designed to be life-saving in the near future.

Keywords: biobank; health; human biological samples; biomedical research; ethnography; caring practices; illness narratives; Portugal (study context)

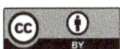

1. Introduction

This article explores the construction of a biobank as a health place. Biobanks, for the collection and storage of biological samples associated with clinical data, have played a major role in the last decades in supporting the development of biomedical research. Moving forward to a post-Human Genome Project Era, laboratory medicine and biomedical research are now focused on genetics and genomics. This turn into genomics was accompanied by the dissemination of large samples as a way of acquiring statistical significance [1], reflecting medicine's biology-centered approach. Conducting such massive research projects implied the study of a large number of samples and clinical data. Biobanks are crucial for this task, providing storage facilities that enable gathering a significant number of samples and their maintenance for long periods of time. Although medical and biomedical research already have a long tradition of samples and data collection from the beginning of the century, currently, these infrastructures have scaled in number and dimension. The size is actually one of the major differences from the previous repositories used by individual doctors and small research teams, which have led to debates over ethical, legal, and social issues [1].

Biobanks collect a wide range of samples such as blood, tissues removed in surgeries or biopsies, saliva, hair, teeth, and feces, among others, and these would be, in most of the cases, given by donors voluntarily[1] aiming to contribute for the advancement of biomedical research. Regardless of their health status, every person could be a biobank donor with different attributes or functions. Biobanks store these large amounts of medical information and biological samples collected in healthcare services to be used in biomedical research. These two contexts—healthcare services and research laboratories—have a significant role in determining the chain of procedures through which samples are collected and organized.

Different countries have been setting up their biobanks differently. From national to local initiatives, biobanks vary in size, shape, and in their governance models [2].

In Portugal, biobanking activities are starting to be established and finding their way into the context of scientific research; however, they are quite under-covered. In fact, the existence of biobanks remains unknown to most medical practitioners and researchers. Currently, the existing biobank initiatives are fragmented and do not correspond to any organized strategy at the local or national levels. Even in institutions that host biobanks, these are more of a project from a small team or group of medical doctors or researchers than an institutional enterprise [3]. Without a dedicated legal framework, biobanks are emerging in hospitals, research institutes, and universities. However, it is not yet entirely clear which characteristics they should have: how do biobanks operate, or under which jurisdiction should they be placed? The latter is key to understanding aspects that may influence the organization model, the funding programs, and the rules that apply to biobanks. Biobanks are often found in a vacuum, making it more difficult to delimit their nature, attributions, or potential. Most of them are organized within a research framework, being settled as research services. Nevertheless, the dependence on healthcare services and the fact that many biobanks were created at hospitals by medical doctors blurs the picture of how these actors and institutions interact when it comes to organizing a biobank.

This research aimed to explore the organization of work in a biobank and to comprehend how it was constructed as infrastructure at the intersection of Health and Science. In the first instance, the rise of biomedicine and its research techniques are discussed, explaining how it enabled the establishment of biobanks. Then, the development of biobanks in Portugal is presented to frame the challenges and the questions posed by this research, reflecting on the role of medical doctors and life-sciences researchers in such an effort. The results are presented reflecting on three main findings: (i) how the work in the biobank makes use of medical categories to organize biological samples and data; (ii) how samples are constructed by a human and what this definition implies in working at the biobank; (iii) how the production of illness narratives based on biological samples contributes to producing practices of care in the context of the biobank. To conclude, these practices are discussed as being crucial to constructing the biobank as a health place.

1.1. Setting the Scene for the Emergence of Biobanks for Health and Biomedical Research

Medicine has always made use of bodies and body parts for studying, teaching, and research. However, in recent decades there has been an increasing need to draw on large sets of human biological samples and produce data in a systematic way to cope with the growing needs of biomedical research.

In order to understand these changes, it might be worth reflecting on the work of Clarke et al. [4]. The authors argued that the turn into biomedicine and biomedicalization was due to a number of transformations that have marked the way of performing, learning, and presenting medicine. In the name of health, life has become an object and an end in itself [4,5]. These transformations were connected mostly to technological developments, such as the appearance of powerful computers and informatics. Computer technology has facilitated the collection and the use of larger amounts of data and the refinement of statistics applied to life sciences. Although these changes began to insinuate themselves after World War II, it is possible to recognize several initiatives of considerable scales, such as the Framingham Heart Study[2] in the United States or the Varmland Health Survey[3], which took place in Sweden. It was at the end of the 20th century that this way of investigating and producing medical-scientific knowledge gained greater visibility through the Human Genome Project. For this reason, it was after this moment that the appearance of more and larger repositories of biological samples to support the intensification of this form of research was rendered more evident. Current research uses large amounts of systematic information, aggregated in databases, as a way to ensure the robustness of scientific evidence in biomedicine and requires an increased storage capacity, both samples and information, requiring technological devices that allow accessing and managing these data [1]. Moreover, it stresses the biological understanding of the disease processes by applying the logic of biology to medical research.

However, the approximation of Medicine to Biology, which had already been hinting since the beginning of the 19th century, had become more evident through the sharing of the laboratory [6]. In this line, Jewson [7] noted that people were no longer the object of medicine; however, the human body has maintained its value as a resource for developing medical knowledge. The influence of Biology progressively extends to language and the way of investigating the body [8]. Against this backdrop, the use of data science becomes more recurrent, as biology has also come to incorporate an important strand of biostatistics and bioinformatics [9]. Statistics as a source of scientific knowledge had already been used in medicine since the early 18th century by collecting information about the state of populations [10,11]. This was even more pronounced in the transition to biomedicine, which brought with it the normality of the body based on statistics. Statistics are produced by comparison with the population considered healthy [11], becoming criteria for defining disease status [12]. The *medical gaze* [13] is now transformed, in the words of Rose [14], into a *molecular gaze*. As noted by Sharp [15], the increased claims for body parts by biomedical researchers contribute to the fragmentation of the medicalized body and, at the same time, promote their commodification. Thus, body parts, namely human biological samples, are still quite useful for the study of physiology and cellular mechanisms, helping to understand disease in biomedical research. The body is, in this paradigm, seen as a complex organization of molecules to be studied. In some cases, genetic testing (both in clinical contexts and self-performed, e.g., direct-to-consumer tests) is defining new ways of dealing with one's body and disease [16], reconstructing self-identity [17], and even mediating the relationship between the nation state and citizens [18–20].

Another important transformation of medical research within this period, signaled by Rose [14], was the emergence of non-medical research professionals conducting research in life sciences. This approach to the life sciences implied an integration of knowledge from other scientific areas and the incorporation of research practices that were not so common in medical practice until then. In this line, the crescent specialization of biobanks is seen by the construction of a specific body of knowledge reflected in scientific articles dedicated to the topic, a scientific journal dedicated to biobanks, and best practices in samples' preservation is a recurring theme at biobanks conferences.

This changing paradigm of biomedical research set the scene for the emergence of greater repositories of samples and clinical data. Biobanks such as deCODE in Iceland and the UK Biobank in the United Kingdom were two big biobanks storing millions of biological samples and clinical data. The appearance of networks such as BBMRI-ERIC (*Biobanking and Biomolecular Resources Research Infrastructure—European Research Infrastructure Consortium*) at the European level that gathers biobanks from all over Europe are also signals of the recent developments in this field.

1.2. The Emergence of Portuguese Biobanks

In Portugal, biobanks are in their early stages. In 2021, there were 16 initiatives: some of them were already in place, and others were just an intention to open a biobank in the near future. Organizing a biobank demands a wide range of resources alongside institutional support. Nevertheless, the low level of recognition of biobanks within the scientific community makes biobanks to be projected by small teams of researchers or medical doctors that mobilize their own resources to organize their own biobanks. Although the growth of initiatives possibly points to a crescent recognition, the existent biobanks are still underused by researchers. In many cases, there is no solid institutional support or a strategic mission that informs the constitution of a new biobank. The absence of a legal framework or a national strategy for biobanks is also problematic—not only because their scope of action is unclear but also because it limits their development. Since biobanks are neither a research project nor a research institution, nor are they considered a health service, they cannot benefit from grants or apply for the more common funding opportunities in the field of healthcare [3]. The lack of specific funding has been seen as a lack of investment in health research. To date, there are some fragmented strategies to stimulate healthcare research, but there has never been a true scientific health research policy in Portugal [21].

In the last 30 years, health research in Portugal has had an impulse through the establishment of relevant research institutions that try to settle upon the intersection of medicine and fundamental research. However, this is a recent and circumscribed phenomenon, and its impact is not yet visible in the biobanks landscape. The investment in health research is poor, with the Health Authorities recognizing the low level of interest in health research [22]. This opened the way for life sciences researchers to develop their research in the health domain. In 2010, it was already clear that doctoral and post-doctoral scholarships in the field of medical and health sciences have come to value mainly biomedical research, where there is no involvement of patients [23].

The management of the biobank itself demands knowledge of laboratory procedures and is mainly carried out by technicians with training in life sciences, and not so much by doctors since many of them do not have the knowledge to operate at this level. This fact is noteworthy since if, on the one hand, doctors seem to be increasingly distant from laboratory research, on the other hand, they still hold leadership positions in these infrastructures [3].

Doctors are still indispensable when it comes to collecting samples through the recruitment of donors. Additionally, considering the legal framework into force that might relate to collecting samples for research [24], only medical doctors could request samples to be used in clinical research. Medical doctors still have a relevant presence in Portuguese society, and they are considered authorities when it comes to health matters [25]. Interestingly, this fact is in line with the expectations of Portuguese citizens reported by Gaskell et al. [26], where 45% place the physician as being an adequate person responsible for protecting the public interest in this field (the highest value of the 27 countries surveyed), followed by researchers (13.2%).

In 2018, there was an attempt to produce an updated legal framework for biomedical research[4], where biobanks could be included and where the most relevant funding agency in Portugal excluded biobanks from its scope of activities, pushing biobanks to the jurisdiction of health authorities. The bill did not come into force; however, these discussions among the possible authorities in charge of biobanks illustrate how difficult it has been to define the domain to which biobanks belong.

Despite these difficulties, some biobank projects have succeeded. However, the heterogenous nature of local and national-level initiatives, and the profusion of actors with changing roles and interests, make it difficult to understand what the biobank attributions are.

2. Materials and Methods

This article reports findings from an ethnographic study [27] performed in a biobank. Latour's advice to follow the actors [28] was considered in order to clarify the workflow of a biobank and the relationships it generates between different social actors. This ethnography was based on the premise of following the samples' trajectory from their collection to storage and their distribution to researchers. Following the samples' path allowed for data collection to focus on the interactions, connections, and relationships that are created and sustained by the biobank activities. As a method, ethnography demands observing and being present (or co-present [29]) to go beyond an immediate observation of practices and to uncover their meanings and how they interrelate.

Observing the biobank daily routine implied spending around two years in the biobank context. Observations made during this fieldwork were systematically registered in a fieldwork diary, which was the main source of data production.

Other researchers used the ethnographic method to study biobanks, such as Argudo-Portal and Domènech in Spain [30]; Stiefel in France [31]; or Stephens, Atkinson, and Glasner in the United Kingdom [32]. Although there are differences in their goals and approaches, their work led to relevant conclusions regarding the biobank's work organization or the way biobanks are organized in wider networks, affirming ethnography as a relevant methodology for the study of biobanks.

The particular biobank where this research was carried out was integrated into a healthcare university campus, sharing the space of a medical university and a university hospital. The biobank was located in a room of one of the leading Portuguese biomedical research institutes. The biobank is conceptualized as a facility of the research institute, and its activities took place across different rooms of the research institute building— the harvesting room, where donors came to give samples; the paper data storage room; and the storage facility. Moreover, part of the facilities needed for the daily work of the biobank were shared with the research units of the institute, such as the washing room, flow cytometry, or the histology laboratory.

Medical doctors and basic researchers shared laboratory spaces within the research institute, and many sample collections were medical doctors' responsibility—these doctors were both medical practitioners and researchers. This biobank stored a diverse range of samples from blood, hair, saliva, aqueous humor, bone, and tumors, among others.

In an exploratory stage of research, the biobank was presented as being organized and dependent on healthcare, despite its location in the research institute. This was made clear by the biobank technical director and the head of the biobank, who was a medical doctor at that time. This idea was embodied in the collection of biological samples in the health services, in the medical responsibility for the biobank, and in the initiation of new collections by doctors. Hence, based on this assumption, it was expected that entering the field would be difficult and experience a possible resistance, as described by ethnographic studies in healthcare settings in Portugal (see, for example, [33,34]). The reality turned out to be different with a very welcoming and straightforward start of the fieldwork in the biobank space, which contributes to a deeper reflection and problematization of the biobank as a "healthcare service".

The permanent staff of the biobank was two biochemists and one clinical analyst technician. Biobank technicians spent an important part of their day going to the university hospital to bring samples to be stored in the biobank. This movement was also a symbolic one when bringing the samples to the biobank; samples were disconnected from the healthcare setting and could be integrated into the biobank circuits. Notwithstanding, the biobank was not totally connected or totally separated from these two worlds of scientific research and healthcare. The daily routine of the biobank staff demanded long hours in the biobank designated space where the storage unit was located. This space comprises a laboratory bench area for preparing samples and an office-like area with computers. It also includes the already mentioned storage space where the freezers were isolated from the other spaces with a false wall and door, the isolated area where procedures considered cleaner were performed (for instance, Peripheral Blood Mononuclear Cells isolation) with specific technical equipment as a laminar flow cabinet.

In this space, contrasting with the colors of the cryogenic tube caps—even considered *photogenic* (fieldnotes)—the biobank atmosphere related to the laboratory idea: an image of brightness, extreme asepsis, and free of contaminants. Despite some minor differences, the biobank was not that different from other laboratory spaces within the research institute, where it was integrated.

The data were generated by setting up the biobank as a place for observation for two years, from 2016 to 2018, considering periods of intermittent observation that allowed them to go from the circumscribed shared space of the biobank to other settings where the biobank technicians developed their activities.

Being at the biobank included the observation of daily routine, including activities such as seminars, conferences, and presentations in health events, among others. It also included being present on biobank open days, when biobank technicians collect samples in public and private institutions in order to recruit donors to obtain control samples for research. This allowed the construction of a place of observation that was not confined to the biobank site. Although other spaces might have been chosen for setting the fieldwork, the biobank was supposed to be referential in the process of sample transformation [35,36] and might eventually be defined as an obligatory passage point [37] in sample trajectory.

The ethnography was preceded by a set of 17 exploratory interviews with biobank coordinators that allowed tracing the map of Portuguese biobanks. The data presented here also refer, when relevant, to the data collected at that stage.

Fieldnotes were the main source of data, reporting not only the daily life in the biobank but also including data generated by watching TV programs, checking the biobank's Facebook profile and posts, news (published mostly on the web), and biobank-produced documents such as posters and leaflets. During fieldwork, interviews were carried out with different actors working closely with the biobank, such as nurses, researchers, scientific committee members, biobank directors, and the former director.

The study was granted authorization by the biobank direction. All actors involved have expressed their consent. The research project was explained to all interviewees, and permission to record and use anonymized data in the dissemination of research results was requested. All the interviews were recorded and transcribed verbatim. Only one interviewee did not allow to record the interview, although they gave permission to use the data. All the material was gathered in MaxQDA version 12 software, enabling a systematic data analysis by themes. All the quotations cited in the text were translated from Portuguese to English by the author.

The next section reports the findings of the research, drawing upon the generated data: fieldnotes and interviews—making use of some illustrative quotes brought directly from the fieldwork diary and the interviews conducted during the fieldwork.

3. Results

3.1. A Medical Framework to Classify Samples

Biobank staff was responsible for the organization and storage of samples. In this regard, classifications recurring to health and illness frameworks were common and central to the work organization. Other management decisions, such as the ones concerning the quality of the samples, the samples to be discarded due to technical conditions, or decisions about sample viability, only depend on the biobank staff's judgment. Samples could, for example, be labeled as infected, diseased, or healthy.

Biological samples were classified according to the part of the body from which they are taken: a bladder, a kidney, a testicle, a carotid artery, a synovial membrane, even if the sample is only part of these organs or anatomical structures. In other cases, they are DNA, RNA, tumors, and cells, according to their typology. These simple classifications reveal different classification systems—some favoring body anatomy, more frequently used in the healthcare sphere, while others are more commonly used in the laboratory sphere. The imposition of reasonably stabilized classification grids also rendered the donor's body into a sample object, which is simpler and easier to manage.

In the day-to-day work, questions about the nature of the samples arise: alive, dead, animal, human, healthy, sick, infected, or not infected are classifications that arise with a certain regularity and that are determinant in or determined by the daily practices of the Biobank. These classifications are, for the most part, changeable and not always obvious. Their complexity is, in many cases, interconnected with essential categories such as dead/living, mortal/immortal, animal/human, or even infected/non-infected, stable/unstable, visible/invisible, healthy/sick. These sets, which apparently constitute opposites, are commonly used in day-to-day life, and throughout the ethnographic observation, it became more evident that they were not necessarily configured as opposing poles but could even coexist in the same sample or in the same reality. This complexity of classifications and articulations also refers to the symbolic domain of the body, to a set of other possibilities that are being created through the biological samples [5,38]. Sometimes the classification of biological samples is clearly determined by the donor; sometimes, it is determined by the analysis of the biological sample itself and its use.

Infected and non-infected is an obvious example of categorization of biological samples, determined a priori by the infected or non-infected status of the donor and imply the medical definition of infection. The classification regarding the infection of the sample is perhaps one of the most obvious and has a direct impact on the processing of biological samples at the Biobank. This classification precedes the entry of the biological sample into the Biobank and is determined by the patient's laboratory tests and then conveyed by the physician. An infected sample designates, in a very general way, samples that may carry in themselves the potential of infecting laboratory technicians in their manipulation, which may lead to the contraction of a certain disease. Thus, biological samples from patients with HIV and hepatitis are considered in this group of infected biological samples. This classification does not depend on systematic verification. Some health services tend to have more patients with these pathologies and are more easily identified; therefore, the biological samples are identified as such. However, in case these pathologies are unknown, the sample is not classified as infected. Therefore, the infection status of the biological sample is not always known to the techniques at the time of entry into the biobank.

On these occasions, the work of the Biobank is completely determined by the categorization attributed in the clinical context to the biological samples. In these circumstances, the encounter with the physician is determinant in the definition of these categories [39,40]. Infection is not macroscopically visible and is not always implicated in disease pathology; therefore, it is necessary to rely on the assessment that is performed in a medical context, admitting that it is not always possible to be in possession of such knowledge.

The contact with biological products, either by spilling fluids or by cutting with the same blade that has already been used in the manipulation of biological material, exposes the Biobank staff to risk, bringing them momentarily closer to the patient's bodily reality.

Another essential category in everyday life is whether the sample is precisely "healthy or diseased". Although this category refers primarily to the status of the donor, it is commonly used to refer to biological samples—a healthy sample is a frequent terminology.

In the health care context, only samples from patients are collected, whereas on days organized by the Biobank, samples are collected from *healthy* people. This option is often called into question as the health status of the healthy is often corrupted with various pathologies.

> "We ask the responsible researcher what kind of control he wants, and they give us the criteria of what is healthy for them. Usually, the ones that are healthy are the ones that don't have the disease under study." Biobank technician, Fieldnotes.

The categorization of healthy or sick seems to refer more to the comparative function that certain biological samples may play in scientific research. Moreover, underlying this classification is the place where the biological sample is collected. If the sample is collected in health care units, it is considered a patient sample, and it is included in collections dedicated to certain projects. If, on the contrary, the biological sample is collected as part of an action for the dissemination and promotion of the Biobank, as happens in the aforementioned open days, that sample is considered healthy. Moreover, it sometimes happens that the declaration of healthy is contradictory to what is considered "healthy" at the laboratory level, reminding us that there are several ways to materialize the disease [41].

> "Look, it was a sample that came supposedly from a healthy control and when I went to do the cell count, there were almost none. That person couldn't be healthy." Fieldnotes.

The healthy and diseased category is often decided a priori, usually not depending on a laboratory analysis for diagnosis or for assignment of such category. Thus, donors who come into contact with the Biobank on open days are naturally integrated into the sample collection of "healthy controls". There is no prerequisite in this case except wanting to donate the biological sample. Various categories are assigned using a medical classification system, which often includes the samples in collections with the name of the pathology "they carry". The medical categories are then transported to the laboratory, and there is not necessarily an immediate or direct correspondence in the classification that is assigned in the Biobank. It should also be added that these categories are not necessarily stable, being regularly redefined in the process of laboratory treatment of the biological samples. Even if the sample is subject to unforeseen conditions, it may still meet the criteria to be used in another way.

Even technical procedures carry medical categories. For example, the implemented system of color classification, with the goal of quickly identifying to which biobank collection a particular sample belongs when opening the freezers. The colored caps of cryogenic tubes indicate, e.g., red for cardiac pathology, black for cirrhosis, transparent for healthy donors, orange for tumors, etc. This is also referred to by Palmer [42] as a way of objectification; it was crystallized in the idea expressed by a journalist who visited the biobank in the news headline "In the biobank, diseases have the colors of the rainbow" (published on 14th October 2017, in a widely read Portuguese newspaper). The metaphor continued throughout the text, enforcing the idea of the absence of the donor and the diseases as being relevant subjects. These classifications enabled a link between health and illness context; additionally, they reduced the multidimensional aspects of the ill-health status of the donor.

The categorization of biological samples often carries the categories assigned to donors, such as infected or non-infected. In other cases, the classifications assigned to the donor and to the sample may be dependent or independent, displaying the donor and sample against each other in the coincidence or mismatch of the categories assigned. Medical categories are thus essential to classify and organize not only samples but to define the work in the biobank.

3.2. Constructing Biological Samples Identities as Being Human

The collection of samples to the biobank regularly encompasses three moments —harvesting, storing, and distributing the samples to biomedical research—around which the biobanking activities are organized. The identity of samples is therefore constructed while they are progressing through this path. The construction of the samples' identity was a constant process of negotiation, and biobank technicians played a relevant role in performing this negotiation in different situations.

The sample collection was additionally accompanied by a collection of lifestyle and clinical data. Usually, medical doctors collect clinical data during medical appointments or pre-surgery procedures. Then, the biobank technicians would pick the samples and clinical data survey, and the informed consent form at the hospital. The biobank staff was rarely responsible for the data and sample collection. They were, in all circumstances, responsible for managing data and samples in the biobank space. When the samples entered the biobank, they needed to be organized and added to the computer system. Both data and samples were collected together, although they entered two different sectors in the biobank software, and the connection between the donor and the samples started to disappear.

Although the linkage between samples and the donor could be replaced, it was partially destroyed at the moment biobank staff entered sample data and donor data into the software. Additionally, pseudonymization was another essential process to silence the connection between donor and data (sample and personal/lifestyle information). The link could only be restored in case the donor asks for withdrawal or if researchers need more data and the donor has consented to be recontacted in this regard. Right before they were no longer identifiable, biobank technicians have the last opportunity to connect the sample to the donor they did not meet, avoiding immediately transforming the sample into an object. Right before they were no longer identifiable, biobank technicians have the last opportunity to connect the sample to the donor they did not meet or had any other previous have not met, then refusing immediately transform the sample into an object.

> *During a technical procedure of processing samples, one technician says to another: "This cannot be like that, please cover the "ruizinho" [allusion to the donor's real name] otherwise he will get a cold." Fieldnotes.*

Not only does the origin of the biological sample seem to be difficult to forget [42], but also the links to the original donor should not be forgotten, although the process of pseudonymization is about to happen. In all the cases, samples were considered to be objects but from a special kind:

> *"I do think it is humanization in the sense of transformation that sample in a human thing". Senior Researcher, interview.*

After samples were processed and stored in the biobank were mentioned as *work material* for researchers. Furthermore, from this moment on, sample management entered a field ruled by principal investigators and medical doctors. Researchers and medical doctors were the ones deciding in which collection the samples were going to be included, in what research they were going to be used and with which researcher samples could be shared, and under which specific conditions. While the Portuguese Legal Framework [24] defines donors as the owners of the biological material, they were no longer responsible for the usage of the sample after they entered the biobanking circuits (unless they desired to withdraw the sample and data). Giving back the property of the samples was also something recalling for the donor—and was not only because it is enforced by law to obtain donor informed consent but also because it was embedded in technician discourses as being the natural and obvious thing to do.

To classify the tissue and cell status, biobank technicians evaluate whether the cells are viable or non-viable and which biological samples could be considered alive or dead. These classifications enable the decision about the quality of samples, type of storage, or type of laboratory analyses that could be performed. The classification relies exclusively on biological material analysis and works apart from donor status. Therefore, biological samples and donors could have different classifications, somewhat ensuring their separation as different entities.

The transformation of samples into human objects was particularly evident when denying samples of possible animal nature. This issue was central in the negotiations of samples' humanness. In some particular cases, such as the case of feces-microbiome preservation, the boundary between two categories was made clear, however allowing the combination of both natures in one entity at the same time.

> *"The problem is that microbiome has human and microbial material, that's why we need to ask two different entities for allowing us to store feces." Biobank technical supervisor, fieldnotes.*

Metzler and Webster [43] mentioned the tendency to consider these entities as human subjects even though their boundaries could be difficult to be considered an asset. If in the precise situation of the microbiome, the boundaries seemed clear, usually they appeared blurred, and the human nature of samples prevails. The boundary was made obvious when the biobank workers were confronted with certain questions about the nature of the samples stored in the biobank.

> *"Here we only have human samples. The closest we have to animal samples are the tumors that we insert in rats and when they grow, they are removed [and kept in the biobank]. But this is still considered as human tissue.—Explained the biobank supervisor to a technician from another biobank who went for a visit." Fieldnotes.*

The boundary between animal and human was again repositioned, though denying the possibility of mixing the natures of the samples again. The boundary was not that clear, but biobank-involved professionals tried, consistently, in diverse moments, to assure the biological samples were human. These biological samples seem to be what Douglas called "a matter out of place" [44]. In this sense, they should be forced to integrate a manageable and already existing category of objects and beings that perfectly fit the previous categorization in action. Therefore, not only the former categories were conserved, but they also enabled the removal of the particular legislation, which provided specific rules to store animal samples. Here, the legal framework does not consider both natures and to what extent these samples should be incorporated into different categories [45].

In addition to the constant denial of a possible animal identity of the samples or avoiding deleting the linkage between the original donor and the biological sample, there were other strategies powered in the daily routine work contributing to setting this human identity.

3.3. Crafting Illness Narratives

The biobank technicians' efforts to defend biological samples stored in the biobank as being human are a result of pushing boundaries that maintain the control and the management rules of the biobank.

Moreover, samples were observed mostly as scientific objects when the link between the sample and other personal data was hidden in order to preserve the donor's identity. Nevertheless, other links are to be created and told.

Kopytoff [46] and Daston [47] suggested that objects could have different biographies, depending on a variety of circumstances, from the object owner's relationship with the object to the cultural setting or the time when it was produced. Similarly, samples also could have their own biography, and biobank workers were involved in their crafting while they processed and stored samples. Samples in themselves were enough to say something about their own trajectory. The sample's appearance could reflect the status of the disease at a given moment. They settled the link between the sample and the donor's disease status. Lawrence [48] described how body parts transformed into relics are embedded in spiritual auras that were passed from the saint to the body part. Here, the donor gives the sample; there is no knowledge or little knowledge about the donor. Thus, she provides the sample with the disease or healthy status, and then all storytelling must be made.

> "For example, this sample, it's not the worst sample at all, but we can see that the patient has been through chemotherapy or radiotherapy [holding a blood tube and looking carefully searching for details]. I could be wrong, but it should be something like that." Biobank technician, Fieldnotes.

In line with Mol [41], this could be another picture of how the disease could be perceived or, in her words, how the disease is enacted. The biological samples enable the construction and projection of the patient disease trajectory. When the biobank staff receives samples from the same donor at different time points, which they call follow-up samples, the narratives turn into more complex stories.

> "In other cases, we have samples from a patient, and we are receiving samples and one day we realize that we are not having samples anymore from that donor and usually is not because he decided to stop giving samples, usually it's because he died ... " Biobank technician, fieldnotes.

The narration is assisted by the biological properties of biological samples in conjunction with personal experiences. Moreover, the biobank staff tended to connect with their own experiences of life, health, and illness, creating a sense of identification with patient trajectory.

> "By the time of my first pregnancy, we were collecting samples for a study with neurotumors and neurological diseases in a pediatrics study. Sometimes I substituted the researcher in duty, doing the medical surveys to parents. I could not remember if the question was there or if it was something that parents mention spontaneously, but I remember so many parents mentioned the labor duration or situations that happen during

labor . . . I started to put all pieces together and started wondering . . . how it is going to be my labor and how it could influence my child health. It was such a hard time." Biobank technician, Fieldnotes.

This contact between biobank staff and donors, especially patients, was rare. When other professionals, such as medical doctors or nurses, collaborate with the biobank in samples or data collection and establish their narratives around the donors' experiences, they often use this contact with the patient in the narrative construction.

"I remember exactly the person [donor]. When I start entering the data [on the computer] "Oh, this one"—because I have the social-demographic data and the profession and helps me to remember. And also, because I'm going there requesting the consent form, after I do the follow up. Then I know who they are and sometimes it's such a pity because some of them died and I really remember them, young people, and makes me wonder . . . " Nurse—researcher, interview.

The narrative inquiry has a long tradition of exploring illness in social sciences [49]. Usually, the narratives are produced by patients but also by health professionals, namely medical doctors, in order to better comprehend the patient's suffering or experience [46]. Here, instead, the biobank staff constructed narratives for their own purposes of making sense of their work in a wider context of health and illness.

3.4. Taking Care of Biological Samples

By entering the categories of human beings, occasionally with a story, the biological samples were then in place of being cared for. Not only biobank staff but other actors involved as medical doctors or researchers acknowledged that humanness in samples should be recalled and have implications when it comes to research. The implications were mainly related to the research practice.

"So, when we use that sample [referring to a human sample] we have the responsibility and an ethical duty of be sure what we are going to do justify the usage of that sample. We are not going to try things because we think that the research project would be more interesting." Senior researcher, interview.

Furthermore, not conducting research with the samples collected was considered non-ethical concerning the donor. In this regard, the samples could not be envisaged as simply as objects collected and stored to be used in the distant future. Additionally, sample discard was strongly discouraged since it would incur a disrespectful practice to the donors who were promised that research would be conducted with their samples. Dignity extended from the human beings to their body parts, as suggested by Palmer [42], reinforcing once again the humanness of biological samples.

In all the aforementioned situations, the concerns about research in biological samples were not orientated specifically to the biological samples but devoted to concerns related to their human nature and the original donors.

In other cases, caring practices only gained shape when the donor was not considered. In the creation of cell lines from a human skin sample, for example, the donor themselves were rarely mentioned. In contradiction to this absence, the samples were compared to babies with some of the features regularly attributed to human babies—such as vulnerability or the need to be nourished and cared for.

"Have you seen them? Our babies? We are creating primary cell lines! And until now they are resisting!

I must change the substrate. I am afraid they die before we finish [the cell line]. The substrate is their food, it has all the nutrients they need. They are still very sensitive; the substrate has antibiotics to prevent infection." Biobank technician, Fieldnotes.

In the biobank's open days, the practice of care expanded outside the biobank's more confined space. The space had to be adapted in order to be functional for the activities they were about to perform, which is usually the sample collection from donors. The outside space was, in fact, more permeable to be changed. Dealing with donors required efforts to transform the space into a comfortable environment, which often included a good-tempered conversation and a jar with sweeties over the table, while donors fulfilled the informed consent and the medical questionnaire. Additionally, transform a regular office room into a waiting room, or transform a shared open space in a health fair into a semi-private space for the samples' collection procedure:

> *We went for a biobank open day. All the time the space has to be organized in order to be functional for the blood collection procedure and for the fulfilment of the medical questionnaire.*
>
> *"I am going to take these chairs out of the room [said one of the biobank technicians to the other]. Doing this, the donors could wait here comfortably, and it will be look more as a waiting room."* Fieldnotes.

In making these space arrangements, biobank technicians organized the space in a way that automatically helped establish the link with healthcare. The created space was closer to a medical doctor's office or a clinic: as the space would be more appropriate for welcoming donors when organized in such a manner. The connection to healthcare was made clearer when a medical doctor highlighted how not collecting samples could even be considered poor-quality healthcare:

> *"Not storing the samples it's certainly not a good service for patients."* Medical doctor, fieldnotes.

Moreover, the recurrent motto in biobank posters and leaflets had an inscribed symbolic meaning. "Help us to save lives" or "finding cures" was recurrent and inscribed in what seems to entail an economy of hope [50,51] that both serve donors as the biobank staff. Particularly, it re-inscribes the work performed in the biobank in the logic of healthcare.

4. Discussion

When biological samples leave healthcare services, they enter the biobank where they are reorganized accordingly to medical classifications or alternatively with categories only attributed in the context of care (as infected).

In this context, samples are transformed into objects of scientific work for the future use of researchers. Nevertheless, despite being considered objects of scientific knowledge, their nature is constantly reconstructed through the work performed in the biobank. The biological samples' identities were not given only based on the assumption the donor was a human being, but they were elaborated recurring to other strategies that enable to consolidate the humanness in biological samples.

Denying animality could be seen as a way to render samples to normal objects, avoiding their troublesome nature [43,52,53], as well as the management of complex issues such as different legal frameworks or laboratory protocols. The constant negotiation of their nature, especially the denial of their possible animal features, was integrated into a set of efforts to restore humanness in biological samples [43]. In a context where the biological sample was often reduced to the sample itself plus the associated diagnosis, considering other aspects was a work of restitution of the social context of the donors, their living conditions, or social relationships [54].

By taking care of biological samples, biobank technicians enforced the importance of the biological samples' humanness. The caring relationship established could invoke an asymmetric relationship where donors are no longer allowed to enter [51]. However, the complete absence of the donor is, in fact, somehow compensated when caring for the samples is into place during work as a reminder of the donor's gift.

In order to construct these narratives, it was needed to recall some information about the patient or the patient trajectory. In this biobank context, sample biographies were mostly based on building up on health and illness experiences. The illness narratives generally used to confer coherence to illness experiences by individuals or health professionals [49,55] were used here with a similar goal by the biobank technicians. The biological sample was a connecting link to a donor; however, the narrative might probably be different from the one donor could tell. Then, recognizing the original donor narrative was not the intention. The aim was instead to promote a sense of identification and empathy with the absent donors.

Therefore, they were able to resignify the biological samples' trajectories while they developed meaningful work practices. Crafting narratives could also be a way of contesting the dehumanization created by biomedicine during the process of objectifying the body through its continuous fragmentation into biological samples [15]. This contestation could even be amplified if it is taken into consideration that the work in the biobank is invisible and usually could not be clearer objectified. In this kind of work, where tasks performed could be reduced to the processing and storage of simple samples, operational work [31] has relatively lower importance when compared to scientific work. The bonds and the emotional and affective relationships emerging in daily work [56] were essential in rescuing the humanness in biological samples. This also strengthens the inscription of the biobank as a healthcare space.

In addition to the rescue of biological samples' humanness, it is important to highlight the role of experiences of health and illness. These experiences work as background, fluid, and changeable, according to the actors' voices that are in action. However, what reunites these different voices is somehow the human features attributed by the biobank technicians. Frequently used *health, diseased, ill*, and *healthy donors* and *patients* are a necessary vocabulary to characterize biological samples. In this sense, health and illness references acted as a layout for sample classification, the motivation of technicians to take care of the samples, and the narrative's construction. Thus, the symbolic language associated with health and illness added a reminder that these activities were intended to result in better human wellness and health.

In shaping the biological samples as things in human objects, the biobank staff allow themselves to portray the biobank as a healthcare space and intrinsically entangled in healthcare system provision. Although French, Miller, and Axler [57] already evidenced the biobank as part of healthcare within an entrepreneurial approach, here, neither the hospital nor the biobank was integrated into such orientation. The biobank is thus connected to healthcare through caring practices of the human biological samples and employing medical categories in samples' classification. These enable the construction of health and illness referential where the biobank develops part of its activities and to what it refers in terms of symbolic practices.

5. Conclusions

This article discussed how the biobank is transformed into a health place, established at the marginal space between science and health.

This entails a reflection regarding the emergence of new professionals in the health field; as the context of healthcare changes, new practices of care develop. However, it seems that the biobank's role is far from healthcare provision, the symbolic action points in the opposite direction.

The work of biobank technicians plays a relevant role in recreating the human identities of samples; however, this identity creation is not a barrier to performing the biobank work but enables it. In addition, the practices of taking care of samples were significant and contributed to transforming daily work into meaningful practices of caring oriented for the benefit of humanity. It is noteworthy that the exploration of other biobanks contexts without such a strong relationship with healthcare services, as the one portrayed in this study, could lead to different conclusions.

However, there are questions that deserve further exploration. When considering the biobank as a healthcare support infrastructure, it is also needed to explore the emergence of new voices and actors in this field. What are their action possibilities, which role they perform, how they interact with the other professionals, and which knowledge is constructed in their practices? Conducting this is essential to address new challenges that are set in the healthcare landscape.

Funding: This research was funded by Fundação para a Ciência e a Tecnologia, grant number SFRH/BD/100779/2014. Part of this manuscript was written during a residency in Fondation Brocher, supported by this institution. The author Brígida Riso is currently supported by European Union's Horizon 2020 under grant agreement no 952377, project ERA Chair iSTARS (Informatics and Statistical Tools for Advancement of Research Success).

Institutional Review Board Statement: The study was approved by the Institutional Review Board of the PhD Program in Sociology of Iscte-Instituto Universitário de Lisboa (Iscte-IUL) in July 2014. All the research conducted at Iscte-IUL respect the national legislation and the fundamental ethical and integrity principles of scientific research.

Informed Consent Statement: Informed consent was obtained from all subjects involved in the study.

Data Availability Statement: The data that support the findings of this study are available on request to the corresponding author. The data are not publicly available due to privacy and ethical restrictions. All the data produced used pseudonyms in order to avoid participants' identification.

Conflicts of Interest: The author declares no conflict of interest.

Notes

[1] Although the term *donor* is not consensual among the social sciences literature about biobanking, here it was chosen as it was the term commonly used by the biobank where the research was conducted. At this stage, in this particular biobank, the options regarding participation of the people entrusting their samples to the biobank, is limited not fulfilling the criteria to be considered research participants.

[2] The Framingham Heart Study is still active, and more information could be consulted at: https://www.framinghamheartstudy.org (accessed on 16 December 2020).

[3] The Varmland Health Survey could be consulted at: https://snd.gu.se/en/catalogue/study/ext0169 (accessed on 16 December 2020).

[4] This legal project was proposed in 2018 in the Portuguese Parliament but has not been voted. More information about this proposal could be consulted here: https://www.parlamento.pt/ActividadeParlamentar/Paginas/DetalheIniciativa.aspx?BID=42877 (accessed on 9 June 2022) (text available only in Portuguese).

References

1. Hoeyer, K. Size matters: The Ethical, Legal, and Social Issues Surrounding Large-Scale Genetic Biobank Initiatives. *Nor Epidemio* **2012**, *21*, 211–220. [CrossRef]
2. Gottweis, H.; Kaye, J.; Bignami, F.; Rial-Sebbag, E.; Lattanzi, R.; Macek, M., Jr. *Biobanks for Europe: A Challenge for Governance*; Publications Office of the European Union: Luxembourg, 2012. [CrossRef]
3. Riso, B. A Saúde Armazenada: O Biobanco na Reconfiguração da Saúde na Sociedade Contemporânea [Stored Health: The Biobank in Health Reconfiguration in Contemporary Society]. Ph.D. Thesis, Iscte-Instituto Universitário de Lisboa, Lisboa, Portugal, 28 July 2021.
4. Clarke, A.E.; Mamo, L.; Fishman, J.; Shim, J.K.; Fosket, J.R. Biomedicalization: Technoscientific Transformations of Health, Illness, and U.S. Biomedicine. *Am. Sociol. Rev.* **2003**, *68*, 161–194. [CrossRef]
5. Webster, A. Bio-Objects: Exploring the Boundaries of Life. In *Bio-Objects: Life in the 21st Century*; Vermeulen, S.N., Webster, A., Eds.; Ashgate: Surrey, UK, 2012; pp. 1–10.
6. Löwy, I. Historiography of Biomedicine: "Bio," "Medicine," and in Between. *Isis* **2011**, *102*, 116–122. [CrossRef] [PubMed]
7. Jewson, N.D. The Disappearance of the Sick-Man from Medical Cosmology, 1770–1870. *Sociology* **1976**, *10*, 225–244. [CrossRef]
8. Pickstone, J.V. *Ways of Knowing—A New Hisotry of Science, Technology and Medicine*; The University of Chicago Press: Chicago, IL, USA, 2001.
9. Webster, A.; Eriksson, L. Governance-by-standards in the field of stem cells: Managing uncertainty in the world of "basic innovation" uncertainty in the world of "basic innovation". *New Genet. Soc.* **2008**, *27*, 99–111. [CrossRef]
10. Armstrong, D. The rise of surveillance medicine. *Sociol. Health Illn.* **1995**, *17*, 393–405. [CrossRef]
11. Lock, M.; Nguyen, V.K. *An Anthropology of Biomedicine*; Wiley-Blackwell: Chichester, UK, 2010.
12. Mol, A.; Law, J. Regions, Networks and Fluids: Anaemia and Social Topology. *Soc. Stud. Sci.* **1994**, *24*, 641–671. [CrossRef]
13. Foucault, M. *The Birth of the Clinic*; Routledge: London, UK; New York, NY, USA, 1989.
14. Rose, N. *The Politics of Life Itself: Biomedicine, Power, and Subjectivity in the Twenty-First Century*; Princeton University Press: Princeton, NJ, USA, 2007.
15. Sharp, L.A. The Commodification of the Body and its Parts. *Annu. Rev. Anthr.* **2000**, *29*, 287–328. [CrossRef]
16. Novas, C.; Rose, N. Genetic risk and the birth of the somatic individual. *Econ. Soc.* **2000**, *29*, 485–513. [CrossRef]
17. Richards, M. Reading the runes of my genome: A personal exploration of retail genetics. *New Genet. Soc.* **2010**, *29*, 291–310. [CrossRef]

18. Busby, H.; Martin, P. Biobanks, national identity and imagined communities: The case of UK biobank. *Sci. Cult.* **2016**, *15*, 237–251. [CrossRef]
19. Fletcher, A.L. Field of genes: The politics of science and identity in the Estonian genome project. *New Genet. Soc.* **2004**, *23*, 3–14. [CrossRef] [PubMed]
20. Tupasela, A.; Snell, K.; Cañada, J. Constructing populations in biobanking. *Life Sci. Soc. Policy* **2015**, *11*, 5. [CrossRef] [PubMed]
21. Guerreiro, C.S.; Hartz, Z.; Sambo, L.; Conceição, C.; Dussault, G.; Russo, G.; Viveiros, M.; Silveira, H.; Barros, P.P.; Ferrinho, P. Política de Investigação Científica para a Saúde em Portugal: II-Factos e Sugestões. *Acta Med. Port* **2017**, *30*, 141–147. [CrossRef]
22. Portugal, Ministério da Saúde. *Plano Nacional de Saúde: Prioridades Para 2004-2010*; Ministério da Saúde: Lisboa, Portugal, 2004. Available online: http://1nj5ms2lli5hdggbe3mm7ms5.wpengine.netdna-cdn.com/files/2015/08/Volume-1-Prioridades.pdf (accessed on 9 June 2022).
23. Parreira, L. Investigação Médica em Portugal: Oportunidades e Constrangimetos. 2010. Available online: http://www.scmed.pt/index.php/publicacoes/101-investigacao-medica-em-portugal-oportunidades-e-constrangimentos (accessed on 9 June 2022).
24. Portugal. Lei n. 12/2005 de 26 de Janeiro—Informação Genética Pessoal e Informação em Saúde [Law no 12/2005, 26th January—Personal Genetic Information and Health Information]. Available online: https://dre.pt/dre/detalhe/lei/12-2005-624463 (accessed on 9 June 2022).
25. Carapinheiro, G.; Serra, H.; Correia, T. Estado, Medicina e Políticas em Portugal: Fluxos e Refluxos de Poder. In *Saúde, Medicina e Sociedade Uma Visão Sociológica*; Alves, F., Ed.; Pactor: Lisboa, Portugal, 2013; pp. 49–74.
26. Gaskell, G.; Stares, S.; Allansdottir, A.; Allum, N.; Castro, P.; Esmer, T.; Fischler, C.; Jackson, J.; Kronberger, N.; Hampel, J.; et al. *Europeans and Biotechnology in 2010 Winds of Change?* Publications Office of the European Union: Luxembourg, 2010. [CrossRef]
27. Atkinson, P.; Hammersley, M. *Ethnography: Principles in Practice*, 3rd ed.; Routledge: London, UK; New York, NY, USA, 2007.
28. Latour, B. *Reassembling the Social*; Oxford University Press: Oxford, UK, 2007.
29. Beaulieu, A. From co-location to co-presence: Shifts in the use of ethnography for the study of knowledge. *Soc. Stud. Sci.* **2010**, *40*, 453–470. [CrossRef]
30. Argudo-Portal, V.; Domènech, M. The reconfiguration of biobanks in Europe under the BBMRI-ERIC framework: Towards global sharing nodes? *Life Sci. Soc. Policy* **2020**, *16*, 9. [CrossRef]
31. Stiefel, L. Étudier le care en infrastructure: Les "petites mains" de la biobanque hospitalière. *Rev. D'anthropologie Connaiss.* **2018**, *12*, 399–427. [CrossRef]
32. Stephens, N.; Atkinson, P.; Glasner, P. The UK Stem Cell Bank as performative architecture. *New Genet. Soc.* **2008**, *27*, 87–98. [CrossRef]
33. Carapinheiro, G. *Saberes e Poderes no Hospital: Uma Sociologia dos Serviços Hospitalares*, 4th ed.; Afrontamento: Porto, Portugal, 1993.
34. Correia, T. *Medicina: O Agir Numa Saúde em Mudança*; Mundos Sociais: Lisboa, Portugal, 2012.
35. Bio-Objects Network. Understanding Biobanks and Their Bio-Objects: Governance Challenges Explored. (n.d.) Available online: https://www.univie.ac.at/bio-objects/pdf_final/Biobankscasestudy1111_FINAL(2).pdf (accessed on 20 June 2018).
36. Stephens, N.; Brown, N.; Douglas, C. Editors introduction: Biobanks as sites of bio-objectification. *Life Sci. Soc. Policy* **2018**, *14*, 6. [CrossRef]
37. Callon, M. Some Elements of a Sociology of Translation: Domestication of the Scallops and the Fishermen of St Brieuc Bay. *Sociol. Rev.* **1984**, *32*, 196–233. [CrossRef]
38. Holmberg, T.; Schwennesen, N.; Webster, A. Bio-objects and the bio-objectification process. *Croat. Med. J.* **2011**, *52*, 740–742. [CrossRef] [PubMed]
39. Canguilhem, G. *O Normal e o Patológico*, 6th ed.; Forense Universitária: Rio de Janeiro, Brazil, 1966.
40. Keating, P.; Cambrosio, A. *Biomedical Platforms: Realigning the Normal and the Pathological in Late-Twentieth-Century Medicine*; K the MIT Press: Cambridge, MA, USA, 2003.
41. Mol, A. *The Body Multiple: Ontology in Medical Practice*; Duke University Press: Durham, NC, USA, 2002.
42. Palmer, C. Human and Object, Subject and Thing: The troublesome Nature of Human Biological Material (HBM). In *Contested Categories: Life Sciences in Society*; Bauer, S., Wahlberg, A., Eds.; Ashgate: Surrey, UK, 2009; pp. 15–32.
43. Metzler, I.; Webster, A. Bio-objects and their Boundaries: Governing Matters at the Intersection of Society, Politics, and Science. *Croat. Med. J.* **2011**, *52*, 648–650. [CrossRef] [PubMed]
44. Douglas, M. *Purity and Danger*; Ark Paperbacks: London, UK, 1966.
45. Schwennesen, N. Bio-Objects: Life in the 21st century. In *Bio-Objects: Life in the 21st Century*; Vermeulen, N., Tamminen, S., Webster, A., Eds.; Ashgate: Surrey, UK, 2012; pp. 117–131.
46. Kopytoff, I. The cultural biography of things: Commodization as process. In *The Social Life of Things: Commodities in Cultural Perspective*; Appadurai, A., Ed.; Cambridge University Press: Cambridge, MA, USA, 1986; pp. 64–91.
47. Daston, L. *Biographies of Scientific Objects*; The University of Chicago Press: Chicago, IL, USA, 2015.
48. Lawrence, S.C. Beyond the Grave—The Use and Meaning of Human Body Parts: A Historical Introduction. In *The Stored Tissue*; Weir, R.F., Ed.; University of Iowa Press: Iowa City, IA, USA, 1998; pp. 111–142.
49. Thomas, C. Negotiating the contested terrain of narrative methods in illness contexts. *Sociol. Health Illn.* **2010**, *32*, 647–660. [CrossRef] [PubMed]
50. Novas, C. The Political Economy of Hope: Patients' Organizations, Science and Biovalue. *BioSocieties* **2006**, *1*, 289–305. [CrossRef]

51. Petersen, A.; Seear, K. Technologies of hope: Techniques of the online advertising of stem cell treatments. *New Genet. Soc.* **2011**, *30*, 329–346. [CrossRef]
52. Hoyer, K. *Exchanging Human Bodily Material: Rethinking Bodies and Markets*; Springer: New York, NY, USA; London, UK, 2013.
53. Svenaeus, F. The Lived Body and Personal Identity: The Ontology of Exiled body Parts. In *Bodily Exchange, Bioethics and Border Crossing: Perspectives on Giving, Sellinf and Sharing Bodies*; Malmqvist, E., Zeiler, K., Eds.; Routledge: London, UK; New York, NY, USA, 2016; pp. 19–34.
54. Martínez-Hernáez, A. Cuerpos fantasmales en la urbe global. *Fractal Rev. Psicol.* **2009**, *21*, 223–236. [CrossRef]
55. Bury, M. Illness narratives: Fact or fiction? *Sociol. Health Illn.* **2001**, *23*, 263–285. [CrossRef]
56. Martin, A.; Myers, N.; Viseu, A. The politics of care in technoscience. *Soc. Stud. Sci.* **2015**, *45*, 625–641. [CrossRef]
57. French, M.; Miller, F.A.; Axler, R. "It's Actually Part of Clinical Care" Mediating Biobanking Assets in the Entrepreneurial Hospital. *TECNOSCIENZA Ital. J. Sci. Technol. Stud.* **2018**, *9*, 133–158. Available online: www.tecnoscienza.net (accessed on 19 February 2019).

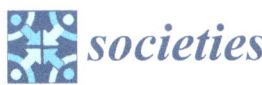

Article

"Mix of Races, Bad Uterus": Obstetric Violence in the Experiences of Afro-Brazilian Migrants in Portugal

Catarina Barata

Instituto de Ciências Sociais, Universidade de Lisboa, Av. Professor Aníbal de Bettencourt 9, 1600-189 Lisbon, Portugal; catarina.barata@ics.ulisboa.pt

Abstract: In this article, I address the issues of obstetric violence and racism in the Portuguese setting of obstetric care. Based on data collected through interviews and participatory artistic creation, I analyze the perception of three Afro-Brazilian migrants about their perinatal experiences of obstetric care in the Portuguese public sector between 2013 and 2019. These women's experiences have much in common with experiences of obstetric violence as narrated by Portuguese, non-racialized women. Despite this, certain aspects of their experience are related to their particular identification as Brazilian, migrant, and Black, such as xenophobic discrimination and their placement in systems of stratified reproduction, including a supposed tendency for birth by caesarean section, as well as self-policing behaviors because of the stereotype of Brazilian women as flirty. I consider a range of manifestations of obstetric violence and racism, from more overt forms to more covert ones, to analyze how, in a country where racism and obstetric violence are only slowly beginning to be recognized as the norm, multiple discriminations intersect and have an impact on the experiences of women of their bodies in pregnancy, birth, and postpartum, including breastfeeding.

Keywords: Portugal; obstetric violence; racism; Brazilian migrants; Black women; obstetric care; childbirth; stratified reproduction

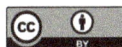

1. Obstetric Violence, Racism and Brazilian Migration in Portugal

Obstetric violence, or the mistreatment of women in the setting of obstetric care, has been framed as a type of gender violence and a violation of human rights, closely imbricated in processes of medicalization and imbued with gendered concepts that devalue of the female reproductive body [1,2]. It assumes many shapes, from overt verbal or physical abuse to subtle psychological abuse and forms of coercion [3]. In Western countries, the most widely discussed form of obstetric violence (OV) is the performance of medical interventions without clinical justification and/or informed consent, relating to highly interventive, technocratic models of care and a structural imbalance in power relations between healthcare personnel, considered authoritative, and the users of services (patients). However, other forms of mistreatment have also been expressed by victims, including abandonment of care or lack of appropriate intervention. Ultimately, what is at stake in OV is the violation of the integrity and autonomy of the woman or birthing person during obstetric care. The consequences of obstetric violence can be devastating, usually related to women feeling a loss of autonomy and of the ability to decide freely about their bodies and sexuality, negatively impacting their quality of life [4]. To date, studies of obstetric violence in Portugal have been scarce [5–7].

Feminist critiques have shown how reproductive medicine, science, and technologies are grounded in racist, gendered, capitalist, and patriarchal ideologies. Social hierarchies rooted in putative embodied racial-ethnic essentialism take different forms across diverse contexts, and they always affect reproduction in multiple ways. Racism functions within reproductive medicine, science, and technology as a mechanism for the perpetuation and mediation of social inequality [8] (p. 725). The consequences of racism in reproduction are relevant not only for maternal and fetal health, but also for the reproduction of inequality across generations, and for how power and inequality are embodied and inherited [9] (pp. 555–556). The concept of stratified reproduction—how "physical and social reproductive tasks are accomplished differentially according to inequalities that are based on hierarchies of class, race, ethnicity, gender, place in a global economy, and migration status and that are structured by social, economic, and political forces" [10] (p. 78)—is helpful to understand social and conceptual arrangements whereby some bodies are deemed more legitimate to reproduce than others. In this article, recognizing the need to take into account in the study of reproduction its constant renewal of racialization, racial privilege, and racial discrimination [8] (p. 726), I consider the nuanced workings of race, racism, and racialization in its relation to preconceived ideas about national origin and stereotypes about Brazilian women migrants in the Portuguese setting.

Because the term obstetric violence does not adequately take into account the contours of racism that materialize during Black women's medical encounters, the term obstetric racism has been recently coined to address the issue of how racism manifests in the provision of obstetric care [11]. According to Davis, "medical racism occurs when the patient's race influences medical professionals' perceptions, treatments and/or diagnostic decisions, placing the patient at risk." [11] (p. 561). The most obvious and measurable consequence of obstetric racism is higher rates of perinatal mortality among racialized minority groups as compared to non-racialized ones, but there are other, more invisible, consequences. Obstetric racism and its most immediate consequences, such as worse perinatal outcomes, have been gradually acknowledged and researched in few countries, such as Canada, the UK, and the USA. Additionally, in Brazil, researchers have identified racial disparities in care during pregnancy and childbirth: when compared with white-skinned women, black-skinned women were more likely to have inadequate prenatal care, to not be linked to a maternity hospital for childbirth, to be without a companion, to seek more than one hospital for childbirth, and less likely to receive local anesthesia for an episiotomy [12]. In the country, health disparities cut across racial lines, the structural dimensions of racism in society thus echoing what happens in the clinical setting [13].

In Portugal, to date, research on racism in obstetric care is practically nonexistent. The few analyses focusing on maternal health care services and migrant populations who are often racialized have identified inequities in access and outcomes between migrants (who are often racialized) and non-migrant populations [14,15][1]. Acknowledging the need to scrutinize an issue that remains largely under-researched, the collective of antiracist activists and researchers SaMaNe has launched an online questionnaire on obstetric racism, the results of which have not been published to date [16].

1.1. Brazilian Migration in Portugal and Racism

Portugal and Brazil have a long history of migration flows in both directions, mainly due to their historical colonial connections [17]. From the 16th century onwards, Portugal colonized and exploited resources in what is nowadays Brazil. It was also a major contributor to the transatlantic market of enslaved people from Africa to the Americas, with massive contingents of people being forcibly dislocated from the coast of West Africa to Brazil. Brazil was the first colonized country to gain independence from the Portuguese colonial power in the 19th century and the two countries maintained privileged relationships throughout, in part due to their linguistic proximity. In the end of the 20th century, the way of the migration flow inverted and migration from Brazil started a constant influx to Portugal that persists. In the second decade of the 21st century, the "wave" of migration was mainly constituted by middle- and upper-class students and entrepreneurs [18]. Currently, Brazilian migrants are the largest foreign resident community in Portugal. In 2020, Brazilian residents accounted for 27,8% of total foreigners, the highest value since 2012 [19].

Several stereotypes accompany Brazilian migrants in Portugal, such as their outgoing ways and communicative capabilities, which have facilitated their insertion in the sectors of the labor market that require contact with customers [17]. Brazilian women have their share of stereotyping in particular: they are seen as hypersexualized and are identified with prostitution, an idea partly shaped by the former colonial ties between the two countries and continuously fed by the media and entertainment industries [20–22]. In the context of obstetric care, health professionals sometimes imply that Brazilian women became pregnant with secondary intentions, such as securing a residence permit or for financial reasons, and ask about the father's nationality [15]. On the contrary, some women tell they felt more respected by the obstetricians when they became pregnant, as motherhood is considered an institution of respectability that contributes to distancing them from the stigma of prostitution [23]. Brazilian women have expressed a certain dissatisfaction regarding the quality of information provided by health professionals and the communication skills of these professionals, in addition to a perception of reduced access to medical specialties. Misinformation about legal rights and inappropriate clarification during medical appointments were frequently reported [24].

In Portugal, racism in institutions and everyday life, although pervasive in all spheres of society, remains largely unacknowledged [25–30]. Forms of "shy racism" prevail: nobody says he/she is racist, but then he/she behaves in ways that in practice have discriminatory consequences [27] (p. 91) [28]. The mainstream discourse on the nation's history perpetuates a narrative of good, exceptional colonization that denies the extreme violence of the foundations of such a sociopolitical and economic regime. Brazil's Gilberto Freyre's myth of "lusotropicalism," according to which the colonization by the Portuguese was founded on miscegenation and was thus less violent than that of other European countries, has its roots deep down in public opinion and discourse, fed by educational materials and public debate [25]. In Portugal, the debate about racism is even today an uneasy matter, because of the silence that has too long surrounded these issues, the lack of information and mental categories to discuss issues, the scarcity of empirical research, and the illusion that there never was and there is no racism in Portugal [29]. The construction of a modern nation-state relies heavily on the construction of corresponding authorized ethno-racial groups [30]. The nation-state, as a machine of production and management of identities, produces a space of belonging that is, at the same time, a place of exclusion. The immigrant is, in relation to that space of belonging to the nation, the "other" national and the "other" racial, the figure of the excluded par excellence [26] (p. 19). Adding to the division between "us" and "them," there is a hierarchical consideration about the value associated to each nationality or group racially defined, and its character more or less desired [26] (p. 22).

1.2. Obstetric Racism?

Analyses of obstetric racism have been absent from ethnographic accounts in the Portuguese setting of obstetric care, as has obstetric violence more generally. In this article, I tackle these issues by analyzing the perception and depiction of the experiences of three Afro-Brazilian women in the Portuguese obstetric care public system, with a special emphasis on birth, but also considering other episodes in their reproductive lives. I analyze the narratives of Diana, Maíra, and Rossana to reveal the racism inherent to reproductive health care. Their birth stories and narratives about obstetric care share many commonalities with the stories told by the average women giving birth in healthcare institutions in Portugal, regardless of their racial identity, class, sexual orientation, age, ability, or migration status. Several forms of mistreatment abound in their narratives, such as being depersonalized and objectified, not being informed or asked for permission, being subjected to painful interventions without clinical justification, being abused verbally, and others. However, there are some particularities to the experiences of these three women that can only be accounted for when race, as well as migration status (more than class), are included in the equation. Systems of stratified reproduction thus become clear: barriers to accessing healthcare, perceptions of xenophobia, ideas conveyed by healthcare professionals about miscegenation producing bodies unsuited for birth and some categories of people being more legitimate for reproducing than others, and condemnation of the exposure of the body for breastfeeding, among other subtleties. Multiple forms of discrimination intersect in these women's experiences, in which racism seems to operate independently of class-based prejudice.

2. Researching Obstetric Violence in Portugal

Data were collected within the framework of a PhD research project in Anthropology. The bulk of research was carried out between 2017 and 2019, but conducting fieldwork "at home" and having an active role as an advocate for women's reproductive rights allowed for continuous observation until 2022. The COVID-19 pandemic declared in March 2020 in Portugal had a great impact on all spheres of society and in the healthcare provision, with several restrictions in place that strongly affected women's experiences of childbirth [31]. I underwent fieldwork in Portugal, with incursions to Catalonia, Croatia, and Slovenia, and maintained multiple virtual connections to other countries as well as continents, through online meetings, seminars, and courses.

I used classical ethnographic methods, such as interviews, participant observation, and focus groups, as well as more experimental ones, such as participatory artistic creation. In the tradition of activist or engaged research, my critical engagement with real-world problems informs my scholarly perspective and I often seek a direct intervention in the setting of the researched subject matter [32,33]. To this end, the project also uses participatory artistic methods for the collection of data and dissemination of results [34]. The artistic strand of the research, the Gallery of Obstetric Experiences, is online and continuously open for contributions[2]. The exploration of difficult birth experiences through artistic creation has proven valuable in accessing invisible dimensions of the lived experience that are often hard to convey through words. The process of creating a depiction provokes a self-reflexive attitude and demands an organization of the experience that often facilitates the identification of the core issues implied, engaging the interlocutor in the problematization of the subject matter at hand. This proves helpful for research, especially when dealing with sensitive matters, such as negative experiences. The participants have expressed how the creative process facilitates a certain therapeutic effect, and the viewers manifest how the materialization of the pieces makes an impactful impression upon them. These and other aspects, such as the potentials and shortcomings of the use of artistic methods in this research, are discussed elsewhere [35].

Participant observation was carried out at birth-related conferences, seminars, and events, such as midwifery and birth conferences, academic seminars, public and political debates organized by political parties or by informal groups within feminist events, childbirth education classes, as well as informal groups and social media groups. I conducted twenty-two in-depth interviews. I interviewed eighteen women who gave birth in Portugal between 1993 and 2019 and self-identify as having suffered OV, initially recruited through an open call or further recruited through snowball sampling. I launched an open call on the Facebook page of the non-governmental organization (NGO) I collaborate with, APDMGP[3], the main birth rights NGO active in the country. I also interviewed a doula who was one of the first activists in Portugal, and three healthcare professionals: a midwife and two obstetricians who have adopted a "humanized" approach in their obstetric practice, and are active voices in the public arena. The midwife also identifies as having suffered OV in her first birth.

I visited two maternity wards in Portugal which are actively shifting to humanized approaches to birth, and in Slovenia to three maternity wards with different degrees of "humanization," where healthcare professionals guided me through and shared their experiences of the process. I organized a collaborative artistic workshop with victims of OV in Portugal, and two focus groups with childbirth activists: one with Portuguese activists of APDMGP, and one with activists from the ten countries[4] attending the European Network of Childbirth Associations (ENCA) meeting in Zagreb in 2019. I analyzed discourses on mass media and online social media. I also had countless informal conversations with mothers, fathers, couples, health professionals, activists, and doulas over a six-year period (2016–2021), mainly in Portugal. All participants have been given pseudonyms in order to protect their identities, except one, who is an artist who signed an art piece for the Gallery and wished to be identified by her real name. Women's rights activism is both a middle-class phenomenon, like other types of activism, and a women-dominated arena, like other issues considered traditionally feminine. My interlocutors were mainly white, educated, middle-class women with liberal professions, with a few exceptions, including the few men who are either obstetricians or activists, and the even fewer women who are racialized.

This article is about the perceptions of obstetric violence of three migrant Brazilian women of mixed African, Indigenous, and European and/or Western Asian descent and is based on data from in-depth interviews and the artwork that one of them produced. They gave birth in five different public hospitals in the two bigger cities of Portugal (two births in Oporto and three in Lisbon) and self-identify as having experienced obstetric violence. One of them identifies as having suffered obstetric racism. They had five births in total: two women had two births and one had one, between 2013 and 2019. Two of these births were considered overall positive, as for their subsequent births the two women invested in getting information and looking for hospitals with a humanized approach. Two interlocutors were recruited through an open call. One of the interlocutors was recruited through snowball sampling. She contacted the researcher in order to contribute to the Gallery of Obstetric Experiences, about which she had learned through an informal group of parents in which a fellow activist of the researcher shared the call for the project. This particular contribution is detailed elsewhere [36].

3. Diana, Maíra and Rossana's Experiences of Obstetric Violence

Diana was employed at a café when I first interviewed her in 2019 and at a cleaning company when I followed up in 2021. She is from the São Paulo hinterland (Southeastern Brazil) and has completed middle education. In Brazil, she attended undergraduate studies in Education for two years, but when she moved to Portugal in 2003, at 19 years of age, she could not afford to pay for her studies and she quit. Her longtime partner and the father of her daughters is Brazilian, from the same hometown as herself. He was jobless in Brazil and they decided to move to Portugal together upon the invitation of his sister, who was married to a Portuguese man and was living in Portugal. This is a common pattern among Brazilian migrants in Portugal, a great percentage of who have friends or family members from their places of origin already living in the country [17] (p. 23) [20]. Diana and António's story fit in the so-called trajectory of couples "ready to go," young and childless couples leaving their country of origin to pursue their life projects elsewhere, with a long-term perspective (Wall et al. p. 616 in [15], p. 41).

Diana had two births in Lisbon, in two different public hospitals. The first was in 2016, when she was 32 years old and had Inês, who was born by vacuum extraction after induction, augmentation, several unconsented interventions, rude treatment by staff, episiotomy, and trial with forceps. The second was in 2019, when she was 35 and had Helena, an eutocic birth[5], after an induction at 40 weeks and five days, due to gestational diabetes in pregnancy. Although there were interventions involved in birth, such as induction, augmentation, and epidural, she felt respected throughout the process and recalls a very positive experience. Like we will see later with Rossana, Diana consciously looked for a different hospital for her second birth, because she wanted to avoid the mistreatment that she experienced in her first birth. Her partner, António, is a truck driver traveling all over Europe, staying away for long periods of time. He could not be present at the second birth because he was working in France, but Diana's best friend was present and filmed it. Diana says he is a very present father and was always very supportive in her pregnancies, in the first birth, and in postpartum. Additionally, his support was fundamental in her realization that she was suffering postpartum depression after her first traumatic birth.

Maíra was raised in Rio de Janeiro state (southeastern Brazil). She holds a PhD in Sociology and is a teacher, educator, performer, and feminist activist. Maíra arrived in

Portugal in 2015 for one year, as a mobility student within her PhD studies program between one university in Central Brazil and one in Lisbon. Later that year, she met her future husband, a Cape Verdean man who has been living in Portugal for two decades and works as a general coordinator at an NGO. The following year, when she was 34 years old, Maíra moved to Portugal to stay. She is part of a very recent "wave" of Brazilian migration to Portugal within the so-called "migration system" between Portugal and Brazil [18], in part constituted by middle and upper-class students, specialized workers, and investors with higher education.

Maíra had one birth in a public hospital in Lisbon in 2018, at 36 years of age. It was an induction at around 41 weeks. Maíra expressed her wish to have a "natural" birth to the team, but synthetic oxytocin was administered intravenously without her consent. Other unconsented interventions followed, such as membrane sweeping (known as *toque maldoso* or "evil touch")[6] performed by the OB/GYN, who was accompanied by a group of students who did not introduce themselves. She later refused to let them perform cervical dilation assessments on her. As Maíra used foul language to express her pain and discomfort because of the intervention that was performed on her without any notice, the OB/GYN threatened to sue her and they exchanged some harsh accusations between each other. Maíra was in labor for four days, before her daughter was born by caesarean section (CS). I detail her story elsewhere, as she produced a piece for the Gallery of Obstetric Experiences [36].

Rossana is from a main city in Piauí state (Northeastern Brazil). She graduated with a degree in Journalism and is a postpartum doula[7], a professional path she chose after becoming a mother. Rossana moved to Oporto in 2012, when she was 23 years old, to marry a Portuguese man from Oporto whom she had met in 2011 on the Internet and who later visited her in Brazil. She enrolled in a Master's degree in Image Design, which she did not complete, as two pregnancies followed (her first daughter Mel was born in 2013 and the second, Aline, in 2016) and she did not find the opportunity to finish her degree. Rossana's trajectory fits in the pattern of migration of young women "long-term new life" (Wall et al. p. 608 in [15], p. 41).

Rossana had two births in two different public hospitals in Oporto. The first one was in 2013, when she was 24 years old. It was a birth with induction at 39 weeks and three days, and it involved a so-called "cascade of interventions"[8] [37], including multiple forms of mistreatment, such as many interventions without information or consent and depersonalized treatment, with health professionals not introducing themselves or "seeing" her, as she describes. She had an unconsented episiotomy and "husband's stitch."[9] After stitching her through a painful procedure, because the effect of the epidural had waned and she could feel everything (but nobody paid attention to her complaints), the physician showed her husband that she had stitched a bit tighter. The second was in 2016, when she was 27. Like Diana, Rossana chose another hospital for the birth of her second daughter. At 40 weeks and one day, she was pressured to be hospitalized for induction, but she negotiated a membrane sweeping with the obstetrician instead. She asked the doctor for a membrane sweeping instead of being immediately admitted and chemically induced, and was able to start labor at home, returning to the hospital for birth one day later. Apart from an OB/GYN who talked disrespectfully when she refused epidural anesthetic (saying "these women come here saying they do not want the epidural, but when it starts hurting, they cry for it"), she describes the whole birth as being very respectful. She handed out her birth plan to the team and it was fully respected. The few interventions there were (two cervical assessments, intermittent fetal monitoring, antibiotics for Streptococcus B) were all done with information, consent, and respect.

In the birth stories of Diana (D), Maíra (M), and Rossana (R), we encounter manifestations of obstetric violence that do not differ from what I have heard from my interlocutors of Portuguese origin and who are racially identified with the normative "white." All three women complained about feeling objectified and subjected to an excess of interventions, detailing their birth processes as pervaded by lack of information, rude treatment by staff, interventions without consent, and other unpleasant features. The topics that came up in the interviews were: induction, augmentation, verbal abuse, lack of privacy, lack of information, lack of consent, threatening and culpabilization, unauthorized manipulations of the newborn (D; M; R); amniotomy, lithotomy, birth companion told to leave the room, Kristeller maneuver, continuous fetal monitoring, frequent vaginal examinations, episiotomy, suturing without anesthetic (D; R); painful vaginal examinations (M; R); discrimination based on personal attributes (being overweight), immediate cord clamping (M; D); undervaluing complaints, refusal to give anesthetic during labor with induction, physical restriction during birth (D); unconsented membrane sweeping, separation from newborn, lack of support in breastfeeding (M); enema, abandonment of care, catheterization, food or drink intake restriction, coercion to take anesthetic during labor, cord traction, "husband's stitch" (R).

Details of these interventions are beyond the scope of this manuscript. All the features enumerated correspond to forms of obstetric violence as classified in the literature [1,3–5]. Any intervention in birth that does not respect the right to self-determination or the integrity and autonomy of the woman, performed without consent or for valid clinical reasons, is considered obstetric violence, which is a form of human rights violation. Some of these interventions are advised against under all circumstances, such as the Kristeller maneuver or the "husband's stitch," and some others are fallback solutions that should only be employed in emergency situations to save lives, and are rarely needed, such as cord traction or episiotomy. All women said that their negative birth experience affected their well-being, perception of self, self-esteem, and sexual life. Rossana said it affected her bonding with the baby and Diana developed postpartum depression that was later diagnosed as being associated with the trauma she suffered during birth.

Apart from all these aspects, which we commonly find in a great amount of facility-based birth stories, there are also particular details in the narratives told by these women that can be considered specific to the situation of Brazilian migrants, informed by racial and national stereotypes.

3.1. System's Constraints—Barriers to Accessing Healthcare

When Rossana found out that she was pregnant, she went to the public health care center of her area of residence, like most women do. Rossana did not have an assigned general practitioner (GP), as she had only recently moved to Portugal, and having a consultation to be seen by a doctor was not straightforward. The administrative assistant at the healthcare center said she was not allowed to have a consultation there, as she was not enrolled in the system. As Rossana declared that she might be pregnant, the assistant became more flexible. Rossana managed to have the first consultation, but she was then told that she could not be assigned a GP there. Instead, she was referred to the hospital, where was assisted by an obstetrician-gynecologist (OB/GYN).

Maternal and infant healthcare in Portugal is a legal, universal right, and every pregnant woman in the country is entitled to full perinatal care for free, regardless of her legal status [15,24]. In the National Health Service (SNS[10]), low-risk pregnancies are attended to at the healthcare center, where a general practitioner (GP) is assigned to pregnant women (and remains her GP afterwards) and prescribes the diagnostic methods, which are done at private clinics at no cost to the patient (paid for by the state). The care is complemented by a nurse, who takes measurements before consultations with the doctor. Hospital care is for high-risk pregnancies and for monitoring the last few weeks of pregnancy, when low-risk pregnant women are referred to the hospital, and is more directed to intervention in pathologies (by OB/GYNs). Whereas at the healthcare center the woman is assisted by the GP assigned to her throughout, continuity of carer is rarely provided for her at the hospital, depending in great measure on the internal policies of each hospital. There is a parallel private sector, in which women are always assisted by the same obstetrician (that they often consciously choose). The intricacies of these two sectors are complex and at many times have had detrimental consequences for the care that women receive at birth [7].

Rossana's case is contrary to what has been identified in the literature as dissatisfaction arising from Brazilian women's concerning lack of access to medical specialties in Portugal [24]. Although Rossana was never refused care, having prenatal care at the hospital, which is for high-risk pregnancies, instead of at the healthcare center, which is for low-risk pregnancies as was her case, could have consequently contributed to her being treated as high-risk. Obstetrical models of care have been associated with a higher risk of interventions and are not considered the golden standard for low-risk pregnancies [38–40]. A discussion about models of care and the need to restructure the Portuguese obstetric care system is beyond the scope of this manuscript. Relevant to our discussion is the fact that Rossana's access to the type of care as it is outlined in the *SNS* was possibly complicated by her legal status as a migrant woman. Although the public sector in Portugal is structurally understaffed, and the system's failure to provide for an assigned GP affects a large part of the population, studies have found that inequalities in access to healthcare exist, and that migrant women are sometimes refused care or demands for payment are made [13,14]. Despite the law, disparities in access to healthcare persist, based on race, socioeconomic status, migration status, and other sociopolitical markers.

3.2. Brazilian Women and the Caesarean Section (CS)
3.2.1. "How Strange, a Brazilian Wanting a Normal Birth!"

At a prenatal appointment, a female obstetrician told Diana that everything seemed on track for a normal birth[11], as she already had a bit of dilation. When Diana showed her enthusiasm for "natural" birth, the obstetrician commented "How strange! A Brazilian wanting a normal birth! They all come here wanting a caesarean!" As Diana confirmed that she wished for a normal birth, the OB/GYN reiterated how rare that is and how Brazilian women always want CSs. Diana quoted the physician: "Ah, that's very rare, because you already come in here demanding a caesarean section." Diana emphasized the employment of the plural of the pronoun (*vocês*) by the physician to underline the fact that she treated her as part of a homogeneous group.

3.2.2. "Mix of Races, Bad Uterus . . . That's Why There Are So Many Caesareans in Brazil"

Maíra describes a midwife as being very affectionate and gentle coming into the room at dawn, on her first day at the hospital. In a very quiet tone and while stroking her head, she said: "Ah, another Brazilian! You are a mix of races; you won't be able to birth your baby. Surrender to the fact that you are having a caesarean section." She added: "Don't you see how many caesareans there are in Brazil? That's because you are a mix of races, your uterus is very bad, because you are a mix of races . . . " On the second day, the nice midwife came back and once again gently repeated how a mix of races make a bad uterus that prevents a woman from having a normal birth, saying that that was the reason why Maíra was still there. She was very nice throughout the interaction. Apparently, the midwife wanted to offer some comfort to Maíra, and she expressed those racist tropes to console her.

3.3. Xenophobia and Stratified Reproduction

Diana said about the birth of her first daughter that she was the most mistreated when she was alone. Her partner was present during labor, except when told to leave in order for the health professionals to carry out interventions, and when Diana had to move to the birth room. Diana says she felt a difference in treatment when she was alone, as if her husband acted as a protective shield, and she thought this happened because she is Brazilian. She told an episode to illustrate the kind of mistreatment she received when her partner was not by her side. When moving from the dilation room to the birth room, she was told to walk on her own feet, and was accompanied by a male midwife. Upon feeling a very strong contraction, she was incapable of moving and abruptly stopped in the middle of the corridor. The midwife "almost hit" her, reproaching her with harsh manners "You have to tell me when you're going to stop, because I'm carrying your drip!" Diana replied that she became breathless on every contraction and was not able to talk.

Diana was convinced that this kind of abuse only happened because she was alone, as the health professionals were more polite to her while her partner was present. She thought this to be connected with her being Brazilian. Two and a half years later, when I asked her to elaborate on this idea, she told me that she had changed her mind and was not so sure whether that was the case. Having heard many awful birth stories in the meantime, she realized the kind of mistreatment she suffered was actually the norm in Portuguese facilities, and she now thinks that this happens regardless of nationality. However, Diana went on to talk about other situations in her life in Portugal when she felt discriminated against for being a Brazilian, especially in the workplace. As for the concept of obstetric violence, she expressed she was familiar with it already in Brazil, but she thought she would never go through it, because in Portugal things were surely different, she thought, "more advanced." Rossana expressed a similar idea, that Portugal being a European country would be expected to be better than Brazil in this regard.

3.3.1. "Control It Now, Alright?"

When asked about discrimination due to her being a foreigner and a Brazilian, Rossana answered that she heard a discriminatory comment from the physician who discharged her from the hospital, after her second birth. The OB/GYN told her, as she performed the physical exam before discharging her, "Now, let's see if you control that, alright?" Rossana interprets that comment as a disciplinary attitude by the doctor, who felt she had the right to tell Rossana how to lead her reproductive choices: it was implicit that she had already "made her contribution to the country's natality rate," Rossana says, and that she should behave now, refrain from "overpopulating" it. She added that she is not sure whether this was because she is a foreigner or because of her age, probably because of both. She was 27 and had two daughters, a pattern not consonant with the national average, with women becoming mothers at 30.7 years of age and having on average 1,4 children[12]. Either way, it conveys ideas of stratified reproduction of which bodies are legitimate to reproduce and which are not [9].

3.3.2. "Beware Not to Have More Children"

Like Rossana, Diana also heard a discriminatory comment from a health professional, after the birth of her first daughter. An older midwife came into the room, bringing the newborn to breastfeed, and asked the mother how the birth had been. Diana answered that it had been awful. The midwife, apparently angry about her honesty, harshly told her, "Well, I also don't want to see you here ever again, beware not to have more children!" This power display was like a punishment for Diana's wrong answer. It was actually a rhetorical question, Diana was not entitled to have an opinion, even more so one that did not fit the inquirer's expectations. The question remains whether the midwife would feel the same right to intrude in Diana's reproductive choices were she a non-racialized, Portuguese woman.

3.4. Ashamed to Breastfeed in Public: The Brazilian Woman as "Piriguete"

Once, at a shopping mall, Diana took her breast out to nurse her four-month-old baby Inês. She heard a Portuguese young woman say out loud, "How awful, that's disgusting!" The woman was alone, so Diana knows she clearly meant her to hear this. Diana immediately felt embarrassed, but she decided not to stop breastfeeding her daughter. She told me that she felt ashamed, because of the stereotype of Brazilian women being *piriguete* (a flirty, promiscuous woman who offers herself sexually): "I get this way, because I'm Brazilian, and there's that stereotype of the Brazilian woman being *piriguete*, that she likes to expose herself, so, in my head, the less I expose myself the better for me." Diana breastfed her first daughter for one year and four months and her second daughter for nine months.

4. Obstetric Violence and Multiple Discriminations

In the birth stories of Diana, Maíra, and Rossana, several elements of what has been defined as obstetric violence abound [3,4]. Their birth stories share many commonalities with the stories told by the average women giving birth in healthcare institutions in Portugal [5–7,35], regardless of their racial identity, class belonging, sexual orientation, age, migration, or ability status. Several forms of mistreatment, such as lack of information, unconsented interventions, objectification of the body, and even verbal abuse concur to make these women's birth experiences paradigmatic of what has been termed and defined as obstetric violence.

Adding to this, these women suffered multiple discriminations based on their national origin, migration status, and categorization of race, more than their class belonging. Ranging from declared forms of racism, such as a midwife telling Maíra that being of "mixed races" meant having as a consequence a "bad uterus" that would make vaginal birth impossible, to more subtle, covert forms of racism, such as disciplinary comments about reproductive choices and preconceived ideas about Brazilian women and their sexual and reproductive habits, informed the clinical encounters of these women with health personnel. All women identified as having suffered obstetric violence. Maíra was the only one to clearly identify having been subjected to racism, because of the racist tropes expressed by the midwife, but the different vignettes discussed before reveal a subtle and covert racism inherent to reproductive health care and policies. In relation to their specific status as migrant Brazilian women, three main themes emerge, related to stereotypes about Brazilian women:

- Identification with caesarean section, either by personal preference or by physical incapacity;
- Being undisciplined breeders;
- Being flirty (*piriguete*).

4.1. Identification of Brazilian Women with Caesarean Section

Multiple stereotypes about Brazilian women pervade public opinion and public discourse in Portugal [20–22] and they also manifest in obstetric care [15,23]. Both Diana and Maíra heard health professionals normalize Brazilian women as naturally prone to deliver by caesarean section, an idea mainly shaped by the high CS rates in Brazil and by the fact that some Brazilian women in Portugal express their wish for an elective caesarean. Brazil stands out among countries with the highest caesarean section rates in the world [41]. According to Morais, Padilla, Rossetto, and Almeida [23], Brazilian women demanding CSs can be seen as an effect of the dominant "caesarean culture" internalized by women in Brazil, who bring these perceptions to their host countries. In highly medicalized systems, the caesarean section as state-of-the-art technology is highly valued. It can also be a strategy they use to avoid not only the fear of vaginal birth, but also the possibility of mistreatment during labor, as they have the perception that their vulnerability as migrants and potential for discrimination as Brazilian is more prone to happen in vaginal birth rather than in CSs [23].

In Diana's case, an OB/GYN takes the woman's preference for CS for granted, and expresses her surprise when Diana tells her otherwise. Diana's individuality is eroded as she is placed within a group, generalized as a Brazilian migrant who is expected to behave in a certain manner. Brazilian women want caesarean sections, or else why would there be so many CSs in Brazil? When discussing the issue of the global rise of CS rates, a common explanation introduced by health professionals is women demanding caesarean sections as a driver for the substantial rise in CS rates globally. However, this thesis has been called into question, as studies show that only a minority of women in a wide variety of countries express a preference for caesarean delivery [42,43]. Additionally, women's choices and preferences do not exist in a void, they are instead embedded in and influenced by sociopolitical contexts [6], and the option for caesarean sections has been shown to be greatly influenced by medical opinion [41,43]. The significant differences in CS rates in public and private sectors also hint at cultural and economic factors influencing this decision, rather than clinical ones [7,43].

In Maíra's case, the midwife offers a simplistic explanation for the high caesarean section rates in Brazil based on race: most Brazilian population is miscegenated, and a "mix of races" produces a "bad uterus"—that is why there are so many CSs in Brazil, she says. She condescendingly urges Maíra to accept her fate as a woman who has no alternative but to have her child via caesarean section, as she is of mixed race. The midwife invokes Maíra's racial status and forces an association between her nationality and the CS to prove the evidence of the outcome she foresees. The surgery is then a "natural" and consequential solution to address a biological problem that "mixing races" brings to women. As a mixed-race woman, Maíra is declared unfit for birth by the healthcare professional, who overlooks all sociological explanations and presents a faulty argument.

As with other processes of stereotyping, the selection of a random characteristic to compose an idea about a whole group is always partial in the information it picks and depending on a generalization whereby heterogeneous groups get reduced to a homogeneous mass of similarity. The identification of Brazilian women with birth by caesarean section is a generalization that, like all generalizations, is based on a detail and simplification from reality, operated through an essentialization. The prejudice according to which Brazilian women are naturally more prone to birthing by CS offers a simplistic explanation of a complex reality, deliberately ignoring all the historical, social, economic, and political reasons that overlap to contribute to the phenomenon. It is also an exercise of stratified reproduction [9], as it classifies a certain category of bodies as being more unsuited for birthing their offspring, in opposition to another kind of body that is able to do so. This adds another layer to the conception of the female body as defective and requiring technological assistance in order to perform reproductive tasks [44].

The so-called "epidemic" of caesarean sections worldwide has been recognized as a public health problem and several reasons have been appointed to explain it, from medical cultures highly reliant on interventionism, financial incentives, personal convenience motivations, and fear of litigation to lead to the practice of defensive obstetrics [45]. The midwife chooses to ignore all this and, by blaming the woman's characteristics instead, puts the onus for what might go wrong on her, exerting a power that has the potential to undermine the laboring woman's confidence. Blaming and culpabilization are common expressions of obstetric violence, with women being coerced into interventions and/or blamed for negative outcomes (potential or real) because of their physical characteristics, their behavior in labor and birth, and not complying to orders by the staff.

4.2. Brazilian Women as Undisciplined Breeders

The concept of stratified reproduction helps us see the arrangements by which some reproductive futures are valued while others are despised, as the inequalities based on hierarchies of class, race, ethnicity, gender, place in a global economy, and migration status deem some human groups more eligible for reproducing than others [10] (p. 78). Both Diana and Rossana were subjected to comments by healthcare professionals, with the assumption that they should be disciplined about their reproductive life choices. In Rossana's case, her class status was overshadowed by her racial status, and her national origin most likely contributed to the shaping of the healthcare provider's framing of Rossana as an undisciplined breeder, as ideas about the Brazilian women as eroticized and disruptive of traditional familiar patterns in the country are conveyed in public opinion [20]. Brazilian women are often confronted with gender and class discriminatory situations that evoke the idea of pregnancy for secondary interests (such as legal regularization) and being questioned about the father's nationality [15] (p. 172, 199, 236), as are other racialized women [16]. Diana also heard comments on her need to refrain from further reproducing after her first birth. The comment proffered sounded like a punishment for Diana being critical of the care that she received during birth.

4.3. Brazilian Women as Flirty

The impact of the stereotypes about Brazilian women extend well beyond the event of childbirth. Diana's self-awareness about her condition as a Brazilian woman leads her to self-police her behavior, to avoid adopting behaviors usually identified with the group she is supposed to belong to. The reproaching comment she heard from a stranger when she exposed her breast to nurse her baby daughter immediately evoked in her mind the stereotype of Brazilian women being flirty and liking to expose themselves, and inhibited her from being at ease breastfeeding in public.

The exotization and erotization of the Brazilian woman is fostered by the media and publicity and entertainment industries, in Portugal but also in Brazil, where certain racialized groups of Black or *mestiças*[13] women are especially subject to these processes of erotization [20]. Brazilian Black feminism has argued that the ideology of *mestiçagem*, associated with the hyper sexualization of Black women, conceals the oppression and sexual violence suffered by enslaved Black women and perpetuates their subaltern condition, linking it to sexuality [21,22]. When arriving in Portugal, Brazilian women are confronted with these preconceptions about themselves as sexually available and as bearers of an exotic and exaggerated sexuality, easily associated with prostitution.

The intersection between gender and race/coloniality seems to be the main intersection to explain the prejudice against Brazilian women in Portugal. Other articulations, such as class, add to the difficulties, but what all the Brazilian women seem to have in common is the stigma of hypersexuality [21] (p.186).

5. Concluding Remarks

In the cases discussed, it is hard to determine whether race or national origin have a stronger bearing on the discriminations that the women have suffered. Apparently, being a Brazilian has predominance over being Black, but the question remains whether it is easier for those involved and for us hearing the stories to identify these situations as xenophobia, because the discourse about Brazilian women is more established and assumed in public opinion and public discourse, rather than the debate about racism.

Despite long standing action by anti-racist activists and work by scholars, the debate about racism in Portuguese society has only very recently received more widespread attention and it is still subject to a lot of disputes in the public arena. Several historical events conspire to make the racist debate difficult in Portugal [25,29]. The myth of lusotropicalism is deeply ingrained in Portuguese society, as is in Brazil the myth of racial democracy, influenced by the ideas of sociologist Gilberto Freyre in the mid-20th century, that has found a fertile ground in both countries [25]. In Portugal, the fascist regime embraced the ideas of lusotropicalism as a way to legitimate colonial power, as it served the purpose of denying the brutality of the colonial power in the domination of native populations. Unlike what happened in other European countries that suffered World War II and started the debate around the inequalities based on the idea of race much earlier, Portugal managed to remain removed from the debate, as its status as a neutral country in the war provided the illusion of not having aligned with state racism [29]. Recently, the debate about everyday racism pervading all spheres of society has been gaining momentum, with the exposure of the ways through which racialized communities are discriminated, excluded, and subjected to stereotypes that are detrimental to their achieving the same educational, housing, professional, material, and symbolic status as other majority, non-racialized communities [27,28]. As the conflation of a national identity with an ethno-racial identity is a central process in the building of modern nation-states, racist ideologies, even if not openly assumed as such, help the hegemonic group maintain its privileges while perpetuating the lack of access of minority groups to de facto equality in society [26,30].

Maíra affirmed that all types of violence are pretty much intertwined, and one cannot be eradicated without eradicating the others. According to her intersectional approach, it is useless to look at racism without looking at gender, at class, and all the categories that work in people's minds and are mirrored in society to hierarchically differentiate and classify people and human groups. As is happening with the debate about racism in Portuguese society, the debate about obstetric violence is finally gaining momentum in the country, after long years of work by both anti-racist and childbirth activists in denouncing the structural dimensions of these phenomena. As the public debates about racism and gender violence provoke discomfort among the groups that benefit from these types of inequality, generating reactions of denial and backlash, it becomes ever clearer that tackling difficult issues requires knowledge about them. The need for research on obstetric violence as well as obstetric racism is crucial to disclose how multiple discriminations intertwine in reproductive healthcare and how so often these forms of violence operate in subtle, disguised, and concealed ways.

Funding: This research was funded by the European Social Fund (ESF) and the Fundação para a Ciência e a Tecnologia of the Ministry of Science, Technology and Higher Education (FCT/MCTES), grant number SFRH/BD/128600/2017.

Institutional Review Board Statement: Ethical review and approval were waived for this study, due to the study being conducted within the framework of the program of PhD studies in Anthropology at the Institute of Social Sciences of the University of Lisbon (Portugal), under the supervision of Chiara Pussetti PhD. All studies developed within the Institute are according to the national legislation and fundamental ethical principles of scientific studies.

Informed Consent Statement: Informed consent was obtained from all subjects involved in the study.

Data Availability Statement: Data from the research was recorded in handwritten form and as such avoids the need for online data protection. Demographic data was anonymized and stored separately from the qualitative data. Identification codes and personal data will be stored in an encrypted file. References to interlocutors in the outputs will be given through codes of identification. Data will not be used for any other purpose other than that purpose for which it was obtained.

Acknowledgments: I thank Beatriz Padilla, Carolina Coimbra, Elsa Peralta, João Vasconcelos, Jucimara Cavalcante, Laura Brito, Maria José Antunes, Monalisa Barros, Sónia Cardoso Pintassilgo, Violeta Alarcão and two anonymous reviewers. Special thanks to all the women who shared their stories with me.

Conflicts of Interest: The author declares no conflict of interest.

Notes

[1] I thank Carolina Coimbra and Laura Brito from SaMaNe collective for bringing these two works to my attention.
[2] Galeria das Experiências Obstétricas: <https://galeriadasexperienciasobstetricas.wordpress.com/>. (accessed on 6 March 2022).
[3] Associação Portuguesa pelos Direitos da Mulher na Gravidez e Parto (APDMGP).
[4] Austria, the Czech Republic, Croatia, Germany, Hungary, Ireland, the Netherlands, Portugal, Spain, and the UK.
[5] Vaginal birth without recourse to instrumental extraction, either by vacuum or forceps.
[6] Health professionals asking women to open their legs in order to do the *toque*—digital vaginal examination to assess cervical dilation—and, with the fingers inside the vagina, sweeping the membranes either to provoke or accelerate labor, without further notice, without asking for permission and without explaining the reasons and risks. It can be a painful procedure and women many times are surprised by the pain it causes, only retrospectively realizing that they were subjected to this procedure and not to the *toque* (which is supposed to be painless) they were expecting.
[7] A doula is a person who provides informational and emotional support regarding perinatal matters. It is a paid service. She is not entitled to perform obstetric interventions.
[8] When one medical intervention leads to another one to contravene the iatrogenic consequences of the previous one and so forth in an endless chain.
[9] An extra stitch done after vaginal delivery to repair a natural tear during childbirth or a cut by an episiotomy. The supposed purpose of the husband's stitch is to tighten the vagina to its pre delivery state, and is done with the idea that it might increase the frequency of the woman's orgasms or enhance a man's pleasure in intercourse. It is neither an accepted practice nor an approved medical procedure and it can lead to painful sex for both partners.
[10] *Serviço Nacional de Saúde*.
[11] "Normal birth" is the emic term for eutocic birth (vaginal, non-instrumental birth), in opposition to dystocic birth either by vacuum extraction, forceps or caesarean section.

[12] Data for 2020, which does not differ from the pattern in the last years: https://www.pordata.pt/Portugal/Idade+m%C3%A9dia+da+m%C3%A3e+ao+nascimento+do+primeiro+filho-805; https://www.pordata.pt/Portugal/Indicadores+de+fecundidade+%C3%8Dndice+sint%C3%A9tico+de+fecundidade+e+taxa+bruta+de+reprodu%C3%A7%C3%A3o-416 (accessed on 9 February 2022)

[13] Terms such as *mestiça*, *mulata* and *cabrita* (crossbred) have their origins in animal reproduction to define the crossing of two different breeds or species, originating a type of animal considered inferior and impure. They are anchored in a historical colonial project that functions to affirm the inferiority of one identity through its attribution to the animal condition. At the same time, the romantization of such terms transforms the relations of power and sexual abuse in glorious sexual conquests, that have resulted in an even more exotic body [28] (pp.12–14).

References

1. Šimonović, D. *A Human Rights-Based Approach to Mistreatment and Violence Against Women in Reproductive Health Services with a Focus on Childbirth and Obstetric Violence*; United Nations: New York, NY, USA, 2019; Available online: https://digitallibrary.un.org/record/3823698#record-files-collapse-header (accessed on 14 January 2022).
2. Sadler, M.; Santos, M.; Ruiz-Berdún, D.; Rojas, G.L.; Skoko, E.; Gillen, P.; Clausen, J. Moving beyond disrespect and abuse: Addressing the structural dimensions of obstetric violence. *Reprod. Health Matters* **2016**, *24*, 47–55. [CrossRef] [PubMed]
3. Bohren, M.A.; Vogel, J.P.; Hunter, E.C.; Lutsiv, O.; Makh, S.K.; Souza, J.P.; Aguiar, C.; Coneglian, F.S.; Diniz, A.L.A.; Tunçalp, Ö.; et al. The Mistreatment of Women during Childbirth in Health Facilities Globally: A Mixed-Methods Systematic Review. *PLOS Med.* **2015**, *12*, e1001847. [CrossRef] [PubMed]
4. Goberna-Tricas, J.; Boladeras, M. (Eds.) *El Concepto «Violencia Obstétrica» y el Debate Actual Sobre la Atención al Nacimiento*; Tecnos: Madrid, Spain, 2018.
5. Rohde, A.M. A Outra Dor do Parto: Género, Relações de Poder e Violência Obstétrica na Assistência Hospitalar ao Parto. Master's Thesis, FCSH–Universidade Nova de Lisboa, Lisbon, Portugal, 2016.
6. Fedele, A.; White, J. Birthing matters in Portugal: Introduction. *Etnográfica* **2018**, *22*. Available online: http://journals.openedition.org/etnografica/5951 (accessed on 10 October 2018).
7. Barata, C. "You're in a Hospital, not a Hotel!": An Ethnographic Perspective on Consumer Culture, Privilege, and Obstetric Violence in Portugal. In *Obstetric Violence: Realities and Resistance from Around the World*; Castañeda, A.N., Hill, N., Searcy, J.J., Eds.; Demeter Press: Toronto, CA, USA, 2022; pp. 159–175.
8. Rapp, R. Race & Reproduction: An Enduring Conversation. *Med. Anthropol.* **2019**, *38*, 725–732. [CrossRef] [PubMed]
9. Valdez, N.; Deomampo, D. Centering Race and Racism in Reproduction. *Med. Anthropol.* **2019**, *38*, 551–559. [CrossRef] [PubMed]
10. Colen, S. Like a mother to them: Stratified reproduction and West Indian childcare workers and employers in New York. In *Conceiving the New World Order: The Global Politics of Reproduction*; Ginsburg, F.D., Rapp, R., Eds.; University of California Press: Berkeley, CA, USA, 1995; pp. 78–102.
11. Davis, D. Obstetric Racism: The Racial Politics of Pregnancy, Labor, and Birthing. *Med. Anthropol.* **2019**, *38*, 560–573. [CrossRef]
12. Leal, M.C.; da Gama, S.G.N.; Pereira, A.P.E.; Pacheco, V.E.; do Carmo, C.N.; Santos, R.V. A cor da dor: Iniquidades raciais na atenção pré-natal e ao parto no Brasil. *Cad. De Saúde Pública* **2017**, *33* (Suppl. 1), e00078816. [CrossRef]
13. Williamson, K.E. The iatrogenesis of obstetric racism in Brazil: Beyond the body, beyond the clinic. *Anthropol. Med.* **2021**, *28*, 172–187. [CrossRef]
14. Machado, M.C.; Santana, P.; Carreiro, M.H.; Nogueira, H.; Barroso, M.R.; Dias, A. *Iguais ou Diferentes? Cuidados de Saúde Materno-Infantil a uma População de Imigrantes*; Laboratórios Bial: Lisboa, Portugal, 2006.
15. Topa, J. *Cuidados de Saúde Materno-Infantis na Região do Grande Porto: Percursos, Discursos e Práticas*; Alto-Comissariado para as Migrações (ACM, IP): Lisboa, Portugal, 2016.
16. Moura, C. "Se é Mais Claro ou Mais Escuro, Perguntam Logo Quem Será o Pai": As Histórias de Mulheres Negras No Parto. Sábado (Lisboa), 10 April 2021. Available online: https://www.sabado.pt/entrevistas/detalhe/se-e-mais-claro-ou-mais-escuro-perguntam-logo-quem-sera-o-pai-as-historias-de-mulheres-negras-no-parto (accessed on 7 October 2021).
17. Malheiros, J. Os brasileiros em Portugal—A síntese do que sabemos. In *Imigração Brasileira em Portugal*; Malheiros, J.M., Ed.; ACIDI, I.P.: Lisboa, Portugal, 2007; pp. 11–37.
18. Fernandes, D.; Peixoto, J.; Oltramari, A.P. A quarta onda da imigração brasileira em Portugal: Uma história breve. *Rev. Latinoam. De Población* **2021**, *15*, 29. [CrossRef]
19. SEF/GEPF. *Relatório de Imigração, Fronteiras e Asilo 2020*; Serviço de Estrangeiros e Fronteiras: Oeiras, Portugal, 2021.
20. Padilla, B. A imigrante brasileira em Portugal: Considerando o género na análise. In *Imigração Brasileira em Portugal*; Malheiros, J.M., Ed.; ACIDI, I.P.: Lisboa, Portugal, 2007; pp. 113–134.
21. Padilla, B.; Gomes, M.S. Empoderamento, Interseccionalidade e Ciberativismo: Uma Análise do "Manifesto Contra o Preconceito às Mulheres Brasileiras em Portugal". *Tomo* **2016**, *28*, 169–201. [CrossRef]
22. Pontes, L. Mulheres brasileiras na mídia portuguesa. *Cad. Pagu* **2004**, *23*, 229–256. [CrossRef]
23. Morais, M.S.; Padilla, B.; Rosseto, C.M.; Almeida, M.A.S. Migração: Saúde reprodutiva e estereótipo. *Cad Saúde Colet* **2021**. ahead of print. [CrossRef]
24. Almeida, L.; Caldas, J. Migration and maternal health: Experiences of Brazilian women in Portugal. *Rev Bras Saúde Matern Infant* **2013**, *13*, 309–316. [CrossRef]

25. Castelo, C. *O Modo Português de estar no Mundo. O Luso-Tropicalismo e a Ideologia Colonial Portuguesa (1933–1961)*; Edições Afrontamento: Porto, Portugal, 2011.
26. Dias, B.P.; Dias, N. *Imigração e Racismo em Portugal: O Lugar do Outro*; Edições 70 e Le Monde Diplomatique: Lisboa, Portugal, 2011.
27. Henriques, J.G. *Racismo no País dos Brancos Costumes*; Tinta da China: Lisboa, Portugal, 2018.
28. Kilomba, G. *Memórias da Plantação. Episódios de Racismo Quotidiano*; Orfeu Negro: Lisboa, Portugal, 2020.
29. Vala, J. *Racismo, Hoje. Portugal em Contexto Europeu*; Fundação Francisco Manuel dos Santos: Lisboa, Portugal, 2021.
30. Silva, M.C.; Sobral, J.M. *Etnicidade, Nacionalismo e Racismo. Migrações, Minorias Etnicas e Contextos Escolares*; Edições Afrontamento: Porto, Portugal, 2012.
31. Lazzerini, M.; Covi, B.; Mariani, I.; Drglin, Z.; Arendt, M.; Nedberg, I.H.; Elden, H.; Costa, R.; Drandić, D.; Radetić, J.; et al. Quality of facility-based maternal and newborn care around the time of childbirth during the COVID-19 pandemic: Online survey investigating maternal perspectives in 12 countries of the WHO European Region. *Lancet Reg. Health-Eur.* **2022**, *13*, 100268. [CrossRef] [PubMed]
32. Hale, C.R. Introduction. In *Engaging Contradictions*; Hale, C.R., Ed.; University of California Press: Berkeley, CA, USA, 2008; pp. 1–30.
33. Ortner, S. Practicing Engaged Anthropology. *Anthropol. Century* **2019**, *25*. Available online: http://aotcpress.com/articles/practicing-engaged-anthropology/ (accessed on 18 June 2019).
34. Pussetti, C. Ethnography based-art. Undisciplined dialogues and creative research practices. An introduction. *Vis. Ethnogr.* **2018**, *7*, 1–12. [CrossRef]
35. Barata, C. The Gallery of Obstetric Experiences: Addressing perceptions of obstetric violence through ethnography-based artistic experimentation. In *Modos de Fazer, Modos de Ser: Conexões Parciais Entre Antropologia e Arte*; Lacerda, R., Fradique, T., Eds.; Etnográfica Press: Lisboa, Portugal, 2022.
36. Barata, C. Body Broken in Half: Tackling an Afro-Brazilian migrant's experience of obstetric violence and racism in Portugal through art making. *(Con)textos* **2022**, *10*, 65–84.
37. Jansen, L.; Gibson, M.; Bowles, B.C.; Leach, J. First do no harm: Interventions during childbirth. *J. Perinat Educ.* **2013**, *22*, 83–92. [CrossRef]
38. Sandall, J.; Soltani, H.; Gates, S.; Shennan, A.; Devane, D. Midwife-Led Continuity Models versus Other Models of Care for Childbearing Women. *Cochrane Database Syst. Rev.* **2016**, *4*. Available online: https://www.cochranelibrary.com/cdsr/doi/10.1002/14651858 (accessed on 1 October 2021).
39. Martin-Arribas, A.; Escuriet, R.; Borràs-Santos, A.; Vila-Candel, R.; González-Blázquez, C. A comparison between midwifery and obstetric care at birth in Spain: A cross-sectional study of perinatal outcomes. *Int. J. Nurs. Stud.* **2021**, *126*, 104129. [CrossRef]
40. Loewenberg Weisband, Y.; Klebanoff, M.; Gallo, M.F.; Shoben, A.; Norris, A.H. Birth Outcomes of Women Using a Midwife versus Women Using a Physician for Prenatal Care. *J. Midwifery Women's Health* **2018**, *63*, 399–409. [CrossRef]
41. Boerma, T.; Ronsmans, C.; Melesse, D.Y.; Barros, A.J.D.; Barros, F.C.; Juan, L.; Moller, A.; Say, L.; Hosseinpoor, A.R.; Yi, M.; et al. Global epidemiology of use of and disparities in caesarean sections. *Lancet* **2018**, *392*, 1341–1348. [CrossRef]
42. Mazzoni, A.; Althabe, F.; Liu, N.; Bonotti, A.; Gibbons, L.; Sánchez, A.; Belizán, J. Women's preference for caesarean section: A systematic review and meta-analysis of observational studies. *BJOG Int. J. Obstet. Gynaecol.* **2011**, *118*, 391–399. [CrossRef]
43. Betrán, A.P.; Temmerman, M.; Kingdon, C.; Mohiddin, A.; Opiyo, N.; Torloni, M.R.; Zhang, J.; Musana, O.; Wanyonyi, S.Z.; Gülmezoglu, A.M.; et al. Interventions to reduce unnecessary caesarean sections in healthy women and babies. *Lancet* **2018**, *392*, 1358–1368. [CrossRef]
44. Martin, E. *The Woman in the Body. A Cultural Analysis of Reproduction*; Beacon Press: Boston, MA, USA, 2011.
45. The Lancet. Editorial: Stemming the Global Caesarean Section Epidemic. *Lancet* **2018**, *392*, 1279. [CrossRef]

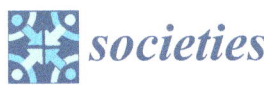

Article

'Focusing and Unfocusing'—Cognitive, Evaluative, and Emotional Dynamics in the Relationship with Human Embryos among ART Beneficiaries

Luís Gouveia * and Catarina Delaunay

Interdisciplinary Centre of Social Sciences, Faculty of Social Sciences and Humanities, University Nova de Lisboa, 1070-312 Lisbon, Portugal; catarinadelaunay@fcsh.unl.pt
* Correspondence: lgouveia@fcsh.unl.pt

Abstract: This article uses data gathered from a study conducted in Portugal to examine the (plural and composite) conceptions that doctors, embryologists, and beneficiaries of Assisted Reproductive Technology (ART) have of the in vitro human embryo. Taking the *sociology of engagements*, developed by Thévenot, as its theoretical lens, the article draws on a total of 69 interviews with ART patients to analyse the plurality of fluid meanings produced about this biological entity, whose status is neither static nor universal. ART beneficiaries are likely to produce plural conceptions of the lab-generated embryo within the framework of different *regimes of engagement*, understood as cognitive and evaluative formats. These various pragmatic regimes, in turn, entail distinct emotional investments. When speaking about their relationship with embryos, beneficiaries therefore express plural emotional experiences, which are articulated using terms such as affection, love, detachment, loss, frustration, hope, mourning, and anguish. Using the theoretical framework of the sociology of engagements, we propose an approach that enables us to produce a detailed record of the connections between the cognitive, evaluative, and emotional dimensions in beneficiaries' relationship with—and decision-making processes about—the embryos, accounting for the plasticity of emotional states linked to the (re)configuration of attributed meanings.

Keywords: in vitro human embryo; ART beneficiaries; regimes of engagement; moral evaluations; emotional states

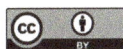

1. Introduction

The birth of the first baby using in vitro fertilization, in the late 1970s, made the creation of humans through assisted reproductive technologies (ART)—in which the embryo is conceived outside the mother's womb [1]—a reality. This technology's development, part of the technoscientification of contemporary medicine [2], is one of the most important innovations of recent decades, and it has provoked controversies over the ontological status of the human embryo. These have led to ethical debates on the use of embryo material for purposes other than those strictly associated with medically assisted reproduction and, specifically, for scientific investigation [3,4].

Reflecting the impact of this technology, a large amount of academic research has been produced. In the social and human sciences, this research has focused particularly on the experience of couples and women who resort to this medical specialty. For example, research has been conducted that examines the embryo as the object of different representations that vary in accordance with the different stages of the fertility treatment. The embryo is neither a static nor a universal biological entity, but it has fluid meanings produced about and statuses conferred on it [5–7]. The human embryo can thus be viewed as child, offspring, potential person, life, viable reproductive product, cluster of cells, lab artefact, or something expendable [4,6]. It can, therefore, be conceptualized in a plurality of ways, both by different ART beneficiaries and by one and the same beneficiary at different points in their therapeutic and personal trajectory [5,8].

The embryo grown in a lab is thus the object of *ontological manipulations* [7,9,10] and of construction and classification using different categories (which are associated with taxonomic structures). These processes of construction and classification are shaped by the embryo's temporal and spatial location, and by what its destiny will be—namely insertion in a parental project, cryopreservation, donation to other couples, use for scientific research, or destruction [11].

Indeed, in vitro human embryos do not differ from spontaneously generated embryos in their biological composition. It is their location outside the uterus at this stage of their existence that makes them susceptible to manipulation, opening up ethical, legal, and moral questions and uncertainties [12]. If medical doctors/embryologists and jurists frame the status of human embryos in medical-scientific and/or legal categories—providing a normative framework for their perspectives on, and interventions related to, the embryo [13]—potential parents are likely to display more plasticity in their ontological relationships with this entity. Their actions and decisions are framed by a plurality of moral principles—a plurality favoured by a cultural context (that of Western societies) in which public discourse around the embryo's status has, so far, not become settled [13,14].

Within this complex web of ambiguous meanings that couples involved in medically assisted reproduction produce, the moral status of the embryo emerges as a central element in these couples' decisions. Academic research into the relationship between these conceptualizations and decision-making processes has focused, particularly, on the context of deliberation about embryos that become surplus following an IVF/ICSI treatment [11,15–17]. However, this production of meanings also occurs at earlier stages of the therapeutic process, starting from the moment of the embryos' creation in the laboratory to their transfer to the uterus. It is this ontological plasticity across the beneficiaries' entire clinical trajectory that this article seeks to address.

Other studies—particularly those in psychology—also focus on ART beneficiaries' emotional experiences. Their ontological manipulations are found to translate into different ways of constructing emotional connections or disconnections with the embryo, as well as emotional states associated with the diagnosis of infertility and engagement in the therapeutic trajectory. In the course of the therapeutic trajectory, a plethora of emotional experiences is, therefore, likely to emerge. These are associated with beneficiaries' experience of infertility as a *crisis* of the parental project [18,19], but they are also linked to the plurality of meanings constructed around the embryo [20,21]. These studies detail oscillations in emotional states throughout the therapeutic trajectory as levels of stress, anxiety, anguish, and depression fluctuate relative to beneficiaries' proximity to the infertility diagnosis and to moments of failure to achieve pregnancy [22–24]. Meanwhile, other studies focus on couples' varying emotional connections with the embryo and how this affects their decisions (as is the case with the choice to destroy or donate spare cryopreserved embryos) due to conceptualizations that transcend strictly instrumental perspectives [17,20].

Again, these studies focus, firstly, on the emotional bonds built around the embryo in the context of the parental project's closure, which relegates the embryo to the status of surplus and requires the parents to decide whether to donate it (to science or other couples) or destroy it. Secondly, the emotional experiences these studies map centre mainly on emotional states associated with the (non-)achievement of pregnancy—falling into categories such as depression, anxiety, or frustration—and coping strategies directed specifically at moments of success or failure during treatments [18,22,24].

This article, by contrast, seeks to understand beneficiaries' emotional experience more broadly. It specifically aims to grasp those oscillations in emotional experience that are not necessarily linked to an infertility diagnosis or to failures in obtaining pregnancy—i.e., to moments of crisis in the parental project. Our focus will instead be on emotional fluctuations and nuances associated with the existing in vitro embryo—fluctuations and nuances that vary according to the different contingencies in patients' therapeutic trajectories, not just their processes of (dis)attachment when deciding on surplus embryos.

Drawing on data gathered by a research project that addresses this ontological plurality of the human embryo, this article introduces a new perspective on this multiplicity of conceptualizations of the human embryo and its associated emotional experiences. Employing a theoretical framework, commonly named *pragmatic sociology* [25–27], we intend to develop a more detailed understanding of how the oscillations in meanings, constructed around the embryo, relate to the different emotions experienced in the course of the therapeutic trajectory (and about the relationship with the embryo in particular)—emotions that change along with these reconfigurations of the moral status conferred on the embryo.

By linking together cognitive, evaluative, and emotional dynamics through this theoretical framework, we intend to highlight the role of emotions in triggering embryos' reclassification, as well as in closing these moments in which the status attributed to this entity is reconfigured. In these processes, the cognitive-evaluative dimension (i.e., categorization and the associated moral judgment) and the emotional dimension of the relationship with the in vitro human embryo affect one another.

Lastly, our analysis aims to provide knowledge about the cognitive-evaluative and emotional dynamics of the beneficiaries who use medically-assisted reproduction technologies, particularly in their relationship with the embryo. The data we have collected support reflection on, and intervention to improve, the quality of information and psychological support provided to beneficiaries in ART centres. We hope this will bring about better management, counselling, and support throughout decision-making processes, involving lab-grown embryos, which involve a heavy emotional load [8,17].

2. Materials and Methods

This article is based on data gathered from an ongoing investigation, in Portugal, into the plurality of meanings produced about the human embryo. The project is named "ETHICHO—Ethico-ontological choreographies: Forms of objectification and evaluation of the human embryo in vitro in the context of Assisted Reproductive Technologies and Scientific Research". It seeks to analyse the plural and composite conceptions that doctors, biologists, and beneficiaries construct around the in vitro human embryo within the context of ART.

Indeed, the embryo is likely to be the object of different representations, which, in turn, rest—according to the theoretical framework we have chosen for this project—on different *regimes of engagement* [25,26], understood as different cognitive and evaluative formats deployed by actors to comprehend their environment [28]—and in this specific case, different formats deployed in order to comprehend the embryo.

To put it as succinctly as possible, this theoretical framework contains a tripartite conceptualization of different regimes of engagement in action, understood as different formats for apprehending a given environment both cognitively (categorization and apprehension of relevant elements in a situation) and evaluatively (in the sense that this categorization and apprehension aims at a given moral good that serves as support to the coordination) [25,26]. The different regimes of engagement in action are located at different positions along an analytical axis that ranges from the general to the particular–i.e., from collective conventions of the public sphere to local and familiar references for action.

In the regime of public justification, action is supported by orders of collective conventions. These collective conventions constitute cognitive and moral frameworks that support the classification of (human or non-human) beings into equivalence classes. Beings within a given equivalence class share a set of common characteristics that confer onto them a partially replaceable character [7]. Each of these conventional constructs–which are moral orders, or orders of worth–is used by actors to evaluate and organize the worth of the various beings in a situation. Each order of worth contains a specific moral perspective for the coordination of human action, in the sense that it concretely expresses a different conception of the common good. The orders of worth most relevant for our purposes in this article are: the *domestic* order of worth, in which tradition/generation/hierarchy constitutes the form of the common good through which the embryo is evaluated; the *civic* order of worth, in which it is the collective interest; the connectionist order of worth, in which it is the project/activity that links individuals; the *industrial* order of worth, in which it is *efficacy*.

Each order of worth identified refers to distinct conceptions of the common good, and consists of a publicly available *grammar* of making the common–a way of reaching commonality and differing through governing practices of criticism and justification [25,26]. The way in which each order of worth is translated into understandings of the embryos is shown throughout the text.

Concerning the remaining regimes, in the regime of engagement in a plan, reality is understood with reference to objectives that form the established plan, with the environment being functionally prepared, and the satisfaction of the accomplished action is the good aimed at. Lastly, in the regime of familiar engagement, action occurs within an area proximate to the actor, supported by this actor's familiarisation with their immediate environment. Comfort and ease are the good aimed at.

These differences, in relationship to the embryo, can thus be distinguished using the architecture of regimes of engagement conceptualized by Thévenot [26–28]:

a. Regime of engagement in a plan: conception of the embryo as an abstract and replaceable resource, within a functional understanding—with the embryo understood as an instrument or a means, mobilized to attain an end (in this case, pregnancy).

b. Regime of public justification: conception of the embryo as falling into a moral class/equivalence category, thus sharing a set of characteristics (e.g., biological properties, insertion in a parental project, etc.) that is common to the beings within this category, through which they are evaluated and ranked, which makes the embryo partially replaceable. However, it is this understanding of the embryo in general terms—using equivalence principles that express senses of justice—that enables the embryo to *rise in singularity* as a criterion to confer *total humanity* [7]. This happens when the embryo is conceived of as a potential child or potential life, as part of an equivalence class associated with the connectionist conventional order, in the sense that it involves a parental/biological reproduction project of the progenitors; as genetic inheritance/offspring, in the sense that it is inserted into a network of kinship/lineage, in the conventional domestic order; as a cluster of cells/biological material, evaluated from the viewpoint of its genetic/morphological quality in the industrial conventional order; as a *gift* for scientific investigation or to other couples in the civic conventional order.

c. Regime of familiar engagement: a conception that singularises the embryo, treating it as a singular, irreplaceable entity—granter of total humanity [7]. This singularisation is very different from a functional or general understanding of the embryo (according to an equivalence principle), which, in this case, is conceived of as a child. This engagement format, in which an irreplaceable status is conferred on the embryo, becomes evident, for example, in the act of giving a name; where the embryo is lost, the non-attribution of this same name to another grown embryo attests to this particularization.

It is important to recognise that conceptions of the embryo are neither fixed nor watertight, but they can draw on different regimes of engagement—sometimes combining them—throughout beneficiaries' therapeutic trajectory. Moments of *disquiet* can occur [27] at any point in this trajectory, opening up the possibility of re-describing the embryo through a different regime of engagement (or combinations of different regimes).

Furthermore, beneficiaries' trajectories are also characterized by fluctuations in the emotional experiences that accompany the meanings produced about the embryos (and the procedures they undergo). In other words, different emotional ambiances/experiences are attached to different cognitive and evaluative operations.

These different regimes of engagement combine cognition, evaluation, and emotion. On the one hand, they presuppose operations of *investment in forms* (i.e., material equipment, relational forms, etc.) that support the comprehension of the environment under a given cognitive and evaluative format [26]. On the other hand, each regime of engagement also involves *emotional investments*—emotional states/ambiences appropriate to the format, according to which the situation is apprehended. These ambiences give authenticity to an actor's engagement with a situation, reinforcing its apprehension according to the cognitive and evaluative format in question [29]. Emotions, therefore, support the interpretation of a situation, according to a given regime of engagement, and are a driving force behind individual and collective action [30].

Each order of worth involves the cognitive apprehension of a given situation in a way that balances its apprehension according to this order of worth and the sacrifice of other forms of apprehension linked to other orders, thus operating in a cognitive economy. But this cognitive apprehension also operates in an emotional economy, to the extent that there is an emotional experience associated with a state of worth and the sacrifice of emotional experiences associated with other orders of worth. Thus emotions participate in a cognitive economy and cognitive operations participate in an emotional economy [29]. This is the case, for example, with the emotional disattachment in the relationship with an embryo from a connectionist or domestic grammar–in view, for example, of enduring moments of failure in the therapeutic plan (such as the loss of embryos in vitro or in utero). This emotional disattachment from the embryo participates in a cognitive re-apprehension of it as, for example, biological material.

We can now describe the emotional dynamics that are associated with each regime of action, and which give each regime its specificity. The domestic grammar presupposes an emotional economy in which warmth is experienced in relationships with other beings—particularly, in this case, the embryo—with these beings' disappearance (in this case, the loss/destruction of the embryo) experienced as an absence whose memory is prolonged in time [29]. The emotional ambiance can, likewise, be characterized by the use of categories such as affection, tenderness, or fondness towards the embryo, as well as sadness, pain, or abandonment in cases of loss or decisions to destroy or donate—categories that confer the typical emotional authenticity of relationships within a family group [29].

However, to identify the forms of engagement–and the corresponding moral and emotional categories–, we need to contextualize how terms are used by actors. This is the case, for instance, with interviewees' use of terms such as mourning or child, terms that might be associated with a familiar engagement with the embryos, but in whose context of use discourse analysis reveals situational dynamics that remain at the level of equivalences–and therefore distant from the genuine singularization that we would expect from familiar engagement.

In the connectionist grammar, emotions towards the embryo are based on its apprehension through categories such as hope and expectation, with the embryo understood as a being integrated into a parental project—therefore, as a potential child. In this grammar, conceiving a child is a project that is more robust and longer lasting than all others (personal, professional, etc.), and it is this robustness and durability that gives the parental project its authenticity [7]. It is the beneficiaries' desire for—and commitment to—the shared parental project that defines their relationship with, and emotional investment in, the embryo, and its loss is experienced as a disruption of this same promise, or expectation, that emotionally links the progenitors to it.

In contrast to the domestic grammar, the industrial grammar is characterized by sobriety. Relational warmth towards the embryo is replaced by the cold calculation of a relationship, mediated by scientific methods and procedures, with the embryo equated to a technical object. With action guided by the passion for efficacy [29], the loss of the embryo is emotionally experienced—in line with a principle of efficiency—as a failure in technical execution and a waste of its potential use as precious material (for reproduction or scientific investigation). The embryo is therefore evaluated according to its level of quality (which grants it industrial worth) and inserted into a larger mechanism, in equivalence with other technical devices.

In the civic grammar, the emotional experience is based on categories such as solidarity and gratitude, which express a connection between the beneficiary and the collective, in the sense that they are contributing to the general interest through impersonal mutuality [3]. This can occur through either scientific development, release, or detachment; the motivation is to help other beneficiaries, with the embryo viewed as a gift.

This grammar is discernible, therefore, in beneficiaries whose therapeutic trajectory leads to the embryo becoming surplus and thus, dissociated from the parental project that led to its creation in the first place. As the embryo is no longer understood through categories such as child or potential child by the beneficiaries, the civic grammar provides a normative framework for reconfiguring meaning around the embryo, enabling a continuous transition, without disruption, by partially preserving the meaning of the previous moral status attributed to it (thus providing ontological continuity). The new status requires an emotional investment in the embryo—albeit of a different nature—that does not fall into the technical distance associated with an understanding of the embryo as a set of cells (industrial grammar). This transfer to the civic grammar—a transfer between orders of worth [31]—provides beneficiaries with a less radical rupture, with the cognitive and moral understanding involved in (and emotional experience attached to) connectionist and domestic grammars, than would a direct transfer to the industrial grammar.

In the regime of engagement in a plan, the emotional ambiance is characterised by distance in relation to the embryo, expressed through categories such as frustration, disappointment, anxiety, anguish, and suffering, which are all emotional experiences related to the non-realization of the pursued goal—and in this case, to the uncertainty about whether the planned action will be accomplished, as well as the failure to achieve pregnancy, both of which are perceived as moments of crisis in the parental project [19]. Thus, these emotions are dissociated from the loss or destruction of the embryo itself and are directly linked to the couple's plan of having offspring.

Lastly, in the familiar engagement regime, categories such as love, protection, care, and bond become central, supporting forms of relation that are based on intimate gestures—gestures that are very different from actions based on the regime of equivalences [32]—and grounded in an understanding of the embryo as a singular being. Within this intense particularizing emotional investment (different from the still-replaceable character associated with the domestic grammar), mourning gains prominence as an emotional category in the case of embryo loss. The embryo's non-development is experienced as a loss that cannot be remedied through replacement by another entity; this is perceived as the loss of a child [7].

Now that we have presented our guiding theoretical-conceptual framework, this article will analyse how these cognitive-evaluative and emotional dynamics are connected to beneficiaries' relationships with the human embryo. More specifically, within this integrated trio of cognition, evaluation, and emotion, emotional experiences are a driving force, triggering (and closing down) reclassifications of the embryo [33]. It is the emotional experience that initiates the process of re-assessing the environment (in this particular case, the embryo) according to distinct cognitive and moral formats; it is the emotional experience that ultimately enables this moment of *test* to be closed down through the convergence between format of engagement and emotional ambiance [33].

Indeed, different points in the therapeutic trajectory tend to be accompanied by different emotional experiences, both individual (experienced by the beneficiary in line with a given regime of engagement) and collective, in the sense that emotions are common to the actors that coordinate action among themselves according to a given grammar [34]. However, it is in situations of disquiet—of questioning the formats of engagement used to understand the embryo—that these emotional experiences become more intense and tangible.

Our aim is to precisely illustrate this ontological and emotional plurality, with a particular focus on the stages of the therapeutic trajectory that are likely prompt beneficiaries to switch between distinct regimes of engagement and, consequently, reconfigure the moral status conferred on the embryo. This is the case in moments of loss (in utero or in vitro) and decision (e.g., donation, destruction, etc.).

The data presented results from interviews with beneficiaries of ART. A total of 69 interviews were conducted, by the same interviewer, between September 2019 and January 2021. The sample was composed of interviewees that had undergone second-line treatments—in vitro fertilization (IVF) and Intracytoplasmic Sperm Injection (ICSI)—which involve the production of embryos in a laboratory.

The interviews were conducted with respondents at different stages of their therapeutic trajectory—during treatment cycles, between cycles, or after already completing the process (with or without a pregnancy). Respondents' treatments took place within a largely similar timeframe: on average, those in the sample started their first treatment cycle in 2016 (standard deviation of 3.4), and their last treatment cycle occurred, on average, in 2020 (standard deviation of 2.9). Furthermore, a significant proportion of the respondents (approximately 20%) were still in treatment at the time of the interview, with a cycle either in progress or due to begin.

Except for five who were born abroad, all interviewees were Portuguese nationals. Only three (female) respondents—all of whom were engaged in a homosexual parental project—went through IVF/ICSI treatment cycles, carried out in clinics located outside Portugal, in a period when the legal regulatory framework for ART in Portugal did not give this group access to treatments.

Concerning this issue, it is important to put into context and refer that, in Portugal, the first law regulating medically assisted procreation techniques, approved in 2006, restricted access to couples in a stable, heterosexual, marital union who had health problems (either infertility or risk of transmitting a genetic condition). However, a subsequent review of this legislation (Law 17/2016) gave all women access to ART, regardless of whether they had an infertility diagnosis, or of their marital status or sexual orientation. Access by male homosexual couples remains prohibited in the present legal framework.

The interviews were conducted both with individual users and with heterosexual and homosexual couples. The great majority of the interviewees were female (nearly 92%) and engaged in heterosexual parental projects (approximately 95%). Only four interviewees were engaged in homosexual parental projects.

The respondents were recruited online (from social networks or forums dealing with infertility) and from a patient association concerned with infertility-related diseases. Most had been through higher education (81.1%), and a significant percentage had done some level of post-graduate study—either master's or doctoral degrees (35%). Since this was a convenience sample—generated through appeals for participation using digital channels—a higher level of representativeness could not be attained either in terms of gender (i.e., male respondents) or in terms of non-heterosexual beneficiaries.

The interviewees were given pseudonyms to ensure anonymity. All interviews were recorded and transcribed verbatim, with analysis conducted using the qualitative analysis software MaxQDA (2018 version).

The interview guide encompassed several themes and sought to cover the different stages of the therapeutic trajectory both before and after completion of the treatments: the formation of the parental project; infertility diagnosis (if applicable) and decision to resort to specialized medical help; knowledge about ART; description of the therapeutic protocol and lived experienced; decision on surplus embryos (if applicable); general conceptions of, and forms of connection with, the created embryos (moral status attributed, moments of change in these understandings, beginning of the construction of an emotional bond, etc.).

With this article's specific goals in mind, we used categorical content analysis to identify the different ontological conceptions and the different emotional experiences—encompassing various emotions at various levels of intensity (*emotional tonalities*)—involved in the interviewees' relationship with the in vitro embryo, at different stages of the therapeutic trajectory.

These different conceptualizations of, and emotional investments in, embryos must be analysed while taking into account the specific characteristics of our sampling process. This process did not seek to ensure a representative sample of participants in terms of sexual orientation, socioeconomic status, ethnic background, etc.; it was mostly restricted to a specific national context, as most respondents were Portuguese nationals and/or had undergone treatments in Portugal. Our analysis, therefore, focuses on capturing the grammatical diversity, and oscillation between grammars, among the study's participants without trying to generalize to other societal contexts or identify patterns according to sociodemographic variables.

3. Results

With the aim of examining these beneficiaries' changing relations with their embryos—which involve oscillations between (and compositions of) the evaluations they make, and associated emotional experiences—we will analyse some interviews in which interviewees' discourse demonstrates, precisely, the multiplicity of regimes of action.

A first perspective is supplied by an interviewee whose therapeutic trajectory was made up of twelve treatment cycles. In total, 24 transferred embryos were generated (classified as viable), along with those that were discarded (the interviewee was unable to provide an exact figure). This long therapeutic trajectory thus serves as a window into the *ontological choreographies* [10] that beneficiaries can develop in their relationship with the embryos, combining different regimes of engagement—understood as cognitive and moral formats—along with plural and composite emotional ambiances.

Here, the interviewee's perspective is characterized by an understanding of the embryos using the category of children, revealing a transition (albeit complete) to a singularizing form of affective engagement with each one:

> Valentina: "From the beginning they were my children ... They were mine, so to speak ... That's why it is so hard for me ... [...] The news took such a toll ... They were my children who disappeared [...]. I sometimes say to my husband 'We've lost twenty-four children' ... That was basically what I felt ... [...] If I have this conversation with my sisters-in-law, with my nieces and nephews, they won't understand this ... This is hard to explain to people who haven't gone through the process ... that to me they were my children too ... Like to them their children are those whom they felt growing in their bellies ... "

Demonstrating an openness to familiar engagement, her discourse shows how the intimate nature of a familiar representation of the embryo is difficult to communicate to those who do not share the same experience ("is hard to explain to people who haven't gone through the process") [27]. This construction of an emotional bond with the embryo in the absence of other *ontological markers* that signal the embryo's rise in singularity [7]—such as the physical symptoms associated with pregnancy ("growing in their bellies")—characterises the particularity of the experience of reproduction using ART.

Although this regime of engagement prevails in the interviewee's relationship with the lab-grown embryos across successive treatment cycles, her description (i.e., the position of the embryo in time and space) goes on to reveal that her representations of these embryos, and the corresponding emotional experiences, are more composite and oscillating:

> Valentina: "But I also ... psychologically filtered that, and we focused only on the ones they said were ... So, if I were to worry ... to focus on everything, this would take an even greater toll ... [...] And, in time, the feelings are complex and you create, we create filters, barriers so it won't ... it won't take as much of a toll, right? So, the focus was on the ones that were viable ... I tried not to think about it, no ... That is, because scientifically they weren't viable, they had genetic problems, that was how I thought ... That was how I had to think [...]. But, there it is, our psychological filter, it's 'Don't think about that anymore, focus

on the others' . . . This is very complex, [. . .] focusing and unfocusing . . . [. . .] to safeguard me from suffering, because . . . It's a very strong pain."

The interviewee uses the focusing-unfocusing pair to describe her oscillation between different cognitive-evaluative formats and their associated emotional experiences. The act of focusing is associated, particularly, with a break from instrumental and biological conceptions of the embryo, through a shift to a familiar form of engagement. This is characterized by a singularizing affect that brings the embryo closer to the status of a child, although it is still inserted in classes of equivalence—be it as a potential child (connectionist grammar) or as part of a kinship network (*domestic* grammar)—that make it partially replaceable. In turn, unfocusing is associated with an inversion in this process of humanizing the embryos and rising in singularity, as the embryos are relegated to the condition of biological material whose genetic quality renders them obsolete in light of the industrial grammar. Detachment therefore follows their classification as technical objects.

In this oscillation between formats of engaging with the embryo, the central role of scientific evaluative devices is highlighted. In particular, the scientific evaluation of the embryo's viability and quality—which, for the laboratory professionals, determines the embryo's industrial worth by identifying its efficacy as a resource—is what grants and reinforces the worth of the embryo as a potential child or progeny/offspring. The interviewee's speech therefore reveals a composition of grammars. Her understanding of the embryo as a child or potential child, and her gradual transition to familiar engagement, find support in objects from the industrial world [25], as she oscillates between emotional connection and disconnection to the in vitro embryo ("the focus was on the ones that were viable").

On the other hand, as the interviewee's language shows, these relational shifts—while still associated with an oscillation in moral status in accordance with the ontological marker in question (viability stemming from the embryo's scientific classification)—are also a way of preserving her engagement in the therapeutic trajectory. It is her desire to avoid "pain"—an emotional experience associated with her conception of the embryo as a child or potential child—that triggers a change in the status she attributes to the embryos evaluated as inviable. These start to be seen as biological material with "genetic problems", with the industrial grammar employed as a convention to support this evaluative judgment.

This dynamic of focusing-unfocusing illustrates the relationship between evaluation and emotion. The cognitive and evaluative operation participates in an emotional economy [29], aiming, in this case, to enable the beneficiary to endure the emotional impact associated with the loss of in vitro or in utero embryos and secure her continuation of the treatment process. It is this non-linearity, throughout the therapeutic trajectory, of the emotional experience (or emotional ambiance)—which is linked to the different cognitive and evaluative formats employed to apprehend the embryo—that is highlighted in the beneficiary's discourse ("the feelings are complex").

Another interviewee describes a similar oscillation in her emotional connection to the embryos—in this case, a weakening of this connection. Here, the accomplishment of the parental project, through a full-term twin pregnancy, leads her to change the status she attributes to the remaining cryopreserved embryos.

Ana: "And then the birth of the twins . . . my memory also began . . . And later I found out I was pregnant [new, spontaneous pregnancy] and so I forgot . . . Then . . . the memory was really very sporadic [. . .]. There was that connection in the beginning, yes . . . But later on, I have to be honest, no . . . no . . . The connection rested with the twins . . . [. . .] . . . That's normal, isn't it? Because they're real . . . ((laughs)), right?"

While, at first, the embryos were conceptualized as a potential child, the interviewee's connection with them is progressively attenuated after achieving the pregnancy with two transferred embryos ("the connection rested with the twins"). In light of the fulfilment of the promise associated with the transferred embryos, from the perspective of the parental project ("Because they're real"), the emotional connection with the remaining ones gradually dissipates over time ("the memory was really very sporadic"). If, in other interviews, the birth of a child leads to the meaning attributed to the remaining embryos being recomposed to reinforce their status as a potential child, in this case, the birth of twins (in addition to the spontaneous pregnancy with a third child) closes the parental project and gradually weakens the emotional connection with the embryos.

However, in this reconfiguration process, the status of the cryopreserved embryos does not return to that of instrument or cluster of cells. The emotional connection with the remaining embryos is reduced to a purely genetic connection, which undermines the embryos' status as a potential child. This is shown by the next excerpt from the same interview:

> Ana: "I remember a situation, when I was already pregnant with [name of the son], who's the youngest . . . I've just remembered . . . The four of us were there, right? I was . . . At that time they even wanted to walk . . . And I don't know why . . . [. . .] One of them came to my belly to cuddle it . . . And I remember saying: 'This is not your only sibling, there are other siblings, but the others–you'll never get to meet them . . . '"

The attribution of the status of sibling is rooted in an overlap between the genetic bond, in the framework of a domestic grammar, and the condition of potential child ("you'll never get to meet them"). Within this cognitive and moral operation, the original category of potential child gives way to the embryo being seen through the lens of a biological/genetic connection. This reclassification of the embryo in the sphere of equivalences—which stems from the closure of the parental project—is accompanied by an attenuation of the emotional experience of affective connection.

On this regard, it is important to stress that the interview data show that the ontological marker of obtaining a full-term pregnancy can bring about other reconfigurations in beneficiaries' conceptualizations of embryos. It can trigger a humanizing singularization of the remaining embryos; favour a transition from viewing them as biological material to considering them a potential child or child (e.g., in the sense that they are perceived as siblings of the already-born child); or prompt the embryos to be seen as a gift to other couples struggling to have a child. Due to space constraints, we can't use excerpts to illustrate this complex non-linear relationship between the completion of pregnancy and the reclassification of embryos that become surplus.

Another interviewee identifies a different ontological marker: he points to the embryo's transfer to the uterus as the moment that prompts a change in the format used to understand the embryo, which is accompanied by a shift in emotional experience:

> Daniel: "Then, there's already . . . The journey can be begun to . . . to paternity . . . And then there's already . . . There's already, always with this feeling of fear, about whether it'll succeed or not . . . And even if it did generate a pregnancy, even then there would still be many, many possible risks of it not working, of having a miscarriage. But there, yes, there is already a small emotional connection, you think that the beginning of everything could be there."

The interviewee's emotional experience is summarized by the central category that he himself uses: "fear" about the pregnancy's realization or non-realization. This category sits within a connectionist grammar that inserts the embryo into the category of potential child—still distant, therefore, from an emotional experience associated with the prospect of losing a being perceived as a child. As the interviewee adds, there is a "small emotional connection", an openness to affective investment in the embryo. However, he still sees this embryo as part of a "journey [. . .] to paternity", and therefore remains in an incipient phase of singularizing engagement.

Along with the transition between grammars used to understand the embryo, the testimony of another interviewee points to the revision—based on the connectionist grammar— of the state of worth [25] conferred on the embryo (initially seen as a potential child) over the course of the therapeutic trajectory. Successive failures to obtain a pregnancy affect the moral status attributed to, and emotional experience of the relationship with, the embryos:

> Bianca: "And everything leads us to believe them to be . . . to be our children, isn't it? To us it was already a . . . A living being, a human being . . . A person. To us, it would already become a person, one day it would be a person, and it is very difficult for us to come to a point and say 'Hang on, this is still nothing.' At the end of the day, it still is nothing, right? It's . . . . It's the beginning of something, but it may not be, and . . . And this is . . . At the time it was very frustrating because we had the embryos, I had everything for . . . for it to go well . . . [. . .]. At the end, it was very difficult because we got to the point where we only wanted a positive pregnancy test, because that was what would make us certain that it was something, and not the embryo."

The experience of successive failures in transferring the embryos leads to a change in the status conferred on them. In this case, an initial understanding of the embryo as potential child ("one day it would be a person") is attenuated, as the in vitro embryo is relegated to a state of lesser *worth* under the same grammar ("the embryo is still nothing").

When we model how the formats of engagement change, in accordance with the different stages of the therapeutic trajectory, the pregnancy test becomes the central device that shifts the ontological status attributed to the embryo: a transition to the state of potential child is prompted by the test's confirmation of the probability of development ("certain that it was something"). Within the connectionist grammar, this stage raises the embryo supported by the pregnancy test to a state of worth higher than that attributed to the embryo not supported by this test [25]. This contrasts with the previous experience of the interviewee, in which the very existence of the embryo precociously granted that same status.

The same interviewee expands on this change in her evaluation of the embryo and her associated emotional experience:

> Bianca: "And this process of accepting that embryos are just embryos is very difficult because we put all our hope in those four or five, and . . . [. . .] And the feeling that we always had about the embryos is that . . . They were people, we spoke of them at home as if . . . Those are our frozen boys there, right? [. . .] For us the embryo was already the beginning . . . right? It was already very important. And this is very difficult, to realize that we had to disconnect, and this process is very . . . extremely hard."

Reiterating the embryo's initial status as a promise since the start of the therapeutic trajectory ("we put all our hope")—i.e., the first stage in a continuum that culminates in the end of pregnancy ("the embryo was already the beginning")—the interviewee's discourse reveals a change in the emotional economy associated with the therapeutic trajectory and, in particular, the relationship with the embryos. Failures lead to a reconfiguration in the format of engagement, which attenuates the status of the embryo as a potential child ("we had to disconnect").

There is, therefore, a revision of the in vitro embryos' state of worth, which brings these beings closer to their biological composition in the way they are evaluated. Consequently, the associated emotional experience is altered: a connection based on hope is weakened, as is the projection of the status of future child onto the embryo ("accepting that embryos are just embryos"). Again, the emotional experience of the loss of embryos ("extremely hard"), intensified by the initial conception of the embryos as potential children ("those are our frozen boys there"), leads to a reconfiguration of the moral status of those embryos generated afterwards.

Another interviewee reveals how the transition from the in vitro to the in utero condition does not constitute a transversal ontological marker. In her case, after the transfer of two embryos, one was lost. However, her discourse demonstrates how this transition of the embryo in space did not translate into a reconfiguration of its status, or of her emotional connection to it:

> Olga: "So, the fact that there was an embryo . . . To me it was already a victory . . . Because . . . I managed . . . It wasn't two, okay, tough luck, it was one . . . But . . . It wasn't . . . It wasn't as if it had been a miscarriage or as if I had lost it . . . Because I think it was so little time . . . that . . . From the time I found out I was pregnant until I was certain it was only one, it was seven days . . . [. . .] When the doctor told me it was just one, that the other hadn't developed, I thought 'Okay, no . . . no problem. I have one, which is more important' . . . So I didn't see it as a loss, no . . . "

The conception of the embryos as a promise or possibility, in this case, translates into an immediate detachment expressed in the interviewee's discourse ("It wasn't two, okay, tough luck [. . .] no problem"). These embryos still have not been singularized, something evident in the interviewee's understanding of them as replaceable in light of the parental project's accomplishment ("I have one, which is more important"). In this case, it seems to be the length of the pregnancy that is preponderant in the construction of an emotional bond and in the gradual transition away from the regime of equivalences. The non-development of the embryo in utero is therefore not experienced as a "loss", in the sense of an emotional experience close to mourning, which is associated with the regime of proximity.

A similar experience can be identified in another interviewee. While the simultaneous transfer of two embryos raised the possibility of a twin pregnancy, the procedure resulted in the loss of one of the embryos and the consequent development of the pregnancy with a single embryo (carried to term). The interviewee's discourse shows how the moment of transfer does not trigger a rise in singularity [7] of the meaning attributed to the embryo.

> Lila: "[. . .] with lightness . . . With naturalness, that is, it was what it had to be . . . Deep down we were ready for the possibility of having two, that is, we knew that . . . in the best or worst case, it would be two . . . It was one, and it was excellent, that is . . . any of the . . . We wanted to have a child so much that any of the possibilities was good for us, and therefore we experienced it as natural . . . [. . .] we didn't feel it was a loss . . . [. . .] Of course, many times we thought 'What if it had been two?' . . . Sometimes we think that, but it's not in the sense of it being a loss . . . "

The realization of the full-term pregnancy through one of the transferred embryos constitutes the attainment of the parental project. In light of this, the loss of one of the embryos translates into an emotional experience described as "lightness" and "naturalness", reflecting the still replaceable character conferred on the embryos, which are understood as possibilities [14,35] associated with a parental project. This remains distant from a humanizing form of engagement that would translate into an experience of *loss* associated with a singularized being ("we didn't feel it was a loss"). The retrospective outlook reinforces this conception. The scenario of twins is understood, precisely, as an unrealized possible outcome of the parental project, which distances the beneficiaries' emotional ambiance from that associated with familiar engagement ("it's not in the sense of it being a loss").

This interviewee's discourse, when discussing a previous failed treatment cycle, also reveals the particular importance they attribute to devices for biomedically evaluating the embryos in prompting changes in the meanings they ascribe to the embryo:

> Lila: "In the first ICSI, it was that hope that . . . that we would make it and that we'd have embryos . . . But the embryos were not high-quality embryos, so, on the day for implanting them they warned us that the embryos were not perfect, that is, we were already a little hesitant . . . But of course, when we found out they hadn't taken hold, of course, then we had a feeling of loss, of . . . That hope

we had created died there. The whole trajectory of the treatment creates a hope that we will have a child, and then, of course, it's lost, isn't it?"

When embryos are understood as a hope, the first indicators of their poor morphokinetic "quality" relegate these beings to a state of lesser worth because they reduce the possibility of generating a pregnancy ("they warned us that the embryos were not perfect"). This evaluation is accompanied by an associated inflection in the beneficiary's emotional experience, characterised by a regression in their nascent construction of a connection to the embryo understood as a potential child ("we were already a little hesitant").

The embryos' transfer to the uterus, and their subsequent failure to evolve, already corresponds to an intensified emotional experience, prompting the interviewee to use the category of "loss" to describe this occurrence. Her utterance highlights an experience still associated with the connectionist grammar, but with the embryo now associated with a different state of worth. This emotional state is associated with the failure of the parental project dependent on the non-evolved embryos, which are inserted into an equivalence class—"hope that we will have a child". It is this hope that was reinforced immediately after the transfer.

On this subject, it is worth to highlight the analytical potential of conceptualizing hope and expectation using the theoretical framework of regimes of engagement. Doing so allows us to avoid essentializing hope [36] by seeing it as immutable, making it possible to consider the temporal patterning of patients' expectations [37] when we examine their experience in healthcare contexts. This theoretical framework encourages us to analyse how the emotional experiences of hope and expectation are intimately connected with the actor's cognitive and moral evaluation of their environment (specifically, the embryo), acquiring different tones–in this case, according to the state of worth conferred on the embryo. Hope and expectation oscillate, shaping how embryos are understood depending on different stages of the treatment (e.g., phase of in vitro development), on vicissitudes (e.g., in vitro or in utero loss of embryos), on circumstances (e.g., classifications of the embryo) and on temporality (e.g., number of treatment cycles) that guide beneficiaries' therapeutic trajectories. Adopting this framework thus enables us to analyze how, from the perspective of a sociology of hope and expectation, entities, thoughts and actions are continuously shaped throughout a patient's clinical path.

We have seen that the revision of the embryo's prior classification occurs with the evaluation of its morphokinetic quality, a positive pregnancy test, or its transfer to the uterus, all of which are ontological markers. However, another specific emotional experience is associated with situations of ambivalence or tension in the formats through which beneficiaries engage with the embryo. This is true for another interviewee who, reflecting on her therapeutic trajectory, recounts the uncertainty experienced in relation to the embryo's moral status. Attached to this uncertainty is an emotional state of anguish, which stems from the tension between the conventional order that guides the professionals' (doctors' and embryologists') approach to embryos in the lab and the meaning she, herself, produces around them, which is connected to a different grammar:

Aurora: "When she [the doctor] told me 'Okay, we have four, four blastocysts, and we'll have to freeze them, because there was overstimulation' ... At that moment I had questions [...] and what I asked her was: 'Do the embryos feel anything when they are frozen? Do they feel anything when they are thawed?' And her response was that they didn't ... My motherly heart said something a little different [...]. And, by the way, this question still remains with me, because I still have three frozen blastocysts ... [...] When I advanced to this treatment, I'll admit, again, that I wasn't ready to deal with that sort of question, I thought it would be something very rational ... That it would be ... A process where those questions would not be relevant because they're microscopic things that you can't see ... However, it was difficult for me for that reason [...], although she'd tell me that the embryos didn't feel ... I still, I still feel some anguish [...] I think that: 'If ... If I loved this embryo that I transferred, and the others ... If

I've loved them since . . . since I knew my eggs had been fertilized, this is worth something . . . This has to mean something.'"

Notwithstanding her reference to her "motherly heart"—which seemingly indicates a domestic grammar, with family relations and personal connection [38] used as a form of argument—the interviewee's discourse predominantly evokes an emotional experience marked by an intense affective investment of love—which comes under the framework of familiar engagement—in her relationship with the embryo. The word "heart" may, therefore, indicate an argument based not so much on a status (mother) associated with a family group, which would connect her to the lab-grown embryo under the conventional *domestic* order, but on an intimate involvement, one that is not accessible to actors that do not share the same experience of emotional investment [27].

This grammar is mobilized in opposition to the discourse of medical practitioners, who are embedded in an industrial grammar that understands the embryo as biological material, subject to a set of technical and scientific devices. Through a familiar form of engagement, the interviewee expresses a feeling of "anguish" about the procedures carried out on the embryo when understood through the industrial grammar (in particular, the laboratory procedures related to the freezing process).

The interviewee herself indicates this mismatch in cognitive and evaluative formats between beneficiary and professionals. She mentions her expectation, at the beginning of treatment, that her engagement format would converge with the environment occupied by beings from the industrial world, with repercussions for the related emotional experience ("I thought it would be something very rational")—something that would be enabled by her non-visualization of the embryo ("microscopic things that you can't see") [7]. This rationality and distancing—which constitute an emotional framework that allows action to be mediated by the resources of technical objects and methods and oriented towards efficiency [29] in the execution of procedures (with procedural success or failure being the focus of the emotional experience)—contrasts with the emotional ambiance that characterises the beneficiary's relationship with the embryo, which is marked by the affective intensity associated with a familiar form of engagement.

Moreover, the interviewee's own description of the emotions, associated with losing the embryo after its transfer to her uterus, reinforces the latter regime of engagement. She mobilizes the category of "mourning" here—a category associated with singularisation that marks the use of a humanizing cognitive and moral format to understand the embryo, one that is far removed from understandings of a technical-scientific nature.

> Aurora: "And when I saw it, to me it was very important to have the image of my embryo, especially for the mourning I'm going through with the miscarriage I had . . . It was very important that I had an image, to me it was important, and it is important. I keep the image of my embryo near me . . . [. . .] It's here on my computer . . . And I like having this image here while I'm in the process of mourning . . . "

While the grammars used by beneficiaries mentioned so far all integrate the embryo into the parental project (whether as an instrument, cluster of cells, genetic inheritance, offspring, potential child, or child), the next excerpt provides an example of the embryo being reclassified in a way that dissociates it from this project—the project that gave rise to its creation. The interviewee describes how the cryopreserved embryos' shift into the category of surplus prompts them to reconfigure their evaluation as potential children under a connectionist grammar. Now that they are surplus, they are given the moral status of gift, and the beneficiary's emotional experience is subsequently recomposed:

> Dalila: "I remember I wrote 'Today I have eleven children . . . But tomorrow I don't know how many they'll be.' But it's like . . . The expectations we had were so low that this didn't . . . Except for the part about the twins, which was very real . . . Of the confirmation of a positive . . . [. . .] The others didn't . . . It was more like something . . . a desire, but not a reality, you know? [. . .] We'd always

authorized them to be studied, and, actually, after it ended [...] [husband's name] said 'No, we won't try again, and it's all going to be studied', and we signed documents ... That all of the embryos that weren't used ... as a life, for us, will be studied to help other people ... "

On the one hand, during the period of in vitro evolution, the interviewee describes the emotional state of "expectation"—associated with connectionist grammar—as connecting the couple to the lab-grown embryos. As she then reports, however, this expectation varied throughout the therapeutic trajectory. It was still "low" in the in vitro stage, given the high chance of failure, and the emotional connection with them as *potential children* remained restrained. It is the "confirmation of a positive" through a pregnancy test that reinforces the state of worth in this connectionist order, simultaneously intensifying the emotional connection with the embryos based on this same expectation. With the ontological marker of the pregnancy test, the embryo ceases to be only a "desire" to become closer to a "reality", and the status of potential or future child is reinforced.

On the other hand, as the interviewee reports, the pregnancy's realization at a later moment in the therapeutic trajectory, and the consequent closure of the parental project, prompts a reconfiguration of the embryos' status. The expectation and hope attached to them gives way to the desire to "help other people"—an emotional experience associated with the *civic* grammar. In this particular case, this solidarity—or sense of civic responsibility [3]—materializes in the form of the remaining embryos' donation for scientific research.

4. Discussion

ART beneficiaries' decision-making processes throughout their therapeutic trajectory are shaped by the interaction between cognition, moral evaluation, and emotion [39]. On the cognitive level, patients must decide and act within an environment composed of information about their prospects of success, the efficacy of technical procedures, and statistical data on health risks (e.g., genetic evaluation of the embryo), amid a context of uncertainty about the pregnancy's realization. These deliberative processes, in turn, incorporate moral judgments, which allow a moral status to be conferred on the lab-grown embryos. Additionally, different emotional responses, both positive and negative (pain, anguish, suffering, joy, etc.), arise in connection with different moments in the therapeutic trajectory [39].

Although many research projects have been conducted on the emotional experiences associated with an infertility diagnosis and the ART trajectory, their conceptual frameworks do not encourage us to look in detail at the plasticity of emotional states, or at how these states relate to oscillations in the embryo's ontological status [40].

Indeed, these studies tend to focus, mostly, on the evolution of beneficiaries' emotional states through categories such as depression, anxiety, or frustration—which are associated with treatments' success or failure—and deploy standardized instruments and questionnaires for clinical observations [24,41]. They include longitudinal studies that analyse how women and couples' emotions change both during and after treatment [42]. Other research is comparative, examining women and couples who experience success versus those that experience failure in achieving pregnancy, as well as the different emotional experiences and coping strategies of male and female members of heterosexual couples [18,22,43]. The decisions and occurrences, involving embryos at different stages of the therapeutic trajectory, are shown to be processes with a heavy emotional load [17,35], one whose effects go beyond the emotional experience strictly associated with infertility and moments of failure in accomplishing the parental project.

Other research suggests that the moral status conferred on the surplus embryos carries little weight in beneficiaries' decision-making processes, or point to a low level of plasticity in ontological constructs: instrumentalising views are thought to predominate, with embryos seen as resources mobilized for reproductive treatment [21,44,45]. Still, other research is based on a duality between emotion and evaluation [6], in which the emotional experience related to decision-making about an embryo (e.g., *disquiet/discomfort* about the prospect of donating embryos relegated to the status of surplus) overlaps with the decisions made (e.g., destruction), without necessarily being accompanied by a resolution at an evaluative level, that is, a definition or reconfiguration of the moral status attributed to the embryo.

By adopting a perspective guided by a sociology of engagements—one that integrates the cognitive, evaluative, and emotional dimensions present in the course of the therapeutic trajectory and related decision-making processes—this article proposes a more detailed analysis of the complexity of such emotional states. This analysis takes into account these states' multiple manifestations, how they oscillate at different moments in the therapeutic trajectory, and their articulation with the cognitive and moral frameworks that guide beneficiaries. This articulation is important because emotional states have an impact on decision-making processes [17]: emotional experiences not only play a part in, but are likely to lead to, the embryo's cognitive and moral re-evaluation (with consequences for deliberations about its fate), with the new status conferred on it leading to emotional appeasement [33,34].

When inserted into the context of ART, the parental project moves away from the intimate, proximal, sphere of the couple [19]; as beneficiaries, they are inserted into a functionally prepared environment, one populated by devices of the industrial world [25] within a framework of technoscientific biomedicine [2]. However, immersion in this context does not necessarily entail the beneficiaries' adhesion exclusively to the cognitive and moral format guided by this composition of regimes of engagement, particularly when it comes to how they conceive of the embryo. Indeed, their actions may be guided by combinations of different regimes of engagement, which are accompanied, in turn, by correlated emotional tonalities.

Given this plurality of beneficiaries' regimes of engagement, the embryo may be understood using various different categories: child, promise/potential, genetic inheritance, offspring, and cluster of cells/biological material. These conceptualizations—which stem from different publicly-available grammars [27]—in turn entail specific emotional experiences that are connected to them.

Therefore, it is particularly in the moments when embryos are reclassified that the emotional states, associated with specific cognitive and moral formats, are most evident. This is because the change in the embryo's status, and the process of re-evaluation on which it is based, increases the emotional ambiance associated with the grammar (or composition of grammars) that supports this reclassification. At the end of a moment of *test*—of the situation's (re)definition according to a regime of engagement (in this case, of questioning how the embryos are classified)—there is emotional appeasement. During these moments of test, however, emotional investments are intensified, shaping the construction of judgments and serving as catalysts for re-evaluation [33]. In particular, the emotions associated with the evaluation of a situation, based on a given regime of engagement, trigger this same exercise of reclassification [29].

These emotional investments, experienced by beneficiaries, are highlighted at specific stages of the therapeutic trajectory—for instance, when the embryo is displaced either in time (e.g., embryonic development stage or the woman getting pregnant) or in space (e.g., transfer into the uterus), or at other moments, such as technical-scientific evaluations (e.g., measurement of the embryo's quality/potential, translated into a probability of achieving pregnancy, or a positive pregnancy test) or biomedical visualization (which make use of technical devices, such as an ultrasound or photos of the embryos).

It is, therefore, the interaction between time, space, clinical judgments, and sensory engagement that determines the different situations in which couples/beneficiaries juggle between different grammars [31] when producing meanings around the embryos. This multi-layered grammatical structure accompanies beneficiaries' subjective progression throughout the clinical path—from the beginning until the end of the parental project—and can change during this path's different moments of success and failure, its setbacks, deadlocks, and restarts. Grammars support the changing meanings (and emotions) around the embryo that influence decision-making in the present, giving new sense to what has occurred in the past and making sense of future possibilities (e.g., when deciding the fate of surplus embryos).

The different stages and contingencies of the therapeutic trajectory are thus liable to trigger reconfigurations in the meanings attributed to embryos, and are accompanied by emotional ambiances associated with the normative format(s) through which the embryo is re-evaluated. Concretely, we can identify three types of key moments of emotional oscillation among the beneficiaries that are associated with changing moral judgments about the embryo:

a. Moments of ambivalence related to the embryo's status (e.g., the execution of clinical procedures on the embryo—such as preimplantation genetic testing—for measuring its quality and development potential, according to an industrial logic; this is in tension with a caring and singularizing connection to the embryo associated with a familiar form of engagement, which generates the emotional experiences of anguish or disquiet);

b. Moments where the embryo's state of worth is revised within the same regime of engagement (e.g., where the embryo's status as hope is strengthened within a connectionist grammar after the evaluation of the embryo's good quality or a positive pregnancy test that reinforces the possibility of achieving pregnancy);

c. Moments where the regime of engagement is revised, leading to a transition between orders of worth or regimes of engagement (e.g., the embryo's transition from being seen as a cluster of cells—in line with an instrumental conception, associated with an industrial grammar combined with an engagement in a plan—to being seen as progeny/offspring within the domestic grammar, leading to the emotional experience of affection or tenderness).

Now, these evaluative and emotional changes in the beneficiaries' relationship with the embryo are more pronounced than those of the professionals involved in the therapeutic plan—in particular, doctors and embryologists. Consequently, tensions and *inhospitable* situations [46] may occur during their interactions. These take the form of dissonances between users and professionals in how they understand the embryo, as well as situations where clinics are unable to accommodate patients' evaluative formats, which diverge from the industrial grammar that predominates in the functioning of ART clinics/units and in the action logics of their staff.

By mapping these patterns of oscillation of emotional ambiances and ontological constructs—which we have tried to do in detail—we have sought to produce a tool for reflecting about the procedures and practices in ART clinics/units. Besides beneficiaries' decision-making autonomy being a normative goal (because it safeguards users' agency without challenging professionals' technical-scientific authority), the beneficiaries we interviewed make critical judgments about their therapeutic trajectory using the grammar of *hospitality* [46].

Participation in an institution/organization implies sharing common objectives and conforming to collective normative frameworks that regulate all activity carried out within it. This is supported by the participants' investment in forms, and particularly, standardized norms that guide actions and perspectives [26]. The grammar of hospitality is one such normative framework that can be used to judge how institutions/organizations function. It is concerned with evaluating these institutions/organizations' capacity to accommodate users' specificities and vulnerabilities. Within the grammar of hospitality, the goal is to facilitate participants' integration in the institution/organization by accommodating singularities/differences and thus, ensuring the ability for each to participate in it.

Questions of hospitality arise around ART units/clinics' ability to accommodate different understandings and modes of connecting with embryos, which can differ from those recognized by the *standardized norms* that regulate the functioning of ART units/clinics as organizations [13]; their ability to better address couples' vulnerabilities, such as the range of emotions that beneficiaries feel towards the embryos, can compromise/affect their decision-making capacity due to their potential emotional charge [17].

The grammar of hospitality is, therefore, mobilized by beneficiaries as a moral foundation for critiquing how the lab-grown embryos are understood and acted upon. Thus, the perspectives conveyed by the interviewees frequently seek greater accommodation by these ART units of ways of conceptualizing the embryo that are dissociated from the biomedical discourse—and the consequent recognition of the fluctuations and plasticity in beneficiaries' emotional states, in relation to the embryo, that are not limited to the stress, anxiety, or suffering associated with the non-achievement of the pregnancy (i.e., engagement in a plan). However, the plasticity of institutions/organizations is constrained by the set of standards that regulate their functioning [26]. If these institutions/organizations are to become more accommodating, then these standards that guide professionals' conduct (that of medical doctors, embryologists, nurses, etc.) need to be improved, so they can better incorporate this plurality of meanings and emotional states around the embryos that beneficiaries can display.

More detailed knowledge about the plurality of meanings likely to be attributed to the embryo—and about oscillations in the associated emotional experiences—also highlights the importance of supplying information to beneficiaries through procedures that go beyond the process of gaining beneficiaries' formal authorization. Concretely, when obtaining informed consent about what happens to the embryo, professionals should follow standard procedures that encourage more continuous follow-up, starting from the moment when beneficiaries decide to move forward with IVF/ICSI. It should be made easier for beneficiaries to communicate the dilemmas that arise for them, as well as the emotional implications of the decision-making processes involving the lab-grown embryos.

Author Contributions: Writing—original draft preparation, L.G.; writing—review and editing, L.G., C.D.; project administration, C.D. All authors have read and agreed to the published version of the manuscript.

Funding: This research was funded by the FCT—Foundation for Science and Technology, I.P., grant number PTDC/SOC-SOC/29764/2017. In addition, this work was funded by national funds through FCT—Foundation for Science and Technology, I.P., within the scope of the project « UIDB/04647/2020» of CICS.NOVA—Interdisciplinary Centre of Social Sciences of Universidade Nova de Lisboa.

Institutional Review Board Statement: The study was conducted according to the guidelines of the Declaration of Helsinki, and approved by the Ethics Committee of the Universidade NOVA de Lisboa (25 September 2019).

Informed Consent Statement: Informed consent was obtained from all subjects involved in the study.

Data Availability Statement: The data presented in this study are available on request from the project administrator.

Acknowledgments: The authors acknowledge the contribution of the professional translator Guilherme Lucas Rodrigues Monteiro and of the professional proof-reader Josh Booth.

Conflicts of Interest: The authors declare no conflict of interest. The funders had no role in the design of the study, in the collection, analyses, or interpretation of data, in the writing of the manuscript, or in the decision to publish the results.

References

1. Dow, K. 'Now She's Just an Ordinary Baby': The Birth of IVF in the British Press. *Sociology* **2019**, *53*, 314–329. [CrossRef]
2. Clarke, A.E.; Shim, J.K.; Mamo, L.; Fosket, J.R.; Fisherman, J.R. Biomedicalization: Technoscientific Transformations of Health, Illness and U.S. Biomedicine. *Am. Sociol. Rev.* **2003**, *68*, 161–194. [CrossRef]
3. Svendsen, M.N. Between reproductive and regenerative medicine: Practicing embryo donation and civil responsibility in Denmark. *Body Soc.* **2007**, *13*, 21–45. [CrossRef]
4. De Lacey, S. Death in the clinic: Women's perceptions and experiences of discarding supernumerary IVF embryos. *Sociol. Health Illn.* **2017**, *39*, 397–411. [CrossRef]

5. Haimes, E.; Porz, R.; Scully, J.L.; Rehmann-Sutter, C. "So, what is an embryo?" A comparative study of the views of those asked to donate embryos for hESC research in the UK and Switzerland. *New Genet. Soc.* **2008**, *27*, 113–126. [CrossRef]
6. Provoost, V.; Pennings, G.; De Sutter, P.; Gerris, J.; Van de Velde, A.; De Lissnyder, E.; Dhont, M. Infertility patients' beliefs about their embryos and their disposition preferences. *Hum. Reprod.* **2009**, *24*, 896–905. [CrossRef] [PubMed]
7. Boltanski, L. *The Foetal Condition. A Sociology of Engendering and Abortion*; Polity Press: Cambridge, UK, 2013.
8. Bruno, C.; Dudkiewicz-Sibony, C.; Berthaut, I.; Weil, E.; Brunet, L.; Fortier, C.; Pfeffer, J.; Ravel, C.; Fauque, P.; Mathieu, E.; et al. Survey of 243 ART patients having made a final disposition decision about their surplus cryopreserved embryos: The crucial role of symbolic embryo representation. *Hum. Reprod.* **2016**, *31*, 1508–1514. [CrossRef]
9. Cussins, C.M. Ontological Choreography: Agency for women patients in an infertility clinic. In *Differences in Medicine: Unraveling Practices, Techniques, and Bodies*, 1st ed.; Berg, M., Mol, A., Eds.; Duke University Press: Durham, UK; London, UK, 1998; pp. 166–201.
10. Thompson, C. *Making Parents: The Ontological Choreography of Human Reproductive Technologies*; MIT Press: Cambridge, UK; London, UK, 2005.
11. De Lacey, S. Decisions for the fate of frozen embryos: Fresh insights into patients' thinking and their rationales for donating or discarding embryos. *Hum. Reprod.* **2007**, *22*, 1751–1758. [CrossRef] [PubMed]
12. Rosemann, A.; Luo, H. Attitudes Towards the Donation of Human Embryos for Stem Cell Research Among Chinese IVF Patients and Students. *J. Bioeth. Inq.* **2018**, *15*, 441–457. [CrossRef]
13. Silva, S.; Machado, H. Legal, medical and lay understanding of embryos in Portugal: Alignment with biology? *Interface Commun. Health Educ.* **2009**, *13*, 31–43. [CrossRef]
14. Delaunay, C.; Santos, M.J.; Gouveia, L. In vitro metaphors: ART beneficiaries' meaning-making on human embryos in the context of IFV in Portugal. *Reprod. Biomed. Soc. Online* **2021**, *13*, 62–74. [CrossRef]
15. Samorinha, C.; Pereira, M.; Machado, H.; Figueiredo, B.; Silva, S. Factors associated with the donation and non-donation of embryos for research: A systematic review. *Hum. Reprod. Updat.* **2014**, *20*, 641–655. [CrossRef] [PubMed]
16. Samorinha, C.; Severo, M.; Machado, H.; Figueiredo, B.; De Freitas, C.; Silva, S. Couple's willingness to donate embryos for research: A longitudinal study. *Acta Obstet. Gynecol. Scand.* **2016**, *95*, 912–919. [CrossRef] [PubMed]
17. Provoost, V.; Pennings, G.; De Sutter, P.; Dhont, M. "Something of the two of us". The emotionally loaded embryo disposition decision making of patients who view their embryo as a symbol of their relationship. *J. Psychosom. Obstet. Gynecol.* **2012**, *33*, 45–52. [CrossRef]
18. Hsu, Y.-L.; Kuo, B.-J. Evaluations of Emotional Reactions and Coping Behaviors as Well as Correlated Factors for Infertile Couples Receiving Assisted Reproductive Technologies. *J. Nurs. Res.* **2002**, *10*, 291–302. [CrossRef]
19. Delaunay, C. L'insupportable et l'incertain. Proximité et détachement dans l'assistance médicale à la procréation avec tiers donneur. *Anthropol. Santé.* **2017**, *15*. Available online: http://anthropologiesante.revues.org/2738 (accessed on 29 December 2021).
20. De Lacey, S. Parent identity and 'virtual' children: Why patients discard rather than donate unused embryos. *Hum. Reprod.* **2005**, *20*, 1661–1669. [CrossRef] [PubMed]
21. Provoost, V.; Pennings, G.; De Sutter, P.; Gerris, J.; Van De Velde, A.; Dhont, M. Patients' conceptualization of cryopreserved embryos used in their fertility treatment. *Hum. Reprod.* **2010**, *25*, 705–713. [CrossRef]
22. Merari, D.; Chetrit, A.; Modan, B. Emotional Reactions and Attitudes Prior to In Vitro Fertilization: An Inter-Spouse Study. *Psychol. Heal.* **2002**, *17*, 629–640. [CrossRef]
23. Hjelmstedt, A.; Widström, A.-M.; Wramsby, H.M.; Collins, A. Patterns of emotional responses to pregnancy, experience of pregnancy and attitudes to parenthood among IVF couples: A longitudinal study. *J. Psychosom. Obstet. Gynecol.* **2003**, *24*, 153–162. [CrossRef]
24. Verhaak, C.M.; Smeenk, J.M.J.; Evers, A.W.M.; Kremer, J.A.M.; Kraaimaat, F.W.; Braat, D.D.M. Women's emotional adjustment to IVF: A systematic review of 25 years of research. *Hum. Reprod. Updat.* **2007**, *13*, 27–36. [CrossRef]
25. Boltanski, L.; Thévenot, L. *On Justification. Economies of Worth*; Princeton University Press: Princeton, NJ, USA, 2006.
26. Thévenot, L. *L'action au Pluriel. Sociologie des Régimes D'engagement*; Éditions La Découverte: Paris, France, 2006.
27. Thévenot, L. What engages? The sociology of justifications, conventions, and engagements, meeting norms. *La Rev. Des Droits De L'homme* **2019**, *16*. Available online: http://journals.openedition.org/revdh/7114 (accessed on 29 December 2021). [CrossRef]
28. Thévenot, L. The plurality of cognitive formats and engagements: Moving between the familiar and the public. *Eur. J. Soc. Theory* **2007**, *10*, 413–427. [CrossRef]
29. Livet, P.; Thévenot, L. Modes d'action collective et construction éthique. Les émotions dans l'évaluation. In *Les Limites de La Rationalité*, 1st ed.; Dupuy, J.-P., Livet, P., Eds.; La Découverte: Paris, France, 1993; Volume 1, pp. 412–439.
30. Kaufmann, L.; Quéré, L. (Eds.) *Les émotions Collectives: En Quête d'un «Objet» Impossible*; Éditions de l'EHESS: Paris, France, 2020.
31. Gajdoš, A.; Rapošová, I. Juggling grammars, translating common-place: Justifying an anti-liberal referendum to a liberal public. *Eur. J. Cult. Polit. Sociol.* **2018**, *5*, 165–193. [CrossRef]
32. Pattaroni, L. Le care est-il institutionnalisable? Quand la «politique du care» émousse son éthique. In *Le Souci des Autres. Éthique et Politique du Care*, 2nd ed.; Paperman, P., Laugier, S., Eds.; Éditions de l'EHESS: Paris, France, 2011; pp. 209–233. [CrossRef]
33. Thévenot, L. Émotions et Évaluations dans les coordinations publiques. In *La Couleur des Pensées. Émotions, Sentiments, Intentions*, 1st ed.; Paperman, P., Ogien, R., Eds.; Éditions de l'EHESS: Paris, France, 1995; pp. 145–174.

34. Genard, J. Une sociologie des émotions «modo aesthetico»? In *Les émotions Collectives: En Quête D'un «Objet» Impossible*, 1st ed.; Kaufmann, L., Quéré, L., Eds.; Éditions de l'EHESS: Paris, France, 2020; pp. 169–203. [CrossRef]
35. Toscano, S.E.; Montgomery, R.M. The lived experience of women pregnant (including preconception) post in vitro fertilization through the lens of virtual communities. *Health Care Women Int.* **2009**, *30*, 1014–1036. [CrossRef] [PubMed]
36. Peterson, A.; Wilkinson, I. Editorial introduction: The sociology of hope in contexts of health, medicine, and healthcare. *Heal. Interdiscip. J. Soc. Study Heal. Illn. Med.* **2015**, *19*, 113–118. [CrossRef] [PubMed]
37. Borup, M.; Brown, N.; Konrad, K.; van Lente, H. The sociology of expectations in science and technology. *Technol. Anal. Strat. Manag.* **2006**, *18*, 285–298. [CrossRef]
38. Lebedev, A.C. Lebedev, A.C. *Le cœur politique des mères*. In *Analyse du Mouvement des Mères de Soldats en Russie*; Éditions de l'EHESS: Paris, France, 2013.
39. Hershberger, P.E.; Pierce, P.F. Conceptualizing couples' decision making in PGD: Emerging cognitive, emotional, and moral dimensions. *Patient Educ. Couns.* **2010**, *81*, 53–62. [CrossRef] [PubMed]
40. Adrian, S.W. Psychological IVF: Conceptualizing emotional choreography in a fertility clinic. *Distinktion Scand. J. Soc. Theory* **2015**, *16*, 302–317. [CrossRef]
41. Mahlstedt, P.P.; MacDuff, S.; Bernstein, J. Emotional factors and the in vitro fertilization and embryo transfer process. *J. Assist. Reprod. Genet.* **1987**, *4*, 232–236. [CrossRef] [PubMed]
42. Slade, P.; Emery, J.; Lieberman, B.A. A prospective, longitudinal study of emotions and relationships in in-vitro fertilization treatment. *Hum. Reprod.* **1997**, *12*, 183–190. [CrossRef]
43. Shaw, P.; Johnston, M.; Shaw, R. Counselling needs, emotional and relationship problems in couples awaiting IVF. *J. Psychosom. Obstet. Gynecol.* **1988**, *9*, 171–180. [CrossRef]
44. Svanberg, A.; Boivin, J.; Bergh, T. Factors influencing the decision to use or discard cryopreserved embryos. *Acta Obstet. Gynecol. Scand.* **2001**, *80*, 849–855. [CrossRef] [PubMed]
45. Holter, H.; Bergh, C.; Gejervall, A.-L. Lost and lonely: A qualitative study of women's experiences of no embryo transfer owing to non-fertilization or poor embryo quality. *Hum. Reprod. Op.* **2021**, *2021*, hoaa062. [CrossRef] [PubMed]
46. Stavo-Debauge, J. *Qu'est-ce que L'hospitalité. Recevoir L'étranger à la Communauté*; Liber: Montréal, QC, Canada, 2017.

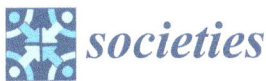

Article

Because You're Worth It! The Medicalization and Moralization of Aesthetics in Aging Women

Chiara Pussetti

Institute of Social Sciences, University of Lisbon, Av. Prof. Aníbal Bettencourt 9, 1600-189 Lisbon, Portugal; chiara.pussetti@ics.ulisboa.pt

Abstract: In this article—based on the fieldwork I conducted in Lisbon (Portugal) between 2018 and 2021, employing in-depth ethnography and self-ethnography—I describe the experience of the medicalization and moralization of beauty in Portuguese women aged 45–65 years. I examine the ways in which practitioners inscribe their expert knowledge on their patients' bodies, stigmatizing the marks of time and proposing medical treatments and surgeries to "repair" and "correct" them. Beauty and youth are symbolically constructed in medical discourse as visual markers of health, an adequate lifestyle, a strong character and good personal choices (such as not smoking, and a healthy diet and exercise habits). What beauty means within the discourse of anti-aging and therapeutic rejuvenation is increasingly connected to an ideal gender performance of normative, white, middle-class, heterosexual femininity that dismisses structural determinants. The fantasy of eternal youth, linked to a neoliberal ideology of limitless enhancement and individual responsibility, is firmly entrenched in moralizing definitions of aesthetics and gender norms. Finally, my article highlights the ways in which the women I interviewed do not always passively accept the discourse of the devaluation of the ageing body, defining femininity and ageing in their own terms by creating personal variants of the hegemonic normative discourses on beauty and successful ageing.

Keywords: ageing; anti-ageing; gender; beauty; cosmetic medicine; body; appearance; aesthetic surgery

Citation: Pussetti, C. Because You're Worth It! The Medicalization and Moralization of Aesthetics in Aging Women. *Societies* **2021**, *11*, 97. https://doi.org/10.3390/soc11030097

Academic Editors: Violeta Alarcão and Sónia Cardoso Pintassilgo

Received: 13 July 2021
Accepted: 10 August 2021
Published: 12 August 2021

Publisher's Note: MDPI stays neutral with regard to jurisdictional claims in published maps and institutional affiliations.

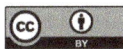

Copyright: © 2021 by the author. Licensee MDPI, Basel, Switzerland. This article is an open access article distributed under the terms and conditions of the Creative Commons Attribution (CC BY) license (https://creativecommons.org/licenses/by/4.0/).

1. You're Worth It!

> "Forever young
> I want to be forever young"
> (Alphaville, 'Forever Young')

When we say: "You're Worth It!" or "These Days, Age is a Choice"—quoting two famous L'Óreal slogans—we are not only enouncing a tagline, we are also proclaiming a moral message. The first slogan has been translated into 40 languages, becoming a global moral imperative that encourages women to control their life and their body, to assume responsibility for the way they look and to believe in their self-discipline every day. The message is clear: you have to do it for yourself. Taking your beauty into your own hands is empowering. Investing in your beauty and in your youth is something no one else can do for you. You deserve to be beautiful, you must love yourself and you have to believe in your self-worth every day, establishing yourself as Glam-ma and not as Grandma. Only if you are thinner, firmer, smoother and younger, will you be better; you will have a more passionate relationship, a better career, more friends and success; you will be happier. Otherwise, if you are unable to 'fix' your aesthetic 'problems' and to 'solve' the signs of bodily ageing, you should consider yourselves to have failed. The age-related bodily changes are redefined as defects or problems that can be improved, repaired or corrected through products and procedures from both the medical–pharmaceutical and beauty industries. In every supermarket, perfumery, pharmacy, beauty salon, shopping mall, hairdresser, and doctors' and gynaecologists' waiting rooms, we find direct-to-women advertising proposing miraculous aesthetic anti-aging products and procedures to restore the lost youth and the beauty of the past. Keeping yourself physically attractive for as long as possible is a question of personal responsibility, but also an expression of self-love and self-esteem, because you deserve it.

In Portugal, the slogan produces a few declinations that always appeal to the self-esteem of women "Because I'm worth it" or "Because I/We/You deserve it", employing feminist values—such as independence, choice, responsibility, empowerment, liberation, radical change and self-worth—to promote the consumption of beauty products as a worthwhile pursuit and expense, a practice which Goldman [1] terms "commodity feminism". This proliferation of moralizing messages in advertising campaigns, asking women to assume responsibility for the way they look, is a key way for major cosmetics brands to build a customer base and reap financial benefit [2–8]. The female body is always problematized, represented as a malleable entity that can be shaped and perfected by the discipline and hard work of its owner. Women's bodies are never perfect enough, and are potentially open to reconstruction: at any age, women are engaged in a project that is always in-progress, trying to correspond to a hegemonic beauty ideal that denies ageing. It is therefore unsurprising that most academic research centred on the body/ageing paradigm focuses on the female perspective. Appearance remains an important issue for women, even as they age: there is a varied body of research on the ways in which women experience and feel towards physical signs of ageing, including white hair and wrinkles [9–13].

Wrinkles, body fat, cellulite, sagging skin, the greying of the hair, skin spots, the loss of firmness, and every other bodily alteration that accompanies aging should be fought with the energetic maintenance of the body with the help of the medical aesthetic, cosmetic, fitness and food industries (protein diets, superfoods and supplements). The inspirational women who front the brand worldwide make the moral imperative of 'self-care, because you deserve' relevant for women of any age, proposing unrealistic beauty standards that ultimately reinforce the sense of inadequacy, increasing women's insecurities. With their imperative tone and the positive verbs denoting transformative actions ('change', 'empower', 'decide', 'make', 'evolve'), these messages encourage women to maintain their beauty at any cost [14–21].

Women are told that they are unstoppable: they can change or obtain anything they so desire, with sheer willpower. It depends entirely on them: with willpower and discipline, nothing is impossible. Women can control the tangible, physical, somatic reality, but also more abstract processes such as 'the ageing process,' 'time', 'gravity' and 'the future'. The battlefield is their body, in an inexorable war against oneself and the natural course of life. The loss of beauty as people grow old, however, is not perceived as a normal consequence of the passage of time. It is rather considered a lack of discipline and will, an inability to dedicate oneself to a goal that requires effort and discipline with dedication and constancy. The age that you show becomes the reflection of your moral qualities, of your lifestyle and of your life choices. Regardless of the circumstances, your appearance reveals your essence.

Even in these very complicated pandemic times, with people staying indoors, scared and confused, covering their face with masks, the desire for facial cosmetic procedures and aesthetic surgery increase. In reaction to this new normal, L'Óreal Portugal launched the campaign "Make up Everyday" ("*Porque Tu Mereces*"), which encourages Portuguese women to maintain their beauty and to combat ageing during the pandemic. To boost this campaign, the brand joined four influencers with an unstoppable routine who are the protagonists of each of the key moments of this campaign—non-stop routine, movie night, meeting and special dinners. If, during the first months of the pandemic, I noticed a certain 'moralization' regarding the consumption of aesthetic interventions and luxury cosmetic items in a moment of global sanitarian crisis, however, the discourse quickly changed.

In Portugal, cosmetics sectors such as hairdressers and beauty salons were the first commercial activities to reopen after the lockdowns. Even more surprisingly, plastic surgery and aesthetic medicine clinics stayed open during the lockdowns. All of the beauty industry has largely proven to be recession-proof. In fact, in Lisbon, we witnessed the opening of at least two new centres during the pandemic in order to respond to customer pressure, investing surgeons and healthcare practitioners in aesthetic clinics. In a recent article, I addressed the impact of the pandemic on our appearance-enhancing practices, highlighting that the social pressure to emerge from the pandemic as a rejuvenated version of oneself resulted in stigma for those who haven't used the time for self-improvement or who haven't the money to pay for the treatments. If the pandemic is not a nuclear aspect of the present paper, I cannot ignore, however, that the fieldwork took place in large part in exceptional times. My interviews highlighted how the lockdown increased the fear of 'wasting time' and of ageing faster and losing wonderful things that previously occupied our time and gave our life purpose. The feeling of lost time during confinement reinforced the desire to restart normal life with a younger appearance. If my fieldwork conditions weren't optimal due to the lockdowns, the pandemic—among immense other things—has nevertheless revealed a veritable epidemic of problematic personal and social issues tied to the obsession with appearance and staying or looking young. Many of the women interviewed expressed fears that the stress of the pandemic would make them look and feel older, claiming that they would be disposed to do anything and to pay any price to get out of the pandemic with a younger and better appearance.

Always during the pandemic period, the Portuguese advertisement for L'Oreal's Age Perfect cream, which contains the slogan "These Days, Age is a Choice", was widely disseminated throughout the country. The campaign works to equate ageing with the look of ageing, to problematize ageing appearance, and to offer marketized solutions to the 'problem' of ageing. According to L'Oreal's brand ambassador, saying that today "age is a choice" means that women can be beautiful, well groomed, active and confident after 60 years of age, investing in maintaining fitness and beauty as ways to boost their self-esteem. One can claim the appearance of youth until later: it is in one's hands; it depends on one's determination not to give up. It means believing that "we deserve it". If, in the United States, Jane Fonda personified the cream Age Perfect, in Portugal the promoters of the brand were singer and actress Simone de Oliveira, and actress and television presenter Lídia Franco. The two ladies represent the so-called "sexygenarians", a category that today encompasses one third of Portuguese women, and represents an important market niche.

The campaign, accompanied by the slogan "It's the difference between a Granma and a Glam-ma", problematizes bodily ageing, and in particular facial ageing (skin, eyes, cheeks, lips), as a serious issue. Beautiful bodies are, overall, presumed to be young bodies, and the look of ageing is considered to be a problem and pathologized. The narrative format of this type of advertising messages is that of 'problem/solution', with ageing as the 'problem' and technologized/scientized/medical/pharmaceutical (even before than cosmetic (of which, more later)) products as the 'solution'. The consumer is persuaded of two important things: (1) that it is undesirable to appear to be ageing, and (2) that she/he must assume responsibility to stay young-looking, controlling, slowing or reversing the effects of ageing.

This article is organized into three parts: (i) a brief premise about the research methods employed and the ideal of ageless beauty from a gender perspective; (ii) a self-ethnographic narrative of the incorporation of hegemonic beauty norms and the desires of eternal youth, based on my life history as a medical cosmetic patient and on my dialogue with other women 'over-fifty'; (iii) a final reflection on the intimate and personal ways in which we incorporate contradictory socio-cultural expectations about how our body should be. Although many of the participating women have narratives similar to mine, each of us has a unique story to tell.

2. The False Hope of the Timeless Beauty

"Will you still love me
when I'm no longer young and beautiful?"
(Lana del Rey, Young and Beautiful)

This article is based on the fieldwork I conducted in the last 36 months with Portuguese middle-class women aged between forty and seventy years old, investigating their anti-ageing practices in the city of Lisbon. I carried out a multimethod research strategy employing in-depth ethnography and self-ethnography. All of the participants were recruited through my personal networks. All of the interviews were recorded and transcribed with the participants' consent, and were conducted under the guidelines, codes of conduct and ethical procedures commensurate with anthropological and ethnographic research standards. Participation in this study was always entirely voluntary, and all of the participants were informed about the contents and objectives of the research, as well as the intended outputs. Regular, unobtrusive contact with the research participants allowed me to build intimate ties to capture a wide range of perspectives, pinpoint the different kinds of experiences and reveal contradictory attitudes.

Even though aesthetic is also an important issue for male subjects, I conducted my interviews predominantly with women. In comparison to women, the heterosexual men with whom I talked did not consider ageing as a problematic process due to the loss of beauty, but rather as a limit on their professional climbing opportunities, sexual potency, or relational choice. While fitness regimes, dietary control, the usage of hair care, shaving or skin moisturizing products and the purchase of consumer goods including clothing, accessories and cosmetics were reported without shame, the issue of beauty rituals remains a very intimate topic, especially for heterosexual men. In my interviews, I noticed an inclination of heterosexual men to value success rather than beauty regarding the social construction of their image. Topics such as hair transplants, masculinization fillers to build a 'powerful profile' as an indicator of leadership competences, or of surgical implants to redefine the chin and to build a strong 'superhero' jawline to achieve a more masculine look are in my opinion incredibly interesting, but unfortunately these are not the theme of the present paper.

I undertook participant observation in private aesthetic clinics, beauty salons and wellness centres, interviewing eight healthcare professionals and 23 middle-class, heterosexual and cisgender Portuguese women who identified themselves as white (adopting the method of theoretical saturation), accompanying them in their aesthetic transformations before and during the lockdown periods. Obviously, ageing is not an issue of concern for middle class 'white' women only. In the last few years, I conducted research and published specifically on the aesthetic labour of immigrants and Afroeuropean women in Portugal, observing the emergence, in the Greater Lisbon Area, of a new market of cosmetic products partly aimed at clarifying the skin and correcting age spots.

If other aesthetic interventions are much more transversal—in relation to social divisions around gender, class, race, ethnicity, social status, sexual orientation, age, or nationality—in the anti-aging and skin clinics of the centre of Lisbon, I only met middle class women who identify themselves as white. Speaking of Portugal as a European 'white' nation—despite decades of immigration, despite the complexity of colonial and post-colonial relations, and despite the presence of non-white Portuguese citizens—in all my interviews with patients and cosmetic practitioners, the ideal beauty appeared as a depoliticized, race-neutral model.

Most of the women I interviewed validated the extensive literature dedicated to the predominance, on a global scale, of a Eurocentered ideal of beauty: white and smooth skin; a thin, tonic, youthful, muscular body; regular lines, big eyes and brilliant long hair [21–27]. In my interviews, I noticed that there are alternative aesthetic models—desirable, however non-hegemonic [28–31]—however, as far as aging is concerned, people's apparent tolerance does not withstand the test of analysis. The aging bodies occupy a unique position in aesthetic norms. The women aged between forty and seventy years old that I interviewed in Lisbon agreed that youth is essential to beauty, and that during their lifespan they are faced with the somatic reality of this process. Confronted with moralizing discourses about fighting the war on wrinkles, they discover that, at the end of the line, aging is inevitable. Losing youth means losing beauty and the power of sexual attraction: they discovered that they are no longer considered beautiful or attractive because they have aged. In Euro-American contemporary "aesthetic economies" [32] (p. 535) the value of a woman depends in large part on attributes (beauty, sexual attractiveness, fertility) that irrevocably fade with age.

As Kathleen Woodward states in her 1999 book, *Figuring Age: Women, Bodies, Generations*:

> Women today begin to experience ageing around the age of fifty, and this process is considered in terms of decay and loss of aesthetic and erotic value, and not in the neutral terms of natural evolution and transformation. [33] (pp. 10–13)

My interviewees confirmed that "beauty is worth riches", "beauty attracts more than gold", that "she who is born beautiful will never be poor", that "beauty is power", and that "she who is beautiful will always be queen". Being attractive was, for many centuries, the only way for women to obtain power and to improve their social position. Despite the legacy of feminist writers like Simone de Beauvoir, whose work *La Vieillesse* first appeared in 1970 [34], and Susan Sontag, who already in 1972 spoke of the "double standard of ageing" [35], which combines gender and age discrimination, more mature women must fight the signs of ageing, attempting to escape time in order to not be relegated to invisibility. Portugal is considered—at the European level—an 'aged country'; a 2010 study by Margarida de Melo Cerqueira showed that:

> From television (series, game shows), newspapers (news reports, comic strips), radio, to various forms of art (cinema, theatre, dance, painting, sculpture, literature), elderly characters are referred to in a derogatory manner, portraying them as having a health problem that weakens them in some way, as being dependent and not very competent. [36] (p. 339)

In order to retain their value, women invest energy, time, effort, money, and physical suffering into attempting to escape time. Many women are willing to suffer physically to be beautiful, to undergo elective cosmetic surgery carrying great health risks, and to develop eating disorders to remain attractive according to society's unrealistic 'forever young' ideal. In order to maintain their social value, they must appear youthful, thin, with well-groomed skin, hair shiny as silk, preferably dyed. Preserving a beautiful youthful appearance for longer is not only an aesthetic, but also rather a moral obligation. "Letting oneself grow old" coincides with "letting oneself go": it implies a lack of discipline, laziness, and sloppiness—all traits of a morally deplorable personality. As I have pointed out in my recently published volume [31], the "body-norm" works as a morality tale that blames those outside the norm for their condition, portraying them as "unruly or negligent" for having bodies that do not measure up. Our apparent 'freedom' of growing older 'naturally' or of gaining weight, refusing cosmetic imperatives, is constrained and shaped by embodied forms of inequality that push us to see ourselves as imperfect, and to find in aesthetic biotechnologies the solution to those imperfections.

Supported by modern medicine, anti-ageing equates old age with physical deformity, disability, illness and dependence [37] (p. 9). Margaret Gullette [38], an important feminist theorist in the study of ageing, calls all of the narratives that invariably associate an individual's ageing with a loss of physical and cognitive function "decline narratives". The newly established "anti-ageing medicine" is confused with self-care practices by including a series of physical procedures that tend to mask the signs of ageing [39] (p. 699), promoting the concept of "age" as a target for biomedical interventions [40]. Paradoxically, while trying to stimulate the idea of an "ageless" appearance, these practices reinforce the fear of ageing [41] (p. 81).

Modern anti-ageing aesthetic medicine offers a panoply of treatments and products which are minimally invasive, low-cost, "lunchtime" and more democratized, which promise to block the passage of time, freezing our beauty to the present. The past fifteen years have been marked by an exponential increase not only in consumption but also in innovation in the anti-ageing industry. The term 'anti-ageing' is everywhere in Portugal (it is common to find the expression in English, together with its portuguese translation '*anti-envelhecimento*'): in drugstores, perfume shops, supermarkets, hairdressers, beauty salons and clinics.

These types of interventions—designated by Abigail Brooks [42] as friends or foes of older women—are part of a double paradigm: if, on the one hand, they provide the chance and freedom of a technological response to alleviate the social pressure imposed on women, on the other hand they accentuate the anxiety of growing old, reconfiguring the ideology that age is something subjective: an attitude, a choice, rather than a biological fact, something that must be actively resisted. Women, in the popularized medical discourse, are encouraged to take control of their body and the ageing process, but have to discipline it according to the sociocultural norms where they are inscribed [43].

Anti-ageing aesthetic medicine is ever more high-performance and high-tech, and it reports details that give a scientific feeling, such as 'Mesoestetic Stem Cells', 'Genomics', 'Regenerative Cellular Reconstruction', 'Receptors for Peptides', 'Molecular Biology', 'Molecular Chemistry Rheology', 'Intercellular Resonance and Amplification', 'PhytoCellTec', 'Celergen' and 'Hydro MN Peptide', and so on. These are designations embedded in the promise of the progress designated to raise hopes for both new anti-ageing solutions and better ageless futures. What makes the anti-ageing industry distinctive is being essentially a 'hope economy' [44] that aims to fulfill what we desire and to provide us products and procedures to pursue a longer, more beautiful and more enjoyable future. These 'regimes of hope' [45] justify any kind of economic investment.

3. Fake Plastic Me

> "He used to do surgery
> For girls in the eighties
> But gravity always wins"
> (Radiohead, Fake Plastic Trees)

3.1. 'Chi Bella Buol Venire Un Po' Deve Soffrire': My Family Legacy

Analytically, by resorting to the intersection between experience in the field, the subjective perception of the ageing process, and the daily confrontation with hegemonic discourses on femininity, youth and beauty, I present through an autobiographical narrative my own transformation into a consumer of anti-ageing aesthetic procedures. Here, my personal experience enters into a dialogue with women of the same age group who have agreed to share their stories with me.

"À quarante-sept ans, je n'avais toujours aucune ride du lion, du front, aucune patte d'oie ni ride du sillon nasogénien, d'amertume ou du décolleté; aucun cheveu blanc, aucun cerne; j'avais trente ans, désespérément" (At forty-seven, I still had no frown lines, forehead, crow's feet or nasolabial folds, bitterness or cleavage; no white hair, no rings; I was thirty, desperately) (Delacourt 2018, p. 169). Like Betty, the protagonist in Grégoire Delacourt's book, I am forty-seven years old and I understand perfectly well what it means to desperately try to appear thirty years old. Ever since I was a little girl, I always used to ask my boyfriends the question that was made famous years later by Lana del Rey: "Will you still love me when I'm no longer young and beautiful?" The idea of one day losing my beauty and growing old seemed terrible to me, and I wondered if I would still be worthy of being loved, desired and appreciated. In my grandmother's house, the mirrors were covered with heavy velvet cloths. In her inability to compare her aged image in the mirror, she repeated to me that my useful time would be short and that, like all the most beautiful and delicate flowers, I would wither quickly.

The ideal of feminine beauty that I was taught to value entails a slender, delicate and sensual frame, with abundant, shiny hair (as long as it is tidy, entwined in complex hairstyles), immaculate porcelain skin, without marks and imperfections. "Fat is cute, beauty is thinness", my grandmother used to recite. She also used to say: "it's no good being young without beauty, nor beautiful without youth". Then she'd look at me eating biscuits and say: "OK, fine, eat your snack! Blessed youth! Youth is already beauty itself!" And, again: "Enjoy now, my granddaughter, because the beauty of youth is a gift that nothing can replace". My parents were proud of me because I was a good student, but also—and perhaps above all—because I was a beautiful child and their friends praised me.

I thus learned that being beautiful was a value and an obligation, and that it goes hand in hand with youth. This association is present in many proverbs, popular sayings and other commonplaces that I have collected over years of research: "youth and beauty are worth riches"; "youth in itself is already beauty"; "beauty and youth are a woman's most important assets"; "youth without beauty is fine, but beauty without youth is not"; "beauty soon runs out"; "beauty has an expiry date"; "beauty is a recommendation letter valid for a short time"; "beauty is fragile like a flower: it is born and quickly dies"; "every beautiful shoe becomes an old slipper"; "growing old is a woman's shipwreck"; "to grow old is to pass from passion to compassion", "desire is linked to beauty, and beauty, to youth"; "beauty and youth are lovers: they stay a little and it will be painful when they go away"; "beauty is like a house: you have to bet on constant restoration".

The world around me taught me that youth was worth even more than beauty. I often heard it said at home, and in my peer group, that "young women are beautiful by themselves"; "when young, everyone is beautiful"; that "the woman was a beautiful lady, but her lover was twenty years younger, of course there was no comparison possible"; that "Marilyn Monroe's luck is that she died young and her beauty remained eternal"; or "poor Brigitte Bardot, she should hide!"

Like the protagonist of Delacourt's novel, I realized from my adolescence onward that getting fat and getting older are the most dangerous enemies of female beauty. I always tried to submit my body to exercise and undergo strict diets, to try to correspond to a model distant from my corporeality. The positive perception I had of my pregnant body was shattered by the comments I received about motherhood as the dramatic end of my girl body and the beginning of a mother's body—generous, welcoming, with breasts that nourish and a gentle embrace that soothes. All very tender, but clearly not sexy. One day, glued on the refrigerator in the kitchen, I met the image of the Venus of Willendorf to remind me of the real shape of my fertile body. In front of my perplexity, my (ex)husband replied that it was an incentive, to give me strength in the battle that I would have had to fight to get back to what I was.

However, if we can eventually recapture an anachronistic teenage body, combat ageing, fight wrinkles, sooner or later we will lose the battle. Like Betty, I grew up amid warlike metaphors, images of restoring and recuperating buildings as well as aesthetic economies, moral imperatives of beauty. Military allegories like "fighting ageing", "fighting wrinkles", "the war against weight", "winning the battle against age", "conquering beauty" have punctuated my entire life, denoting the idea of effort and suffering linked to the work that goes into preventing, maintaining, delaying, reversing or masking the effects of ageing.

"*Chi bella buol venire un po' deve soffrire*" (translated from the Italian: "whoever beautiful wants to become, must suffer a little") recited my grandmother, when she combed and braided my hair. "A woman has to suffer to be beautiful, pain is the price of beauty; a woman is made to suffer, to endure pain, to close her mouth, to shape her body". This was the legacy my family passed on to me: beauty has risks and takes work, but I had to be beautiful at any cost. The conquest of the aesthetic ideal usually entails economic efforts, strict rules and routines, and even health risks. My body was mouldable and controllable. It depended on my discipline to stay in control, shaping me to better match up with the hegemonic beauty norms. To take my experience seriously means understanding the reality of a looks-based culture, exposing the entangled relationship between physical attractiveness, identity as a woman and social value. I grew up cultivating my physical appearance as a gift, a positive value and a possible resource from a very young age. The project of being beautiful occupied a big part of my life and somewhat constituted my identity—a woman who draws attention. Maintaining a youthful, attractive appearance was a strategy to maintain my identity, to not vanish in a kind of social invisibility, with my reflex hidden by velvet curtains.

3.2. I Want to Look Like Me Forever: The Gullible Anthropologist

My interviews highlight that the visible signs of ageing—such as wrinkles, sagging, a lack of muscular toning, or grey hair—are more threatening and problematic for women than for men, and that female rituals aimed at rejuvenation begin significantly earlier. Ageing is thus a phenomenon experienced within a broader system of gender inequality, in which the loss of youth in the female body is considered a loss of social value.

While it is very true, as Radiohead say in the song 'Fake Plastic Trees', that "gravity always wins", it is also true that women are encouraged to undertake aesthetic activities, interventions or procedures to try and counter the physical law of gravity. Their social identity is located on the surface of their bodies. Daily make-up; hair, eyelash and eyebrow maintenance; manicures and pedicures, waxing, intermittent diets and fasting, exercise, facial gymnastics, expressive re-education, yoga and pilates, cosmetic products for face and body, teeth whitening, aesthetic medicine and plastic surgery are just some of the weapons one can use to fight the battle against time. The range of products and services which are available to slow down ageing and preserve beauty is almost endless.

Most of the women I interviewed conform to the hegemonic, Euro-American ideal of beauty: thin, white, regular lines, and skin almost without imperfections. We have to consider that this youthful and attractive appearance is always presented as the result of a lifetime of effort and economic investment in the prevention of ageing and the maintenance of beauty. Throughout the ethnographic process I was urged, by the people I interviewed, to intervene quickly to counter the dramatic effects of ageing, to soften the cartography that wrinkles already drawn on my face, and I was often scolded for not having thought about prevention, in advance.

On the one hand, I assimilated a whole lexicon akin to banking or the stock market: invest, value, lose value, preserve capital, monetize, trade, write off. After hearing so much talk about investment, I tried to calculate my monthly expenditure on beauty (considering also gym costs and a certain type of dietary care), and realised with some surprise that I spend something close to a quarter of my salary. On the other hand, I incorporated the discourse concerning the accountability (or lack of care) about the ineluctable process of ageing.

Here, I refer to an interview with Clara, 51 years old:

> Many women think they are powerful and well-adjusted, because they do nothing against ageing, grey hair, fat, face falling off . . . They even try hard to be seen as feminists, against the dictatorship of beauty: but it's all a façade! They are lazy, careless, negligent and slovenly women who don't value themselves. They have not *self-esteem* and self-respect: they let themselves go, they are a real failure. (*Clara, 51 years old, beautician*)

Along with the words of Ana (46 years old):

> *Yes, I spent a lot of money on fillers and botox, and luxury creams such as La Prairie, so what? Maybe you spend more on a Chanel bag. But you get that bag of lard on your belly, which is an old woman's [belly]. Each person decides how to grow old. You don't want to strive to be better? You don't want to make an effort to be better? Then don't do anything. Then you'll see what your life will be like: old, ugly, sloppy, alone.* (Ana, 46 years old, designer)

According to Armanda, 54 years old, all the effort is worth it:

> *Looking at me it's easy to say: this woman has gone crazy with this diet, sport, aesthetics stuff. And they still say . . . ah, but you're lucky, you have good genetics. Lucky? Do you know what I have? I have strength, will, constancy and the ability to endure pain and sacrifice. Not luck! Being in shape, being well groomed involves constant commitment. Vanity has a high price. But idleness, yeah, that is wasting your life.* (Armanda, 54 years old, entrepreneur)

Finally, Catarina, 56 years old, stated that:

What I would like to explain to you, and what I even tell my own daughter, is that having good genetics helps, yes, but sooner or later beauty will leave you all the same, if you don't help yourself. You age ... but it is not true that against time nothing can be done. Nothing here, in my body, happened by chance: it's pain, sacrifice, effort, regimes, and a lot of money invested. I've been in menopause for eleven years, but nobody believes me, and you know what? ... Neither do I, because I still look like a woman of forty, forty-five. But my life since then has been a constant battle against nature. Why do I have to let myself grow old and lose this battle? I have done, and continue to do, everything in my power, sacrificing money and time just for me. If you want to, you can. And if you're still fit and beautiful after sixty, know that you owe that only to yourself, to the work and sacrifice of a lifetime. Because life is long ... but as an old person it is long, not as a young one. Preserving the body is not the frantic pursuit of "à la recherche du temps perdu". It is more like fighting so that time leaves no marks: it is war! (Catarina, 56 years old, counsellor)

My interviewees have in common a consideration of themselves as physically attractive and sexually desirable women, and they are used to receiving positive feedback and being socially appreciated. None of them accepts the loss of her value and social impact, or being cast aside. They are afraid of feeling disconnected from their ageing bodies. They don't want to look old, because they don't feel old, as if there was a gap between their exterior appearance and their inner and true selves.

Cristina, 62 years old, explained to me:

I look tired, I look sad, but I feel as if I had thirty years. Sometimes, I see my image reflected in a showcase and I think: But who is that lady? It feels like she's not me. I don't recognize myself. I don't look to myself like the image I have in my mind. My ideal self is younger Cristina. My real self is who I am at present. I don't want to look in the mirror and see my mother. I would like to see me. The young, beautiful and sexy me. The dissociation I feel is this, between what I think I am and what I appear. And then come others, and my relationship with others. Which has to do with my personality. I don't see myself at all as a typical, traditional sixty-year-old woman. I feel better with younger people. I find younger people more attractive, physically speaking. It is consistent with my view of life, of the world, of people, with my profession as a teacher: for me it is very easy to relate to younger people. In mental terms, for me it is perfectly natural. One day you will understand: you will be old enough to don't recognize yourself anymore in the mirror. (Cristina, 62 years old, teacher)

Maria, 64 years old, confirmed this sensation of dissociation:

My face is what I see in the mirror. My self image. My self-perception of myself depends on the face, where I see the traits of my personality that, despite age, remain the same. That's why I make aesthetic changes to my face: to continue to correspond to the mental state that hasn't changed, because it's my way of being. I want to continue to correspond to myself. To recognize in the mirror the person I think I still am. To rediscover myself in the average of the person I am, between my mental image of myself and the biological reality in terms of appearance. (Maria, 64 years old)

It happened suddenly. By participating as an ethnographer in all arenas of the beauty market, constantly confronted with hegemonic discourses on youth and beauty, I became increasingly attentive and permeable to the ways in which my interlocutors in the field commented on my appearance. In every interview taking place in aesthetic and cosmetic medicine clinics, the professionals held up a mirror in front of my face, directing my attention to the imperfections of my skin texture, the enlarged pores, the lack of youthful radiance and glow, the expression wrinkles, the marionette, the bar code, the crow's foot. Only hyaluronic acid and botulinum toxin filling could soften the signs and bleakness of ageing.

Abruptly, I looked at my image reflected in the doctor's mirror and realised that I was no longer young. Still attractive, yes, but "the expiry date was approaching", as my former mother-in-law later commented. It was a real shock. Until recently, I found it curious when people addressed me in the street calling me "madam", because it seemed obvious to me that I was still considered a girl, with that typical naivety of young people who believe they will be so forever. However, during fieldwork, consumers, professionals and colleagues constantly reminded me that the time of youth was gone and that lost beauty would never return.

> *For you to change your place of work would be complicated. The university today thinks like a corporation: they are much more willing to hire younger people, [rather] than forty-seven-year-old women. It's like in relationships. The MILF (corresponding complete terms for acronyms: Mother I'd Like to Fuck) is no longer in fashion. Now is the time of the WHIP (corresponding complete terms for acronyms: Women Hot, Intelligent and in their Prime) And okay, the young girls. Those are an evergreen.* (Simão, researcher, 31 years old)

> *It is like in the dating apps!—explains Isabel, 32 years old—It is worth lying about your age. Everybody lies about height, weight or age. If you're a woman over 45, listen to me: change your age in your Tinder bio. It is better to erase something like mmm 10 years?* (Isabel, 32 years old)

I was talking with Simão, a colleague in his thirties, and Isabel, a PhD student, in an informal conversation in the college canteen, comparing professional and social opportunities and discussing the power of sexual attraction. A few months later, in an academic job application in which I placed first, on an equal footing with a colleague in his thirties, I discovered that Mauro was right, and the final choice was explained to us on the basis of age. In the same period, I had a date with a 33 years old boy and I realized that I was not comfortable to reveal to him, i.e., that I already have 47 years. The Portuguese slogan of ERA®, the famous real estate agency, comes to mind: "It's Gone!". My Goddesses of the universe, it happened: "I'm Gone!". I began to seriously worry.

In the course of the fieldwork, I approached dermatologist doctors, spent a lot of time in aesthetic clinics, and created relationships of trust. I then asked the research subjects what I could do to block this ageing process. The answers I got from these professionals surprised and scared me even more:

> *I would say that you should have had this concern at least ten years ago. You should have thought about prevention. The ideal was to intervene before the structure collapses. What's more, a woman with your profession: classes, conferences, and public exposure. And divorced to boot. Look, competition at work and in love is tough! Keeping a youthful appearance is a strategy to maintain a competitive advantage, my dear.* (Miguel, dermatologist)

> *Chiara, the face . . . the face is like a calling card. You can tell you haven't used sunscreen . . . see these little spots? They're not freckles, no. They're ageing spots. For women, I always say that caring for the facial skin is an obligation. If we then want to be accomplices of the disgrace . . . that's something else!* (Pierre, dermatologist)

> *If you had asked me, I would never have told you not to intervene, even if you had made an appointment at twenty or thirty years old. It's called prevention, you know what it is, right? You should have intervened to prevent the appearance of the first expression lines, before wrinkles create marks. And then, yes, our work becomes more difficult and we no longer achieve that result. Now we can try to treat, to attenuate: but the damage is already done.* (Sofia, dermatologist)

In that mirror, which was a constant presence in my interviews, I began to examine my face in detail and to notice details that the medical eye, with the force of its authority, had transformed for me into defects that needed to be corrected. I might even have remembered to put on moisturizer or sunscreen, but suddenly I felt irresponsible and careless. I explained that I didn't want to change my appearance, that I don't like "botoxed" faces, "duck-billed" lips, cheek fillers that create a "cat cheek" effect. The doctors reassured me about "natural" results, presenting several alternatives:

> *On your face it would just be baby botox, don't worry, or a biorevitalisation. It could even be something very soft like micro-needling. Nothing invasive. Radiesse maybe, or*

> *Sculptra. It would just be softening, you're still yourself, but an improved version of yourself. Like you've had a lot of rest on holiday.* (Manuel, dermatologist)

> *This would be to brighten, refresh the skin a little, tone it up. It's just a few injections, it's not hard. Here we have to replace the lost volume with hyaluronic acid . . . but Botox (botulinum toxin) you can't escape: you don't want to have those awful glabellae, which make you look angry and very masculine. Let's put a little bit on the eyebrows to open up the eye and take away that tired look.* (Miguel, dermatologist)

> *None of the hyaluronic acid fillers that then look all the same, all puffy. Absolutely not. for volume, only collagen stimulators so your body reacts and does its job again. These are new generation products. Like Radiesse. The name says it all, doesn't it?* (Pierre, dermatologist)

> *Fillers and botulinum toxin are the most common, but it is the last thing I advise. You can also use your body's resources, your own blood. Let's do Platelet Rich Plasma, which stimulates cell growth factors and promotes collagen synthesis. In my opinion, it would be radiofrequency before, vitamin mesolift after. And I recommend botox, hyaluronic acid and sculptra, in a unique session. In winter you should think about a good peel or ablative laser resurfacing, for those enlarged pores on your forehead, which are really awful.* (Sofia, dermatologist)

I became lost in this panoply of possibilities and contradictory advice. Only one message came through loud and clear: "I deserve and must value myself", "love myself", "take care of myself" and "be a better version of myself". With one injection, I can look less tired, more relaxed, like I'm coming back from a long holiday. My life is still stressful, of course, but I can exhibit an air of youth, rest and repose. Gradually, I came closer to my subjects' perspectives, seeing my body through their lenses. I went from observer to observed, and began to incorporate a medical view that pathologized the signs of my ageing.

When I decided to get my first 'baby botox', I entered into an ethical and intellectual conflict. How could I participate in the same discourse that I critically analyse, that of the aesthetic dictatorships over women's bodies, the myth of perfection at any cost? Feminist sociologist Dana Berkowitz reported an analogous reflection on the conflict experienced between her activism denouncing the dangerous consequences of beauty culture and her consumption of botulinum toxin, speaking of "cognitive dissonance" [20] (p. 95). I would say more about the confluence of the different roles required of me. Chiara/anthropologist is the one who discusses the social construction of gender, the power relations implicit in aesthetic hierarchies, and the disciplinary practices that shape the female body. Chiara/woman is the one who nevertheless replicates in her daily life all of the micro-practices that constitute the performance of femininity, who wishes to preserve the beauty and the power of attraction of youth, who is afraid of losing value with age. Clearly, figuring myself as a consumer proved to be useful during fieldwork, from the phenomenological point of view of sharing experience with my interlocutors and for the privileged ties I created in the field.

Botox and hyaluronic acid filling are almost painless procedures, which carry some risks and of which the effects are not immediate. The first changes appear within a fortnight. I observed the small changes in my face, hardly perceptible, except for the blockage of the corrugator and procerus muscles, between the eyebrows (in the glabella). After a week, I had the sensation of looking more rested and relaxed, with a more open and smoother look. Not exactly younger, but certainly more beautiful and luminous, to the point that I reduced the use of make-up, as I do when I'm on holiday. With a few injections, I had achieved the same effect I was trying to create by altering my digital photos with skin beautifying filters, to soften wrinkles and dark circles. The only problem is that the effect is ephemeral and transitory, and after four or five months everything returns to the initial state. The desire then immediately arises to reinject the products to recover that distended aspect. I had heard many times about addiction and compulsive use of fillers and Botox, and suddenly I realised how difficult it would be for me to stop now. There, I was already in the process of becoming addicted.

The "shelf life" of my botox expired during the confinement period, due to the COVID-19 pandemic. As soon as the deconfinement was announced, I called my dermatologist to immediately schedule the next treatment. I was told that I could be put on a waiting list, because requests had increased exponentially, and the clinic's phone kept ringing. The cosmetic, aesthetic medicine, hairdressing, and beauty salon sectors reopened on 4 May 2020, a fortnight before all of the other services. All of the people I spoke to were eager to perform some kind of aesthetic service as the first stage of their return to social life. I then confirmed my botox and filler sessions, the beautician, and the hairdresser straight away. Aesthetic medicine had already entered into the normal routines of my beauty regime, such as hair maintenance, waxing, manicures and pedicures. The only question was: would I talk about it publicly or not? Would I admit to it, write about it? Would I assume that I have a chemical as well as a digital body, that I embody liquid biotechnologies, along with the models of beauty they represent, underpinned by the aesthetics industry and the multiple power relations involved?

4. Conclusions: Freedom of Choice and Its Contradictions

"I wanna have control

I want a perfect body

I want a perfect soul"

(Radiohead, Creep)

The anti-ageing products on the market show the smiling faces of women who manage to cheat time. The names of the facial creams allude to treatments in aesthetic medicine (fillers, botox, laser), or incorporate terms belonging to the scientific fields of biology, genetics and biotechnology: "Cell Renewal", "Repairwear", "Biotechno-performance", "Revitalizing Supreme", "Replumping", "Regenerating", "Treats Wrinke Lifting", "Laser Focus", "Recovering Filler", "Lift Repair Extreme", "Lift-designer", "Sculpting-lift", "Botulin Effect", "Cellular Boost YouthFX", "DNAge", "LASER X3", "Genefique" and "Hyaluronic Filler Extreme". Their effectiveness is largely symbolic: substances such as collagen or hyaluronic acid are large molecules that do not penetrate the dermis, nor do they alter the volume and structure of the skin. Consumers have changed the way they buy and use anti-ageing cosmetics products: they talk about beauty therapy, self-care routines, health and natural products, preferring to buy products labelled "cruelty-free" "clean" "hypoallergenic" "nontoxic", "organic", "paraben-free" and "natural". Consumers want to know more about key ingredients, looking for example at the percentage of vitamin C, niacinamide, zinc, retinol or hyaluronic acid.

Almost all of the women interviewed, however, admitted to spending a lot of money on anti-ageing creams and serums for the face, and reported devoting much more time and energy to the face than to the body, with the exception of slimming products.

> *Age can be seen mainly in the face. The body is easier to hide: it's enough to wear the right clothes to camouflage flabbiness. For example, after forty, I recommend wearing shirts with three-quarter or long sleeves. It is necessary to hide the 'goodbye muscle', the one that wobbles when you wave goodbye. You know, the 'bat wings'. The rest, we have no way of disguising. And the face is the first thing we see of a person, where our attention is focused. The wear and tear caused by the sun, the wrinkles, the spots, the irregularities, the loss of tone in the jaw line, the jowls, the drooping eyelids . . .*
> (Catarina, 54 years old, ex-model)

> *I need, first of all, to feel good when I look in the mirror. I need to have moments of satisfaction—or at least prolong a moment of well-being in my most visible part, which is my face. I want to meet expectations, mine in the first place. Not other people. Is it to please my partner? I've never had any problems with my body. I like using my body. But*

there is a contradiction. I feel relaxed, but I am aware that something has changed and now I want less and less light in the bedroom . . . (Inês, 60 years old, teacher)

I've never liked old people. Imagine what it's like to see in the mirror that I'm starting to look like an old woman myself. I don't want to indulge in the ease of accepting old age; I want to continue to feel good about myself. To accept ageing is precisely to age. I want to grow old in a lazy way. Like those who always talk about illness, oh my god! I can't stand it. If there's one topic that's completely unsexy, it's talking about illness. I don't want to relate to people who are completely sloppy and relaxed. They're already beaten out of life. And I'm not like that. It's a question of aesthetics, but also of coherence with what I am. (Cristina, 65 years old, chartered accountant)

Even it's not difficult for interviewees to talk about beauty rituals involving creams or serums, the conversation becomes more arduous when we move on to less-light interventions, from the surface of the skin to deep procedures, commonly known as "minimally-invasive" procedures (botox injections, fillers, peelings, tensor threads, ablative laser treatments). At first, most of the people interviewed hid their recourse to aesthetic medicine and—even in the face of evidence—answered that they had never done anything, and that perfect skin depended on a balanced diet and a daily intake of two litres of water to hydrate the tissues.

The reasons for shyness in confessing to aesthetic interventions are multiple: from the attempt to create the illusion of a total "naturalness", to shame about the money spent for "vanity"; from embarrassment in revealing one's real age to the stigma that this search for beauty can create in more critical or militant feminist contexts. Even the few women who spoke calmly about the aesthetic procedures carried out always gave "morally acceptable" reasons to justify this choice: personal and family issues (separation, divorce, illness, the psychological need to take care of oneself, low self-esteem, or even relationships with younger partners); professional issues (the importance of image at work, public relations, media exposure); even clinical (botox to reduce migraines, laser for sun exposure damage, vaginal rejuvenation to increase sexual pleasure, blepharoplasty to improve eyesight, rhinoplasty to breathe better). My decision to reveal the aesthetic manipulations of my face to the informants obviously had an impact on the fieldwork. The sharing of the experience immediately created a greater ease in the telling of stories and desires, providing an atmosphere of complicity and trust. There were even proposals and invitations from friends and colleagues to accompany them for various rejuvenation treatments.

I do tell what I do . . . to my daughter, my sister, you and some gay friends, who are super supportive. If someone insists, like: did you do something? At first I don't say anything, but then, if they insist a lot, I don't deny it at all. But I'm not the one who has to tell everyone that I do this or that. Only people close to me know. But I feel a degree of pride in telling you. I even feel a certain feminine empowerment. I do it because I want to, because I can, because I am the one who sets my priorities and because I want to feel good about myself. I do it with a lot of determination. (Joana, 56 years old, entrepreneur)

I feel a contradiction regarding telling. To my students, for example, I couldn't tell them. We come from different historical, political and cultural backgrounds. I was born during the period of repression; I lived through the April 25th revolution, with a communist father who always taught me to take responsibility for all my attitudes, good or bad. There are many layers. The aesthetic question has to do with a whole life story. I live in a constant contradiction: is it for others or for me? But, at the end of the line . . . it is for me. (Sara, 60 years old, teacher)

To remain youthful and attractive brings you advantages, to be young and beautiful is not a disgrace, it is a privilege. I pity the people who don't understand that, if you ask me. In certain jobs it is necessary to look beautiful, in others less so, of course. University, for example, is a world somewhat apart. There are women who criticize those who make aesthetic alterations because of a dimension, which I would define as ideological. Who are these people who criticize the option to get aesthetic interventions? What is their background? (Claudia, 60, researcher)

Thus, I already joined, such as the women who had the generosity to share their experiences with me, the club of those Berkowitz calls "body entrepreneurs" [46] (p. 95)—that is, people who strategically improve their own appearance to increase their social, cultural and economic power, and the chances of professional success and in love relationships. Beauty, like youth, has an effective social value. Extending the privileges associated with beauty and youth means preserving one's own body capital to ensure social capital (social integration, the power of sexual attraction), symbolic capital (status and prestige) and economic capital (better salaries, professional mobility). Both are, however, ephemeral privileges and involve hard work, maintenance, and much economic investment, as well as suffering. At the same time, cosmetic procedures and choices are informed by cultural, economic and political structures and material inequalities. With amped-up betterment messaging on social media about getting in shape and staying young and beautiful, we know that we have to "improve" and "fix" our body, using drastic measures to keep up. The social pressure to maintain a youthful, attractive appearance results in stigma for those who have not the money to pay for the treatments. Attractive bodies are produced, regulated and disciplined on the basis of power relations experienced not as "obligations" but as aspirations, desires and values, encouraged and legitimized by various discourses—medical (care, control and prevention), moral (personal valuation, responsibility, willpower) and social (the globalization of virtual images of beauty, youth and success). The economy of anti-ageing is linked to segmented marketing: the personalization of enhancement products is clearly addressed to people based on gender, social class, economic status, age, education and profession. The pressure for women to conform to the dominant aesthetic standards is extremely high and entails unrealistic demands, considering the natural process of aging. For this reason, women make decisions about their bodies, assuming possible risks not on the basis of health problems but on the basis of the forever-young beauty ideals proposed by consumer culture. The access to anti-aging technologies is not equal for all, reproducing and contributing to the amplification of social inequalities. The body appearance carries with it a dense history of meanings regarding race, class, gender, sexuality, disability and age. The technologies of self-improvement in our contemporary era are, using Donna Haraway's words, "knowledge-power processes that inscribe and materialize the world in some forms rather than others" [4] (p. 7). These knowledge–power processes reinforce the body-norms that end up excluding the most vulnerable people in society. In our very unequal world, this means that a wide swath of humanity is largely excluded from these technologies of self-improvement, as the more desirable technologies become branded as luxury items limited to those with access to the best health care systems, or to those with the purchasing power to buy the ideal body. None of the women I interviewed, exploring the ways we age, can be judged a superficial person for spending energy and money trying to maintain her beauty, wanting to look "like her" again. In fact, there is nothing superficial about body appearance or beauty, and that's why they matter so much. So, no—age, today, is not a choice. Or, at least, it is not an equal choice for everyone; we do not all have access to the same resources or the same possibility to choose: a certain configuration of the social order restricts the ability and freedom of choice of certain individuals or groups, even when we are talking about access to beauty or the preservation of a youthful appearance.

Funding: This research was funded by the project EXCEL, "The Pursuit of Excellence: Biotechnologies, enhancement and body capital in Portugal" (PTDC/SOC-ANT/30572/2017), financed by the Portuguese Foundation for Science and Technology and coordinated by Chiara Pussetti (Website: www.excelproject.eu, accessed on 10 July 2021).

Institutional Review Board Statement: The Ethics Board of the Institute of Social Sciences of the University of Lisbon supervises the project, according to the ethical requirements of the European Research Council. The Ethic Board is aware of and complies with European and national legislation and fundamental ethical principles, including those reflected in the Charter of Fundamental Rights of the European Union and the European Convention on Human Rights and its Supplementary Protocols. The participation in the study will be entirely voluntary and all participants will be informed that they can withdraw from the study at any time and with no consequences to them. The confidentiality of information supplied by research participants and the anonymity of respondents will be respected. Demographic data collected as part of the project (name, age, gender, family status, etc.) will be anonymized and will be stored separately to the qualitative data collected. All participants will receive a clearly formulated document of informed consent in advance—written in a language and in terms they can fully understand—describing the aims, methods and implications of the research, and the nature of their participation.

Informed Consent Statement: Informed consent was obtained from all of the subjects involved in the study.

Data Availability Statement: Data from the research was recorded in handwritten form and as such avoids the need for online data protection. Demographic data was anonymized and stored separately from the qualitative data. Identification codes and personal data will be stored in an encrypted file. References to informants in the outputs will be given through codes of identification. Data will not be used for any other purpose other than that purpose for which it was obtained.

Acknowledgments: I am grateful for the opportunity to collaborate with the editors of this special issue. I would like to sincerely thank the reviewers for taking the time to read my paper, and for their very generous comments and feedback. In the fieldwork process, I have benefited from the support of many people and I am particularly thankful to the women who shared with me their intimacy with intellectual generosity. I want to thank my daughter, Sole, who warms my heart.

Conflicts of Interest: The author declares no conflict of interest.

References

1. Goldman, R. *Reading Ads Socially*; Routledge: London, UK; New York, NY, USA, 1992.
2. Sullivan, D. *Cosmetic Surgery: The Cutting Edge of Commercial Medicine*; Rutgers University Press: Bew Brunswick, NJ, USA, 2001.
3. Pitts-Taylor, V. *Surgery Junkies: Wellness and Pathology in Cosmetic Culture*; Rutgers University Press: Piscataway, NJ, USA, 2007.
4. Berkowitz, D. *Botox Nation Changing the Face of America*; New York University Press: New York, NY, USA, 2017.
5. Blum, V.L. *Flesh Wounds–The Culture of Cosmetic Surgery*; University of California Press: Berkeley, CA, USA, 2003.
6. Furman, F.K. *Facing the Mirror: Older Women and Beauty Shop Culture*; Routledge: London, UK; New York, NY, USA, 1997.
7. Hurd Clark, L. *Facing Age: Women Growing Older in an Anti-Aging Culture*; Rowman and Littlefield: Toronto, OH, USA, 2010.
8. Hurd Clark, L.; Griffin, M. Visible and invisible ageing. Beauty work as a response to ageism. *Ageing Soc.* **2008**, *28*, 653–674. [CrossRef]
9. Baker, L.; Gringart, E. Body image and self-esteem in adulthood. *Ageing Soc.* **2009**, *6*, 977–995. [CrossRef]
10. Brooks, A. *The Ways Women Age*; New York University Press: New York, NY, USA, 2017.
11. Winterich, J.A. Aging, femininity and the body; What appearance change mean to women with age. *Gend. Issues* **2007**, *24*, 51–69. [CrossRef]
12. Wolf, N. *The Beauty Myth: How Images of Beauty Are Used against Women*; Random House: London, UK, 1991.
13. Gannon, L. *Women and Aging: Transcending the Myth*; Routledge: New York, NY, USA, 1999.
14. Weitz, R. *The Politics of Women's Bodies: Sexuality, Appearance and Behaviour*; Oxford University Press: Oxford, UK; New York, NY, USA, 1998.
15. Gibson, M. Bodies without Histories. Cosmetic Surgery and the Undoing of Time. *Aust. Fem. Stud.* **2006**, *21*, 51–63. [CrossRef]
16. Gimlin, D. *Cosmetic Surgery Narratives. A Cross-Cultural Analysis of Women's Accounts*; Palgrave Macmillan: London, UK, 2012.
17. Sayre, S. Facelift Forensics: A Personal Narrative of Aesthetic Cosmetic Surgery. In *Advances in Consumer Research*; Arnould, E.J., Scott, L.M., Eds.; Association for Consumer Research: Provo, UT, USA, 1999; Volume 26, pp. 178–183.
18. Jones, M. *Skintight: An Anatomy of Cosmetic Surgery*; Berg: Oxford, NY, USA, 2008.
19. Heyes, C.; Jones, M. (Eds.) *Cosmetic Surgery. A Feminist Primer Burlington*; Ashgate: Surrey, UK, 2009.
20. Beghin, J.C.; Teshome, Y. *Perfecting Beauty under the Knife: The Determinants of Global Cosmetic Surgery Consumption*; Working Paper No. 14017; Iowa State University Department of Economics Ames: Ames, IA, USA, 2014.
21. Colebrook, C. Introduction: Special Issue on Beauty and Feminist Theory. *Fem. Theory* **2006**, *7*, 131–142. [CrossRef]
22. Satzewich, V. Whiteness Limited: Racialization and the Social Construction of "Peripheral Europeans". *Soc. Hist. Hist. Soc.* **2000**, *33*, 271–289.
23. Zhang, L. Eurocentric Beauty Ideals as a Form of Structural Violence: Origins and Effects on East Asian Women. *Deliberations* **2013**, *1*, 4–12.
24. Heyes, C. All cosmetic surgery is "ethnic": Asian eyelids, feminist indignation, and the politics of whiteness. In *Cosmetic Surgery. A Feminist Primer Burlington*; Heyes, C., Jones, M., Eds.; Ashgate: Surrey, UK, 2009; pp. 191–205.

25. Mire, A. Skin Trade: Genealogy of Anti-ageing 'Whiteness Therapy' in Colonial Medicine. *Med. Stud.* **2014**, *4*, 119–129. [CrossRef] [PubMed]
26. Poitevin, K. Inventing Whiteness: Cosmetic, Race and Women in Early Modern England. *J. Early Mod. Cult. Stud.* **2011**, *11*, 59–89. [CrossRef]
27. Saraswati, L.A. Cosmopolitan whiteness: The effects and affects of skin whitening advertisements in a transnational women's magazine in Indonesia. *Meridians* **2010**, *10*, 15–41. [CrossRef]
28. Pussetti, C. From Ebony to Ivory 'Cosmetic' Investments in the Body. *Anthropol. J. Eur. Cult.* **2019**, *28*, 64–72. [CrossRef]
29. Pussetti, C. La Gazzella, P. La gestione dell'apparenza razziale nella industria della moda. *Off. Della Stor. Mag.* **2020**, *29*, 8–39.
30. Pussetti, C. 'Ethnic' aesthetic medicine and surgery: Biopolitics, bioeconomies and bioethics of 'racial' transformation. In *Entrecruzares bioéticos*; Barbosa, A., Fernandes, I., Eds.; Centro de Bioética da Faculdade de Medicina da Universidade de Lisboa: Lisboa, Portugal, 2020; pp. 153–183.
31. Jarrín, A.; Pussetti, C. (Eds.) *Remaking the Human: Cosmetic Technologies of Body Repair, Reshape and Replacement*; Berghahn Books: Oxford, NY, USA, 2021.
32. Jarrín, A. Towards a Biopolitics of Beauty: Eugenics, Aesthetic Hierarchies and Plastic Surgery in Brazil. *J. Lat. Am. Cult. Stud.* **2015**, *24*, 535–552. [CrossRef]
33. Woodward, K. *Figuring Age: Women, Bodies, Generations*; Indiana University Press: Bloomington, IN, USA, 1999.
34. Beauvoir, S. *La Vieillesse*; Éditions Gallimard: Paris, France, 1970.
35. Sontag, S. The Double Stand of Ageing. *Saturday Rev. Lit.* **1972**, *39*, 29–38.
36. Cerqueira, M.M. Imagens do Envelhecimento e da Velhice: Um Estudo na População Portuguesa. Ph.D. Thesis, Universidade de Aveiro, Aveiro, Portugal, 2010.
37. Gilman, S.L. *Creating Beauty to Cure the Soul–Race and Psychology in the Shaping of Aesthetic Surgery*; Duke University Press: London, UK, 1998.
38. Gullette, M. *Aged by Culture*; University of Chicago Press: Chicago, IL, USA, 2004.
39. Higgs, P.; Leontowitsch, M.; Stevenson, F.; Jones, I.R. Not just old and sick–the 'will to health' in later life. *Ageing Soc.* **2009**, *29*, 687–707. [CrossRef]
40. Mykytyn, C.E. Medicalizing the optimal: Anti-ageing medicine and the quandary of intervention. *J. Ageing Stud.* **2008**, *22*, 313–321. [CrossRef]
41. Gilleard, C.; Higgs, P. *Culture of Ageing: Self, Citizen and the Body*; Prentiss Hall: Oxford, UK, 2000.
42. Brooks, A. Aesthetic anti-aging surgery and technologies: Women's friend or foe? *Sociol. Health Illn.* **2010**, *2*, 238–257. [CrossRef] [PubMed]
43. Bordo, S. *Unbearable Weight: Feminism, Western Culture and the Body*; University of California Press: Berkeley, CA, USA; Los Angeles, CA, USA, 2003.
44. Franklin, S. Ethical biocapital. In *Remaking Life and Death: Toward and Anthropology of the Biosciences*; Franklin, S., Lock, M., Eds.; School of American Research Press: Santa Fe, CA, USA, 2003; pp. 97–128.
45. Moreira, T.; Paolo, P. Between truth and hope: On Parkinson's disease, neurotransplantation and the production of the 'self'. *Hist. Hum. Sci.* **2005**, *18*, 55–82. [CrossRef]
46. Haraway, D. *Modest_Witness@Second_Millenium.Femaleman_Meets_Oncomouse: Feminism and Technoscience*; Routledge: New Yor, NY, USA, 1997.

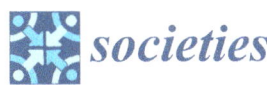

Review

Attitudes and Practices towards HPV Vaccination and Its Social Processes in Europe: An Equity-Focused Scoping Review

Violeta Alarcão [1,2,*] and Bilyana Zdravkova [1]

1 Centro de Investigação e Estudos de Sociologia, Iscte—Instituto Universitário de Lisboa, Avenida das Forças Armadas, 1649-026 Lisboa, Portugal
2 Instituto de Saúde Ambiental, Faculdade de Medicina, Universidade de Lisboa, Avenida Professor Egas Moniz, 1649-028 Lisboa, Portugal
* Correspondence: violeta_sabina_alarcao@iscte-iul.pt

Abstract: The sociological understanding of the human papillomavirus (HPV) vaccination offers the possibility to understand society better as the processes that shape health beliefs and influence HPV vaccine decisions relate to gender, power, and identity. This research aimed to locate, select, and critically assess scientific evidence regarding the attitudes and practices towards HPV vaccination and its social processes with a focus on health equity. A scoping review following the Preferred Reporting Items for Systematic Reviews and Meta-Analyses extension for scoping reviews (PRISMA-ScR) and the recommendations made by the Joanna Briggs Institute was undertaken. Medline and Scopus were searched from their start date until December 2021. The review followed the Population/Concept/Context (PCC) inclusion criteria: Population = General population, adults and adolescents, Concept = Empirical data on determinants of HPV vaccination, Context = Studies on attitudes and practices towards HPV vaccination and its social processes with a focus on gender, class, and ethnic/racial inequalities. Of the 235 selected articles, 28 were from European countries and were the focus of this review, with special attention to socio-economic determinants in HPV vaccine hesitancy in Europe, a region increasingly affected by vaccination public distrust and criticism. Barriers and facilitators of HPV vaccine uptake and determinants of immunization were identified. Given the emphasis on health equity, these data are relevant to strengthening vaccination programs to promote vaccination for all people.

Keywords: HPV vaccination; sexual health; health disparities; equity

Citation: Alarcão, V.; Zdravkova, B. Attitudes and Practices towards HPV Vaccination and Its Social Processes in Europe: An Equity-Focused Scoping Review. *Societies* **2022**, *12*, 131. https://doi.org/10.3390/soc12050131

Academic Editor: Gregor Wolbring

Received: 29 July 2022
Accepted: 15 September 2022
Published: 18 September 2022

Publisher's Note: MDPI stays neutral with regard to jurisdictional claims in published maps and institutional affiliations.

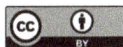

Copyright: © 2022 by the authors. Licensee MDPI, Basel, Switzerland. This article is an open access article distributed under the terms and conditions of the Creative Commons Attribution (CC BY) license (https://creativecommons.org/licenses/by/4.0/).

1. Introduction

The sociological understanding of the human papillomavirus (HPV) vaccination, which varies between and within countries [1], offers the possibility to better understand society as vaccination processes, and in particular, vaccination against HPV—a widespread and sexually transmitted viral infection responsible for approximately 70% of cervical cancer cases in the world [2]—are constructed within social, cultural, and institutional contexts that produce normative notions on rights and responsibilities of health citizenship. The distinctive fact about the HPV vaccine's target being sexually transmitted links it to longstanding controversies around sex, gender, and young women's bodies and sexual behaviors [3,4]. Cervical cancer can serve as an example of the systematic disadvantages that women experience due to social and sexual inequalities and enables us to understand how gender intersects other social hierarchies such as class and ethnicity/race to (re)produce social inequalities in health [5,6]. Although both men and women are at risk of developing HPV-related cancers, social campaigns regarding vaccination against HPV are aimed mainly at the prevention of cervical cancer for women [7]. The promotion of HPV vaccination is surrounded by feminization and moralization processes, influencing the understanding of HPV vaccination and the accessibility of vaccination as preventive health behavior. The stigma associated with HPV vaccination due to the stereotypical perception of the HPV vaccine as a facilitating agent of immoral sexual behaviors influences not only the decision-making process but also the discrimination against those who get the vaccine, serving as social control for girls and women [8]. This adds to the fact that knowledge about sexually transmitted infections (STIs) is frequently obtained from social campaigns, media, and the Internet, due to an absence of comprehensive sexuality education programs, which accentuates health disparities among underserved and disadvantaged populations (e.g., sexual and gender minorities) [9].

HPV vaccination coverage rates are affected by social norms (including of one's family, friends, healthcare professionals, and religious or community leaders) [10]. Social sciences research has been describing the processes through which individuals receive and manage medical definitions and interventions for their bodies, such as marketing from pharmaceutical industries and professional claims of knowledge [8,11–15]. Trust in doctors, nurses, and other health professionals, in the healthcare system and the pharmaceutical industry, and patient-centeredness in care, influence health-related beliefs and HPV vaccine decision making [16–20]. It is important to better understand the social determinants of vaccination and the system-level barriers to HPV vaccine uptake [21]. Among the existing theoretical frameworks to help define vaccination behaviors, the 5As' practical taxonomy for the determinants of vaccine uptake focusing on access, affordability, awareness, acceptance, and activation seemed to be most adequate [22].

A literature review represents an opportunity to look at how intersecting gender, age, class, ethnicity/race, and other social inequalities in different contexts shape health care decisions.

The HPV vaccine coverage rates have been suboptimal in some European countries, particularly in Eastern Europe, but also in Ireland, France, and Denmark. Variations can be partly explained by contextual and implementation factors, such as vaccine delivery (schools or public or private health systems), depending on the country and immunization program [10]. Moreover, vaccination is increasingly suffering from public distrust and criticism in Europe. The existing literature suggests the need for reviews looking specifically at socio-economic determinants in HPV vaccine hesitancy to support the development of context-specific interventions to improve confidence in HPV vaccination [10]. Therefore, this review aims to characterize the existing research on attitudes and practices toward HPV vaccination and the social and cultural construction processes involved in the understanding of the HPV vaccine to cancer prevention in Europe with a focus on health equity. The overarching research goal was to identify the social determinants of HPV under vaccination among diverse populations while exploring the following:

1: What are the barriers and facilitators of HPV vaccine uptake (based on the 5As) [23]?

2: What are the determinants of HPV vaccine uptake across gender, age, ethnicity/race, and population diversity?

3: Which practices and policies related to HPV vaccination can contribute to improving uptake and coverage routine to promote health and reduce health inequities?

2. Methods

2.1. Study Design

A scoping review was conducted to map and characterize the types of available evidence related to the social determinants of attitudes and practices towards HPV vaccination, and to identify knowledge gaps.

The review was undertaken following the Preferred Reporting Items for Systematic Reviews and Meta-Analyses extension for scoping reviews (PRISMA-ScR) [24] and the recommendations made by the Joanna Briggs Institute (JBI), a global organization promoting and supporting evidence-based decisions that improve health and health service delivery [25].

2.2. Search Strategy

A systematic literature search was performed using Medline (via PubMed), and Scopus electronic databases, with combinations of the search terms, tailored to the syntax and functionality of each database. Searches were conducted on 14 December 2021 with no date range limitation. The following search query was used: "HPV vaccination" OR "Papillomavirus Vaccines"[Mesh] OR HPV OR "human papillomavirus" AND (("Vaccination Hesitancy"[Mesh]) OR "Vaccination Refusal"[Mesh] OR "Attitude to Health"[Mesh] OR "Patient Acceptance of Health Care"[Mesh] OR "Health Knowledge, Attitudes, Practice"[Mesh]) AND ("Health Equity"[Mesh] OR "Social Justice"[Mesh] OR "Intersectional Framework"[Mesh] OR Intersectional* OR "health disparities" OR "Gender Equity"[Mesh] OR "Ethnicity"[Mesh] OR "Racial Groups"[Mesh])). Only English-written documents were considered eligible for inclusion.

2.3. Inclusion and Exclusion Criteria

The Population (or participants)/Concept/Context (PCC) method recommended by JBI to identify the main concepts in the primary review questions was used for the search strategy and the definition of inclusion criteria [25]: P (Population = General population, adults and adolescents), C (Concept = Empirical data on determinants of HPV vaccination), C (Context = Studies that report on attitudes and practices towards HPV vaccination and its social processes with a focus on gender, class, and ethnic/racial inequalities). All publications based on empirical studies (regardless of research design) were included. The exception was intervention studies, which were excluded, because of their distinguished features compared to observational studies. Book chapters, book reviews, vignette studies, study protocols, commentaries, guidelines, and editorials were also excluded.

Each relevant record was reviewed independently by the two authors, who screened titles and abstracts, and, when needed, full texts. A final decision was obtained for each record and uncertainties were resolved by discussion between the two authors.

2.4. Data Extraction and Synthesis

For all the included articles, the following data were extracted: (1) author(s) and year of publication, (2) country and setting, (3) population (sample size, gender, age, nationality/ethnicity, and diversity), (4) rationale and aim, (5) design and methods, (6) HPV outcome(s), (7) overall results, (8) overall limitations, (9) and overall recommendations. Information regarding the journal's title, publication quartile, and domain of work (i.e., the domain with the highest quartile in the year of the study publication according to the Scimago Journal & Country Rank) was also collected.

Methodological quality or risk of bias of the included articles was not appraised because it was not relevant nor necessary to the scoping review objectives [25].

Results were synthesized using a thematic approach on the relevant themes related to the barriers and facilitators of HPV vaccine uptake, and its social processes, with a focus on gender, class, and ethnic/racial inequalities.

3. Results

A total of 533 articles were identified, 291 in PubMed and 241 in Scopus. After duplicate removal ($n = 75$), 458 articles remained for screening. Of these, 224 were excluded because they were not empirical studies (i.e., literature reviews, study protocols, or commentaries/letters) or were intervention studies or did not focus on HPV vaccination attitudes or practices, or the study population was only health professionals. As a result, 234 publications could be included, with publication dates ranging from 2007 to 2021. Most of the studies ($n = 175$; 75%) were conducted in the United States of America (USA), and only 28 articles (12%) were conducted in European countries and were selected to be included in this review for mapping the state of the art and to reveal the specific trends in the field in Europe. A flow diagram providing the number of articles included and excluded at each stage is provided in Figure 1.

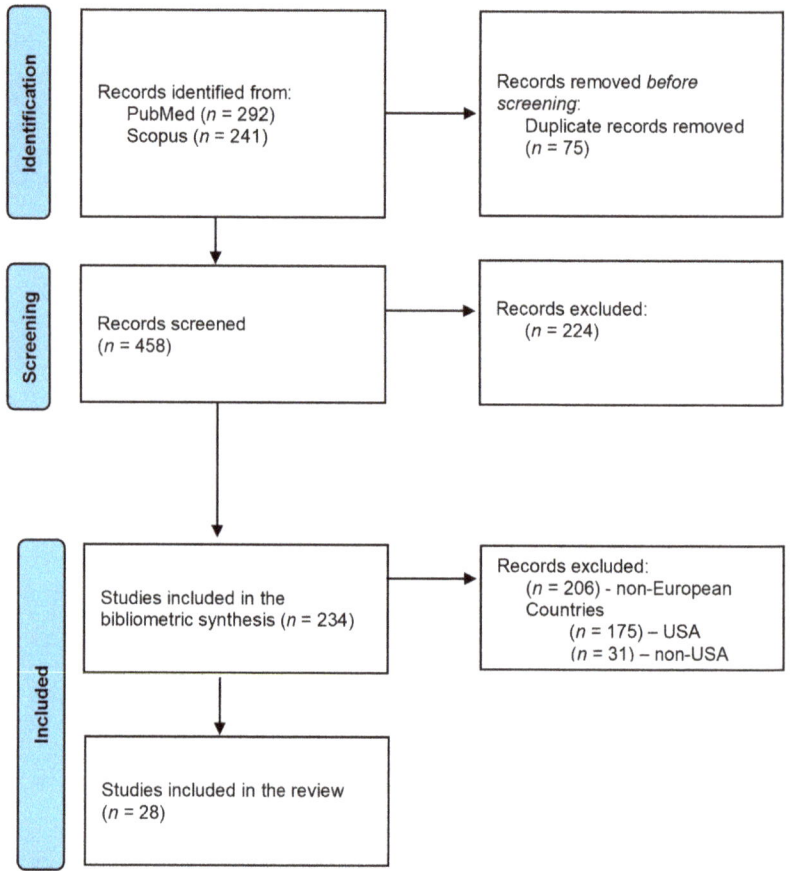

Figure 1. PRISMA 2020 flow diagram of the selection of the articles.

3.1. Who Is Being Studied and How?

The first publications (*n* = 2) were issued in 2008 (Table 1). The number of articles published each year ranged from zero articles in 2010, 2011, and 2013 to four articles in 2009, 2015, 2017, and 2018. All publications were in journals with an impact factor, and the majority ranked in the first quartile (21/28). Four articles were published in journals in the second quartile, and three articles in the third quartile. All articles were published in the medical and health sciences subject area, and one was also classified in social sciences (the journal of *Medical Anthropology Quarterly*).

Studies were conducted in 10 countries. Eleven studies were conducted in England [26–36], the first two publications in 2008, four in 2009 (the year that the government immunization program began with HPV vaccination of girls aged 12–13 years), and the last in 2020. All articles provided data concerning the role of ethnicity in HPV vaccination uptake.

Three studies were conducted in Romania [37–39], in 2012, 2016, and 2019, all focusing on Romanian parents/guardians' vaccine hesitancy.

Three studies were conducted in the Netherlands [40–42], in 2014, 2015, and 2017, aiming to assess inequalities in vaccine uptake; one included a qualitative study with an intersectionality framework to capture the perceptions of migrant women from Somalia concerning cervical cancer prevention [42].

Three studies were conducted in Sweden [43–45], in 2014, 2017, and 2019, with different study designs and populations. The first study used individual interviews with parents who refused their daughters from receiving the HPV vaccination. The second study investigated HPV vaccination status in female adolescents and related sociodemographic factors, individual beliefs and knowledge about HPV prevention, and sexual experiences. The last study aimed to investigate inequities in HPV vaccine uptake 10 years after its introduction in the country, where three different delivery modes of the vaccine have existed since 2007.

Moreover, three studies were conducted in Denmark [46–48], one in 2015 and two in 2018, all using data from the Danish childhood immunization program.

Finally, five countries had one publication each, with different populations and approaches. The study conducted in Greece in 2020 focused on the vulnerable population of Roma women [49], while the study conducted in Poland in 2021 focused on Polish men [50]. Research conducted in Norway [51] and Spain [52] was centered on adolescent girls and parents, and the Italian study investigated factors related to HPV vaccination refusal in young adult women without starting or completing HPV vaccination [53].

The majority of the articles had as the main outcome HPV vaccination uptake and its determinants ($n = 19$), while others focused only on HPV vaccination intentions ($n = 9$). Twenty-two articles used a quantitative approach, mostly with a descriptive design, while six articles used a qualitative approach with individual interviews and focus groups.

Table 1 presents more details on the characteristics of the studies.

3.2. Barriers and Facilitators of Vaccination Uptake

All the included articles referred to barriers or facilitators of vaccine uptake. Access, acceptance, and activation were the most frequent themes, and awareness and affordability were less frequent. Barriers and facilitators to HPV vaccine uptake subthemes were identified and are summarized in Table 2.

- Access and Affordability

Demographic and socioeconomic status were common barriers to HPV vaccine uptake in different European countries [35,41,48,49]. Specific barriers were also reported for people with refugee/migrant or ethnic minority backgrounds [48,49,52]. For example, Spencer et al. combined the use of the index of multiple deprivations and census ethnicity data to explore the links between HPV vaccination and cervical screening uptake with deprivation and ethnic composition of the area of residence in a deprived region in England. Results revealed that girls from the most deprived areas were less likely to complete the three vaccine doses. The authors concluded that there is a group of women from disadvantaged backgrounds and with a higher concentration of ethnic minorities who miss both cervical screening and HPV vaccination [35].

Several socioeconomic predictors of HPV vaccination were found in a cohort study based on the national HPV childhood vaccination program in Denmark. Ethnicity was found to be a strong determinant of initiation and completion of HPV vaccination. A social gradient regarding education, income and employment status was also observed, where decreases in vaccine coverage were associated with girls whose mothers were more disadvantaged [48]. A cross-sectional study in the Netherlands also found that vaccination uptake was higher in low urbanized settings and among girls without a religious background [41].

Table 1. Characteristics of the studies.

Author, Date	Journal, Quartile	Area of Expertise	Country	Population	Methods, Study Design	HPV Outcomes
Alberts et al., 2017 [40]	*BMC Public Health*, Q1	Medical and Health Sciences	The Netherlands	Parents/guardians of daughters (n = 1309) from different ethnic groups	Longitudinal study Database of the Youth Health Service of the Public Health Service of Amsterdam Self-completion questionnaire	Determinants of HPV vaccination intention and uptake
Amdisen et al., 2018 [46]	*Vaccine*, Q1	Medical and Health Sciences	Denmark	Girls who were residing in Denmark between their 12th and 13th birthday (n = 161,528)	Register-based cohort study Data from the Danish Vaccination Register were linked with demographic data from the Danish Civil Registration System	Determinants and uptake of the first dose of the HPV vaccine (HPV1)
Conroy et al., 2009 [26]	*Journal of Women's Health*, Q1	Medical and Health Sciences	England	Girls and women aged 13–26, of black, white, or other ethnicity (n = 262)	A baseline survey, linked with demographic data, gynecological history, and attitudes associated with vaccination at follow-up	Determinants of HPV vaccination uptake and follow-up
Craciun and Baban, 2012 [37]	*Vaccine*, Q1	Medical and Health Sciences	Romania	Romanian mothers aged 30–50 who decline vaccine of their daughters, aged 10–11 (n = 24)	Data from the project "Psychosocial, Political and Gendered Dimensions of Preventive Technologies in Bulgaria and Romania: HPV Vaccine Implementation", Semi-structured interviews and focus groups	Determinants of HPV vaccination intention
Forster et al., 2015 [27]	*BMC Public Health*, Q1	Medical and Health Sciences	England	Girls aged 15–16, of White, Black, Asian, or another ethnicity (n = 2163)	Data was collected through surveys from an ethnically diverse sample of girls from twelve London schools	Determinants of HPV vaccination status
Forster et al., 2017 [29]	*Psycho-Oncology*, Q1	Medical and Health Sciences	England	Ethnic minority/White British parents of girls (36–62) (n = 33)	Data from parents was collected via interviews and analyzed using Framework Analysis	Determinants of HPV vaccination intention and uptake

Table 1. *Cont.*

Author, Date	Journal, Quartile	Area of Expertise	Country	Population	Methods, Study Design	HPV Outcomes
Grandahl et al., 2014 [43]	*Acta Paediatrica* Q1	Medical and Health Sciences	Sweden	Parents who refused their daughters from receiving the HPV vaccination, aged 10–12 (n = 25)	Data from parents was gathered via interviews	Determinants of HPV vaccination intention and uptake
Grandahl et al., 2017 [44]	*PLoS One* Q1	Medical and Health Sciences	Sweden	Upper secondary school students, boys and girls aged 16 (n = 832)	Cross-sectional study Data from the project Prevention of HPV in a school-based setting Health Belief Model (HBM) and reports of cross-sectional studies	Determinants of HPV vaccination follow-up uptake and status
Hansen et al., 2015 [51]	*Preventive Medicine* Q1	Medical and Health Sciences	Norway	Girls and parents of Norwegian nationality (n = 90,842)	Data collected from national registries for all Norwegian girls eligible for routine school-based HPV vaccination and their registered mother and father were merged	Determinants of HPV vaccination uptake and follow-up
Marlow et al., 2008 [31]	*Journal of Medical Screening* Q1	Medical and Health Sciences	England	Women aged 25–64, of white or non-white ethnicity (n = 994)	Random sampling of postcode address Self-reported cervical screening and intention to accept an HPV test; In a subsample (n = 296) with a young daughter's self-reported willingness to accept HPV vaccination	Determinants of HPV vaccination intention
Marlow, et al., 2009 [30]	*Vaccine*, Q1	Medical and Health Sciences	England	Female students, aged 16–19, of White, Black, Asian, or another ethnicity (n = 367)	Participants from two further-education colleges reported on acceptability and attitudes (based on the Health Belief Model) after reading information about HPV	Determinants of HPV vaccination intention

Table 1. Cont.

Author, Date	Journal, Quartile	Area of Expertise	Country	Population	Methods, Study Design	HPV Outcomes
Marlow et al., 2009 [32]	Journal of Epidemiology and Community Health Q1	Medical and Health Sciences	England	Ethnic minority women (n = 750) and white British women (n = 200), aged 16–55+	Cross-sectional study with quota sampling to ensure adequate representation of ethnic minority women and a comparison sample of white British women	Determinants of HPV vaccination intention
Marlow et al., 2009 [33]	Human Vaccines Q3	Medical and Health Sciences	England	Black/Black British (n = 10) and Asian/Asian British mothers (n = 10) of daughters at least 16 years old	Face-to-face interviews	Determinants of HPV vaccination intention
Miko et al., 2019 [38]	Medicine Q3	Medical and Health Sciences	Romania	Romanian parents/guardians (n = 452)	Cross-sectional survey based on the Matrix of Determinants for Vaccine Hesitancy designed by SAGE	Determinants of HPV vaccination intention
Moller et al., 2018 [47]	European Journal of Cancer Prevention Q1	Medical and Health Sciences	Denmark	Refugee girls (n = 3264) Danish-born girls (n = 19,584)	Register-based cohort design Data from the National Danish Health Service, identifying all contacts for HPV immunization in the ordinary and catch-up HPV immunization program	Determinants of HPV vaccination uptake
Mollers et al., 2014 [41]	BMC Public Health Q1	Medical and Health Sciences	The Netherlands	Girls aged 16–17, Dutch, Turkish, Moroccans, Surinamese, Antilleans, Arubans, and other (n = 2989)	Nationwide online questionnaire with knowledge and other variables associated with vaccination status	Determinants of HPV vaccination status
Navarro-Illana P. et al., 2018 [52]	Gaceta Sanitaria Q2	Medical and Health Sciences	Spain	Adolescent girls and their parents, aged 25–60+, (n = 1278)	Cross-sectional study on knowledge and attitudes related to HPV infection and vaccine	Determinants of HPV vaccine intention and uptake
Pop, 2016 [39]	Medical Anthropology Quarterly Q1	Medical and Health/Social Sciences	Romania	Parents from South Romania, women (n = 43)	In-depth semi-structured interviews,	Determinants of HPV vaccination intention

Table 1. Cont.

Author, Date	Journal, Quartile	Area of Expertise	Country	Population	Methods, Study Design	HPV Outcomes
Restivo et al., 2018 [53]	International Journal of Environmental Research and Public Health Q2	Medical and Health Sciences	Italy	Women aged 18-21 without starting or completing HPV vaccination (n = 141)	A cross-sectional study using a telephone questionnaire, with items on HPV infection and vaccination knowledge based on the Health Belief Model framework	Determinants of HPV vaccination intention and uptake follow-up
Reszka et al., 2021 [50]	Journal of Preventive Medicine and Hygiene (JPMH) Q3	Medical and Health Sciences	Poland	Hetero and homosexual men, aged 14-39 (n = 169)	Cross-sectional study with open-ended, close-ended, and nominal, multiple-choice questions	Determinants of HPV vaccination status
Riza et al., 2020 [49]	International Journal of Environmental Research and Public Health Q2	Medical and Health Sciences	Greece	Vulnerable population of Roma women aged 18-70 (n = 142 in 2012; n = 122 in 2017)	Cross-sectional study, interviewer-administered questionnaire based on the behavioral model for vulnerable populations	Determinants of HPV vaccination status
Rockliffe et al., 2017 [34]	BMJ Q1	Medical and Health Sciences	England	Data from 195 schools obtained for girls from diverse ethnic backgrounds uptake rates	Uptake rates for the three recommended vaccine doses from 2008 to 2010 from schools combined to census data related to the postcode of each school for the ethnic characterization of the resident population	Determinants of HPV vaccination uptake
Salad et al., 2015 [42]	International Journal for Equity in Health Q1	Medical and Health Sciences	The Netherlands	Somali women aged 17-21, (n = 14); Somali mothers, two groups, aged 30-46 and 23-66 (n = 6)	Semi-structured interviews; thematic content analysis	Determinants of HPV vaccination intention
Schreiber et al., 2015 [48]	Journal of Adolescent Health Q1	Medical and Health Sciences	Denmark	Girls in childhood immunization program (n = 65,926)	Data obtained by linkage to Statistics Denmark and the Danish National Health Insurance Service Register	Determinants of HPV vaccination status uptake and follow-up
Spencer et al., 2014 [35]	BMJ Q1	Medical and Health Sciences	England	Mothers; daughters, aged 12-13	Index of Multiple Deprivation scores and census ethnicity data	Determinants of HPV vaccination status and initiation

Table 1. Cont.

Author, Date	Journal, Quartile	Area of Expertise	Country	Population	Methods, Study Design	HPV Outcomes
Stearns et al., 2020 [36]	*International Journal of Environmental Research and Public Health* Q2	Medical and Health Sciences	England	Men who have sex with men, ethnicity mostly white 84% (n = 115)	Cross-Sectional Survey Design	Determinants of HPV vaccination status and uptake
Walsh et al., 2008 [28]	*BMC Public Health* Q1	Medical and Health Sciences	England	Participants mix of social class and ethnicity aged 16–54 (n = 420)	Street survey with semi-structured interview questionnaire Setting: three areas of Birmingham to target a mix of social class and ethnicity	Determinants of HPV vaccination intention
Wang et al., 2019 [45]	*Preventive Medicine* Q1	Medical and Health Sciences	Sweden	Girls born between 1990 and 2003 (n = 689,676)	Cumulative incidence of receiving the first dose of the vaccine	Determinants and uptake of the first dose of the HPV vaccine (HPV1)

In Southeast Europe, a cross-sectional study in Greece with various groups of vulnerable women found that nationality was related to knowledge and attitudes on cervical cancer etiology and the HPV vaccine, with native women demonstrating higher knowledge than migrant and Roma women. The findings also indicated that Roma women faced higher levels of marginalization and social exclusion compared to legalized migrant women [49]. Additional factors associated with limited knowledge on risk factors for cervical cancer and erroneous attitudes and perceptions on cervical cancer prevention (Pap smear and HPV vaccine) included older age, low educational level, housing conditions, and lack of insurance coverage [49]. The lower uptake of the HPV vaccine among refugee girls is a challenge to immunization programs in raising ethnically diverse societies [47].

Socioeconomic factors and education were among the identified facilitators of vaccine uptake [43], in addition to factors such as country of origin and time of residence as predictors of uptake in migrant populations [47]. Routine school-based vaccination and free-of-charge vaccination were also identified as providing equitable delivery, yet needing to be complemented with information campaigns designed to optimize the uptake of the HPV vaccine by reducing disparities in some socio-economic disadvantaged sub-groups with lower vaccine uptake [45,51]. A nationwide cohort study in Sweden, for example, compared three delivery modes of the vaccine and concluded that free-of-charge school-based HPV vaccination was the most effective and equitable delivery mode, including high-risk groups for cervical cancer [45].

A qualitative Swedish study among parents who did not consent to their daughters receiving the HPV vaccination showed that parents went through a complex decision process, in an equation of the perceived risks and benefits of the vaccine, leading to the choice to vaccinate, or not to. Reasons for HPV vaccination refusal relate to the belief that it was better for the daughter's health and well-being. Given the private and intimate nature of the HPV vaccination (perceived as a behavioral vaccine), some parents chose not to vaccinate based on the fact that the common good of herd immunity was of minor interest compared with the best interests of their daughter. Another key reason for declining HPV vaccination was the perceived absence of sufficient knowledge about HPV and the vaccine. Parents rated the information received from the school health system unsatisfactory and preferred to postpone vaccination. Levels of trust in vaccinations, healthcare providers, and governments also were found to affect the complex HPV vaccine decision process [43].

There were less data on vaccine affordability. A study among vulnerable women in Greece pointed out the need to increase access by way of enlarging insurance coverage and reviewing screening recommendations. Improved healthcare delivery systems, towards more direct patient care, reduced delayed care, and appropriate preventive health services, were highlighted to reduce non-financial barriers to vaccination [49].

Enabling factors identified, such as insurance coverage for HPV vaccination, echo the ability of the person to navigate the healthcare system and in obtaining social benefits. Interventions to increase uptake in catch-up age groups must safeguard that vaccine costs are included [26].

- Awareness and Acceptance

Lack of information/knowledge or perceived need were frequently cited barriers to vaccination [27,29,32,37,39,42,43,49,50]. One cross-sectional study among young adult women in Italy showed that participants with more concerns about the safety and efficacy of HPV vaccination were less likely to be vaccinated. Results seem to indicate the need for delivering accurate and clear information about vaccine efficacy and safety to boost HPV vaccination coverage [53]. An exploratory study in Poland on the knowledge about HPV infection and HPV-related cancers also found that the danger is poorly understood among men. The authors suggest that healthcare professionals need to broaden their knowledge about the specific health needs of underserved populations such as LGBTQ+ communities to prevent health disparities [50].

Table 2. Barriers and facilitators of vaccination uptake.

	Barriers	Facilitators
Access	• Demographic and socioeconomic status (Mollers et al., 2014; Riza et al., 2020; Schreiber et al., 2015; Spencer et al., 2014) [35,41,48,49] • Place of birth/origin (Navarro-Ilana et al., 2018; Riza et al., 2020; Schreiber et al., 2015) [48,49,52]	• Socioeconomic factors, background, education (Grandahl et al., 2017; Møller et al., 2018) [44,47] • Routine school-based vaccination and free-of-charge (Hansen et al., 2015; Wang et al., 2019) [45,51]
Affordability	• Lack of resources/insurance coverage (Riza et al., 2020) [49]	• Insurance coverage for HPV vaccination (Conroy et al., 2009) [26]
Awareness	• Lack of information/knowledge or perceived need (Craciun, Baban, 2012; Forster et al., 2015, 2017; Grandahl et al., 2014; Marlow et al., 2009; Pop, 2016; Reszka et al., 2021; Riza et al., 2020; Salad et al., 2015) [27,29,30,32,33,37,39,42,43,49,50]	• Supplying correct information on vaccine efficacy and safety (Restivo et al., 2018) [53]
Acceptance	• Public concerns over safety (Amdisen et al., 2018; Craciun, Baban, 2012; Forster et al., 2015, 2017; Grandahl et al., 2014; Marlow et al., 2008, 2009; Miko et al., 2019) [27,31,32,34,37,38,43,46] • Cultural, religious, and social barriers (i.e., Sex-related concerns) (Forster et al., 2017; Marlow et al., 2009; Salad et al., 2015) [29,33,42] • Mistrust in healthcare/government (Grandahl et al., 2014; Forster et al., 2017; Miko et al., 2019; Salad et al., 2015) [29,38,42,43] • Ethnicity and/or religion (Marlow et al., 2009; Mollers et al., 2014; Riza et al., 2020; Salad et al., 2015; Walsh et al., 2008) [28,32,41,42,49] • History of an abnormal Pap test (Conroy et al., 2009) [26]	• Past childhood vaccination uptake (Alberts et al., 2017) [40] • Advice from nurse or other healthcare professionals (Navarro-Ilana et al., 2018) [52] • Normative belief that one's parents, partners, and clinicians endorsed HPV vaccination (Conroy et al., 2009; Møller et al., 2018) [26,47]
Activation towards vaccination uptake	• Lack of information or practical support from health-care professionals (Craciun, Baban, 2012; Forster et al., 2015, 2017; Grandahl et al., 2014; Marlow et al., 2009) [27,29,30,37,43]	• Provider recommendation (Grandahl et al., 2014; Navarro-Ilana et al., 2018) [43,52] • Catch-up vaccination initiatives (school) (Hansen et al., 2015; Wang et al., 2019) [45,51] • Culturally tailored community-based interventions (Alberts et al., 2017; Forster et al., 2017; Marlow et al., 2009, Riza et al., 2020; Salad et al., 2015; Stearns et al. 2020) [29,32,36,40,42,49]

Mollers et al. found that vaccinated girls in the Netherlands were less likely to have a religious background, and amongst those who professed religion, vaccinated girls were more often Catholic while unvaccinated girls were more often Protestant Christian. Moreover, no differences were found in terms of sexual risk behavior and knowledge of HPV infection and transmission, while differences were found in contraceptive use, the number of lifetime sexual partners, and opinions on the use of condoms after HPV vaccination and the protection of vaccination against all HPV types [41].

A six-month follow-up study conducted in 2006 shortly after the HPV vaccine was licensed in England found that young women with a history of an abnormal Pap test were less likely to have received the vaccine. This fact was confirmed by others [51]. On the contrary, identified predicted factors for HPV vaccination included the belief that one's parents, partners, and clinicians recommended HPV vaccination [26].

A survey in Spain also pointed out that advice from the nurse and physician was the key factor in HPV vaccination [52]. This result adds to the understanding that social norms predict HPV vaccine intent and uptake [47].

Among the facilitators, the intention was a strong predictor of uptake, together with past childhood vaccination uptake. Furthermore, HPV vaccination intention and uptake are based on similar determinants in the different ethnic groups, meaning that interventions based on similar behavior change methods (e.g., psychological inoculation or peer modeling) could be designed with added actions to reach different ethnic populations [40].

- Activation towards vaccination uptake

Nurses and doctors lead the health processes of healthcare users, and the uptake of their recommendations [43,52]. Catch-up campaigns may improve immunization coverage with doctors' and trusted individuals' endorsements and promote vaccination as normative [47].

In the case of vulnerable populations, interventions to increase the prevention of cervical cancer, routine examination with the Pap test, and HPV vaccination need the healthcare delivery systems to be adapted accounting for cultural, social, and religious diversity [49]. Ethnic disparities in HPV vaccination may be understood in light of the levels of concern about the vaccine [29]. Interventions to increase immunization should be culturally tailored and community-based [29,33,40,42,49].

3.3. Attitudes and Beliefs about the HPV Vaccine

There are diverse health beliefs and objections to vaccination. Mollers et al. found that vaccinated and unvaccinated girls in the Netherlands were comparable in most sexual risk behaviors and had similar scores on knowledge of HPV infection and HPV transmission, but they differed for characteristics such as contraceptive use, the number of lifetime sexual partners, and their opinions on the use of condoms after HPV vaccination and the protection of vaccination against all HPV types. Sexually active vaccinated girls were more aware of the risk of HPV infection when engaging in unprotected sex [41].

Some studies mentioned the role of religious and cultural prohibitions on sex before marriage as a barrier to vaccination, related to low levels of awareness in some minority groups [35]. For some families, the HPV vaccination was not considered compatible with their life values. Building self-confidence in girls to delay sexual debut was chosen among other alternative methods of prevention [43].

Besides moral concerns, some studies indicate that there is a group of parents who consider that the vaccine is not necessary and/or serves the interest of the government or pharmaceutical companies. In this case, HPV vaccine decline is linked to the belief that vaccines are unnatural. Other reasons include the belief that vaccinations are used for population control [43]. A qualitative study in Romania points out that mothers' main reasons for not vaccinating their daughters are the belief that the vaccine represents an "experiment that uses their daughters as guinea pigs", the belief that the vaccine embodies a conspiracy theory to reduce the population, and mistrust in the health system [37].

4. Discussion

This study described barriers and facilitators of HPV vaccine uptake and identified determinants of under-immunization, reviewing data on European countries, where HPV vaccination has been gradually introduced in the national immunization programs since 2007. Given the chosen focus on health equity, these data are relevant to strengthening vaccination programs to promote vaccination for all people.

Health policies and practical implementation processes of HPV vaccination vary across European countries, as shown in Table 3, with information on HPV national immunization programs of the 10 countries covered in this review (Denmark, Greece, Italy, Netherlands,

Norway, Poland, Romania, Spain, Sweden, United Kingdom). In most countries, the HPV vaccine is administered in public health clinics, while countries such as Norway, Sweden, and the UK have established school vaccination programs, and Spain offers a combination of school and/or health centers depending on the region.

Four of the analyzed countries (Italy, the Netherlands, Norway, and Poland) recommended gender-neutral vaccination, i.e., vaccination in all girls/women and boys/men, and one (the United Kingdom) for men from specific subgroups (men who have sex with men). However, information concerning HPV vaccination coverage rates is missing in men, indicating the need for better surveillance [54,55].

Access to and acceptance of HPV vaccination are key factors influencing vaccine uptake, therefore requiring multilevel action. Access barriers were the country of origin related to the sociodemographic status, and cultural beliefs [52]. Local delivery of HPV vaccination and organizational factors are central to reducing cervical cancer inequities [35], such as the role of school nurses in increasing HPV vaccine uptake among vulnerable groups [56].

A recent study that reviewed HPV vaccination coverage in 31 European countries has concluded that structured vaccination programs targeting females early in adolescence and free-of-charge vaccine administration were more frequently observed in countries with high vaccination coverage rates. Facilitating access to HPV vaccination by increasing onsite vaccine availability, sending invitations and reminders to attend for vaccination, and relying on schools as the main setting to administer the vaccine could also be important factors to achieve higher vaccine uptake [54].

The findings of this review have shown that besides HPV vaccination policies and practical implementation, HPV vaccination is also influenced by sociocultural factors and individual characteristics.

Religion has been shown to influence the vaccination decision-making process with certain religious or ideological groups being linked to anti-vaccination movements and outbreaks of vaccine-preventable diseases [57]. Some parents perceived their daughters to be too young to be vaccinated and to be sexually active. A more flexible vaccination schedule with the option of offering vaccinations later and providing more adequate and comprehensive explanations about the virus and the vaccine could be strategies to improve vaccine uptake [43].

Interventions aimed at increasing HPV vaccine coverage should be focused on raising health professionals' HPV awareness to better inform patients about HPV infection and vaccination [52]. The dissemination of culturally adapted and unbiased information, together with the opportunity to talk about the vaccine with healthcare professionals, could contribute to trust in public government recommendations and increase vaccine coverage [43]. As the COVID-19 pandemic has revealed, the success of public health campaigns relies on trust in leaders, experts, and medical professionals, however social determinants like race, class, and gender influence vaccines attitudes and beliefs, on the one hand, and also the state, on the other, because interactions with the state are multifaceted, bureaucratic, and can be coercive. Further investigation on attitudes toward immunization among marginalized populations is needed to identify alternative practices from dominant narratives that could better inform inclusive public health outreach [58].

Table 3. Status of HPV national immunization programs in the 10 EU/EEA countries under analysis (Denmark, Greece, Italy, Netherlands, Norway, Poland, Romania, Spain, Sweden, United Kingdom).

Country	Year of Introduction	Age Targets for Vaccination in Years (Female, Male)				Delivery	HPV Vaccination Coverage Rate (Most Recent Year)	HPV Vaccine Funding
		Primary		Catch-Up				
		Female	Male	Female	Male			
Denmark	2009	12		<18		Health Council	F-58% (2019)	Full

From 1 January 2014 to 21 December 2015, any girl or woman born between 1993 and 1997 was eligible for HPV vaccination. From 1 February to 31 December 2018, boys aged 15 to 20 who are attracted to boys could receive free HPV vaccination. From 2019, both boys and girls in Denmark are eligible for HPV vaccination.

Country	Year	Female	Male	Female	Male	Delivery	Coverage	Funding
Greece	2008	11–18		11–14 (2nd) 15–18 (3rd)		Health Council	No data available	Full (Partial for boys *)

HPV vaccination is provided free of charge to girls aged 11–18, as a 2-dose scheme for those aged 11–14, and as a 3-dose scheme for those aged 15–18. * It is also provided at no cost to boys aged 11 to 18 who are members of high-risk populations, such as those who are immunocompromised.

Country	Year	Female	Male	Female	Male	Delivery	Coverage	Funding
Italy	2008	11–12	11–12 (from 2015, some regions)	Differs by region	-	Health Council	F-50% M-5% (2017)	Full

In all Italian regions, girls up to the age of 12 are offered free HPV vaccination. Some regions have extended the vaccination offer to girls of other ages. Some areas also provide free HPV vaccination to people living with HIV. Most regions also consider a lower payment for ages that are not included in the primary target. Male vaccination became free in six regions in 2015.

Country	Year	Female	Male	Female	Male	Delivery	Coverage	Funding
Netherlands	2009	12–13 (until 2021) 10 (from 2022)	10 (from 2022)	-	-	Health Council	F-46% (2019)	Full

An HPV vaccination catch-up campaign was organized in 2009 for girls born between 1993–1996 (13–16 years old then). Since 2010, 12-year-old girls born in 1997 or later were eligible to receive the HPV vaccination as part of the National Immunization Programme. Since 2021, boys are offered the vaccination as well and in 2022 vaccination for children can be taken at the age of 10. To give boys the opportunity to protect themselves against HPV, a catch-up campaign took place 2022 which will continue in 2023 too. Boys born in 2004, 2006, 2008, 2009 and 2012 received an invitation, and girls from these years who had not yet been vaccinated against HPV. Adolescents born in 2005, 2007, 2010, 2011 and 2013 will be invited starting 2023. The vaccination is free and voluntary.

Country	Year	Female	Male	Female	Male	Delivery	Coverage	Funding
Norway	2009	12	12	≤25 (2016–2018)	-	School (7th grade)	F-88% (2018)	Full

Women born in 1991 or later have been offered free HPV vaccination for two years, beginning on November 1, 2016. As part of the childhood immunization program, the government provided HPV vaccine to all 7th-grade boys in the 2018–2019 school year.

Table 3. Cont.

Country	Year of Introduction	Age Targets for Vaccination in Years (Female, Male)				Delivery	HPV Vaccination Coverage Rate (Most Recent Year)	HPV Vaccine Funding
		Primary		Catch-Up				
		Female	Male	Female	Male			
Poland	No data available—absence of a national program	11–12	-	-	-	No data available	No data available	None

HPV vaccination has been recommended in the national immunization program for girls aged 11 to 12 years since 2008. The expert committee, formed in 2010 at the initiative of the Polish Pediatric Society, also recommended HPV vaccines for girls aged 13 to 18 who had not previously been vaccinated. This vaccination was not included in Poland's mandatory immunization program. Due to the additional cost of prophylactic HPV vaccination in primary healthcare centers, the coverage of Polish teenagers vaccinated against HPV is said to be between 7.5% and 10%. Some districts have decided to fund prophylactic HPV vaccination programs.

Country	Year of Introduction	Primary Female	Primary Male	Catch-Up Female	Catch-Up Male	Delivery	Coverage Rate	Funding
Romania	2013	11–14	-	-	-	Health Council	No data available	Full

The Romanian Ministry of Health launched a school-based immunization campaign in 2008, offering free HPV vaccination to girls aged 10–11. Only 2.6% of the girls were vaccinated, hence the program was terminated. An information campaign was launched in 2009, followed by a second vaccination program aimed at 12–14-year-old girls. A catch-up program was also offered, in which adult women could get the vaccine for free through their healthcare provider. Despite the vaccine's availability, uptake remained low, and the school-based program was terminated at the end of 2011. In April 2013, the program was relaunched for the third time. HPV vaccination is included in the National Vaccination Programme under the category 'Vaccination of Population at Risk,' and is intended for girls aged 11 to 14. The National Health System does not fund the program.

Country	Year of Introduction	Primary Female	Primary Male	Catch-Up Female	Catch-Up Male	Delivery	Coverage Rate	Funding
Spain	2007-8	12	-	-	-	School and/or health center (depending on the region)	F-73% F-85% (2018)	Full

In 2007, the Inter-Territorial Council of the National Health System, the coordination body for the various health services approved a recommendation to begin routine HPV vaccination in Spain. To vaccinate a cohort of girls aged 11 to 14, with a preference for age 14, and a deadline for implementation in 2010. Following that, each autonomous community developed its implementation plan, with the first three communities launching in 2007, and the rest following in 2008. Since 2015, as agreed by the Interterritorial Council, HPV vaccination is recommended for girls aged 12 in all regions. Since 2018, HPV vaccination has also been recommended for the following risk groups: those with warts, hypogammaglobulinemia, immunodeficiency, and myelokathexis (WHIM) syndrome (a primary immunodeficiency); women with solid organ and hematopoietic transplants up to the age of 26; people living with HIV (with a 3-dose schedule and up to the age of 26); sex workers up to the age of 26 (3-dose schedule). Since 2019, females up to the age of 18 have received catch-up vaccination.

Country	Year of Introduction	Primary Female	Primary Male	Catch-Up Female	Catch-Up Male	Delivery	Coverage Rate	Funding
Sweden	2012	10–12	-	<18	-	School (5–6th grades)	F-84% (2019)	Full

In 2010, the HPV vaccine was included in a free national vaccination program for girls born in 1999 or later who are in the fifth or sixth grade. However, due to procurement delays, vaccinations did not begin until 2012. During the same period, all counties provided free catch-up vaccinations to girls between 1993 and 1998. According to a child vaccination regulation update (HSLF-FS 2016:51), all girls should now be offered HPV vaccinations up to the age of 18. The vaccination will soon be available to boys as well (starting from those born in 2009).

Table 3. *Cont.*

Country	Year of Introduction	Age Targets for Vaccination in Years (Female, Male)				Delivery	HPV Vaccination Coverage Rate (Most Recent Year)	HPV Vaccine Funding
		Primary		Catch-Up				
		Female	Male	Female	Male			
United Kingdom	2008-12	11–13	No data available	<18	No data available	School (8–10th grades) Health Council (catch-up)	F-84% (2019)	Full

Vaccination programs, along with the year they begin, differ slightly by region. Girls who missed their first HPV vaccination can get a catch-up vaccination up to the age of 18. There was a catch-up period at the beginning of the program for girls born between 1991 and 1995. As of 2019, the United Kingdom has made HPV vaccination available to both boys and girls.

Source: European Centre for Disease Prevention and Control. Guidance on HPV vaccination in EU countries: focus on boys, people living with HIV and 9-valent HPV vaccine introduction, 2020. Stockholm: ECDC; 2020. Authors compilation.

4.1. Strengths and Limitations of the Research

The results of this review should be interpreted in light of its limitations. First, only two different databases were consulted for locating papers with no additional search strategy, such as searching references of the included papers or references of literature reviews identified during the screening process. This may have limited the inclusion of more articles from the social sciences field, although Scopus is among the largest databases, with a wide global and regional coverage of scientific journals. A strong point, nevertheless, is that the search strategy was comprehensive and followed the recommendations made by the Joanna Briggs Institute (JBI) [25], such as the Population/Concept/Context method, to identify the main concepts and the definition of inclusion criteria.

The second limitation is that only the studies conducted in European countries were included in this review, with no inclusion of comparisons with other contexts for a broader mapping of the state of the art regarding the attitudes and practices towards HPV vaccination and its social processes. Given the great variability in terms of the social, cultural, and institutional vaccine contexts and national vaccination programs, efforts were made to add more knowledge about the European contexts, that were less investigated, to better identify tailored and evidence-informed strategies.

Finally, all articles, independently of the study design or quality, were included to jointly present findings, which may also be considered a limitation. However, this review aimed to summarize the scientific evidence regarding the barriers and facilitators with a focus on health equity; therefore, all identified articles were included to facilitate the overview of the key factors influencing vaccine uptake.

4.2. Recommendations for Research and Action

This review is not representative of the European region, considering that included studies came from only ten countries, largely focusing on Western Europe. Given that all EU/EEA countries have introduced HPV vaccination in their national programs, and many countries have recently changed or are changing to a gender-neutral HPV vaccination [59], there is a need for more data on HPV vaccination with disaggregated data for diversity, which is rarely collected by national data. Monitoring HPV vaccination uptake and policies at a European level, as well as sharing experiences between countries, could contribute to the success of HPV vaccination programs and address health inequities [54].

Certain subpopulations were not well reported and did not reflect on how different intersecting identities place people at multiple disadvantages, such as LGBT people, different migrant and ethnic minorities, and several other vulnerable and most at-risk-identified populations. This indicates a need for HPV vaccine uptake datasets in Europe that disaggregate by diversity to monitor HPV vaccination inequalities. Sub-analyses on vulnerable populations could be conducted with disaggregated data from general population studies.

Joining vaccination strategies with other recommended healthcare services for populations burdened by HPV infection and HPV-related diseases, such as LGBT people, could increase vaccination in these populations where HPV vaccine acceptability tends to be high [9].

Action plans to address specific perceptions and barriers towards HPV vaccination should be co-designed with the most at-risk-identified populations and inclusive catch-up initiatives could be considered drawing on new models of good practice in vaccine delivery employed during the COVID-19 pandemic [23].

Author Contributions: Conceptualization, V.A.; methodology, V.A.; analysis, V.A. and B.Z.; writing—original draft preparation, V.A.; writing—review and editing, V.A. and B.Z. All authors have read and agreed to the published version of the manuscript.

Funding: This research received no external funding.

Institutional Review Board Statement: Not applicable.

Informed Consent Statement: Not applicable.

Data Availability Statement: Not applicable.

Conflicts of Interest: The authors declare no conflict of interest.

References

1. Bruni, L.; Saura-Lázaro, A.; Montoliu, A.; Brotons, M.; Alemany, L.; Diallo, M.S.; Afsar, O.Z.; LaMontagne, D.S.; Mosina, L.; Contreras, M.; et al. HPV vaccination introduction worldwide and WHO and UNICEF estimates of national HPV immunization coverage 2010–2019. *Prev. Med. (Baltim)* **2021**, *144*, 106399. [CrossRef] [PubMed]
2. World Health Organization. *Global Strategy to Accelerate the Elimination of Cervical Cancer as a Public Health Problem*; World Health Organization: Geneva, Switzerland, 2020.
3. Carpenter, L.M.; Casper, M.J. A tale of two technologies: HPV vaccination, male circumcision, and sexual health. *Gend. Soc.* **2009**, *23*, 790–816. [CrossRef]
4. Casper, M.J.; Carpenter, L.M. Sex, drugs, and politics: The HPV vaccine for cervical cancer. *Sociol. Health Illn.* **2008**, *30*, 886–899. [CrossRef] [PubMed]
5. Bozhar, H.; McKee, M.; Spadea, T.; Veerus, P.; Heinävaara, S.; Anttila, A.; Senore, C.; Zielonke, N.; de Kok, I.M.C.M.; van Ravesteyn, N.T.; et al. Socio-economic inequality of utilization of cancer testing in Europe: A cross-sectional study. *Prev. Med. Rep.* **2022**, *26*, 101733. [CrossRef]
6. Perehudoff, K.; Vermandere, H.; Williams, A.; Bautista-Arredondo, S.; de Paepe, E.; Dias, S.; Gama, A.; Keygnaert, I.; Longatto-Filho, A.; Ortiz, J.; et al. Universal cervical cancer control through a right to health lens: Refocusing national policy and programmes on underserved women. *BMC Int. Health Hum. Rights* **2020**, *20*, 21. [CrossRef]
7. Logel, M.; Laurie, C.; El-Zein, M.; Guichon, J.; Franco, E.L. A Review of Ethical and Legal Aspects of Gender-Neutral Human Papillomavirus Vaccination. *Cancer Epidemiol. Biomarkers Prev.* **2022**, *31*, 919–931. [CrossRef]
8. Siu, J.Y.M.; Fung, T.K.F.; Leung, L.H.M. Social and cultural construction processes involved in HPV vaccine hesitancy among Chinese women: A qualitative study. *Int. J. Equity Health* **2019**, *18*, 1–18. [CrossRef]
9. Meites, E.; Wilkin, T.J.; Markowitz, L.E. Review of human papillomavirus (HPV) burden and HPV vaccination for gay, bisexual, and other men who have sex with men and transgender women in the United States. *Hum. Vaccin. Immunother.* **2022**, *18*, 2016007. [CrossRef]
10. Karafillakis, E.; Simas, C.; Jarrett, C.; Verger, P.; Peretti-Watel, P.; Dib, F.; de Angelis, S.; Takacs, J.; Ali, K.A.; Celentano, L.P.; et al. HPV vaccination in a context of public mistrust and uncertainty: A systematic literature review of determinants of HPV vaccine hesitancy in Europe. *Hum. Vaccin. Immunother.* **2019**, *15*, 1615–1627. [CrossRef]
11. Clarke, A.E.; Shim, J.K.; Mamo, L.; Fosket, J.R.; Fishman, J.R. Biomedicalization: Technoscientific Transformations of Health, Illness, and U.S. Biomedicine. *Am. Sociol. Rev.* **2003**, *68*, 161–194. [CrossRef]
12. Giami, A.; Perrey, C. Transformations in the medicalization of sex: HIV prevention between discipline and biopolitics. *J. Sex Res.* **2012**, *49*, 353–361. [CrossRef] [PubMed]
13. Conrad, P. The Shifting Engines of Medicalization. *J. Health Soc. Behav.* **2005**, *46*, 3–14. [CrossRef] [PubMed]
14. Reich, J.A. Vaccine Refusal and Pharmaceutical Acquiescence: Parental Control and Ambivalence in Managing Children's Health. *Am. Sociol. Rev.* **2020**, *85*, 106–127. [CrossRef]
15. Mamo, L.; Pérez, A.E.; Rios, L. Human papillomavirus self-sampling: A tool in cancer prevention and sexual health promotion. *Sociol. Health Illn.* **2022**, *44*, 218–235. [CrossRef] [PubMed]
16. MacArthur, K.R. Beyond health beliefs: The role of trust in the HPV vaccine decision-making process among American college students. *Health Sociol. Rev.* **2017**, *26*, 321–338. [CrossRef]
17. Harrington, N.; Chen, Y.; O'Reilly, A.M.; Fang, C.Y. The role of trust in HPV vaccine uptake among racial and ethnic minorities in the United States: A narrative review. *AIMS Public Health* **2021**, *8*, 352–368. [CrossRef] [PubMed]
18. Caso, D.; Carfora, V.; Starace, C.; Conner, M. Key Factors Influencing Italian Mothers' Intention to Vaccinate Sons against HPV: The Influence of Trust in Health Authorities, Anticipated Regret and Past Behaviour. *Sustainability* **2019**, *11*, 6879. [CrossRef]
19. Cooper, D.L.; Hernandez, N.D.; Rollins, L.; Akintobi, T.H.; McAllister, C. HPV vaccine awareness and the association of trust in cancer information from physicians among males. *Vaccine* **2017**, *35*, 2661–2667. [CrossRef]
20. Fenton, A.T.; Elliott, M.N.; Schwebel, D.C.; Berkowitz, Z.; Liddon, N.C.; Tortolero, S.R.; Cuccaro, P.M.; Davies, S.L.; Schuster, M.A. Unequal interactions: Examining the role of patient-centered care in reducing inequitable diffusion of a medical innovation, the human papillomavirus (HPV) vaccine. *Soc. Sci. Med.* **2018**, *200*, 238–248. [CrossRef]
21. Holman, D.M.; Benard, V.; Roland, K.B.; Watson, M.; Liddon, N.; Stokley, S. Barriers to human papillomavirus vaccination among US adolescents: A systematic review of the literature. *JAMA Pediatr.* **2014**, *168*, 76–82. [CrossRef]
22. Thomson, A.; Robinson, K.; Vallée-Tourangeau, G. The 5As: A practical taxonomy for the determinants of vaccine uptake. *Vaccine* **2016**, *34*, 1018–1024. [CrossRef]
23. Crawshaw, A.F.; Farah, Y.; Deal, A.; Rustage, K.; Hayward, S.E.; Carter, J.; Knights, F.; Goldsmith, L.P.; Campos-Matos, I.; Wurie, F.; et al. Defining the determinants of vaccine uptake and undervaccination in migrant populations in Europe to improve routine and COVID-19 vaccine uptake: A systematic review. *Lancet Infect. Dis.* **2022**, *22*, e254–e266. [CrossRef]

24. Tricco, A.C.; Lillie, E.; Zarin, W.; O'Brien, K.K.; Colquhoun, H.; Levac, D.; Moher, D.; Peters, M.D.J.; Horsley, T.; Weeks, L.; et al. PRISMA Extension for Scoping Reviews (PRISMA-ScR): Checklist and Explanation. *Ann. Intern. Med.* **2018**, *169*, 467–473. [CrossRef] [PubMed]
25. Peters, M.D.J.; Marnie, C.; Tricco, A.C.; Pollock, D.; Munn, Z.; Alexander, L.; McInerney, P.; Godfrey, C.M.; Khalil, H. Updated methodological guidance for the conduct of scoping reviews. *JBI Evid. Implement.* **2021**, *19*, 3–10. [CrossRef] [PubMed]
26. Conroy, K.; Rosenthal, S.L.; Zimet, G.D.; Jin, Y.; Bernstein, D.I.; Glynn, S.; Kahn, J.A. Human papillomavirus vaccine uptake, predictors of vaccination, and selfreported barriers to vaccination. *J. Womens. Health (Larchmt)* **2009**, *18*, 1679–1686. [CrossRef] [PubMed]
27. Forster, A.S.; Waller, J.; Bowyer, H.L.; Marlow, L.A.V. Girls' explanations for being unvaccinated or under vaccinated against human papillomavirus: A content analysis of survey responses. *BMC Public Health* **2015**, *15*, 1278. [CrossRef] [PubMed]
28. Walsh, C.D.; Gera, A.; Shah, M.; Sharma, A.; Powell, J.E.; Wilson, S. Public knowledge and attitudes towards Human Papilloma Virus (HPV) vaccination. *BMC Public Health* **2008**, *8*, 368. [CrossRef] [PubMed]
29. Forster, A.S.; Rockliffe, L.; Marlow, L.A.V.; Bedford, H.; McBride, E.; Waller, J. Exploring human papillomavirus vaccination refusal among ethnic minorities in England: A comparative qualitative study. *Psychooncology* **2017**, *26*, 1278–1284. [CrossRef]
30. Marlow, L.A.V.; Waller, J.; Evans, R.E.C.; Wardle, J. Predictors of interest in HPV vaccination: A study of British adolescents. *Vaccine* **2009**, *27*, 2483–2488. [CrossRef]
31. Marlow, L.A.V.; Waller, J.; Wardle, J. Sociodemographic predictors of HPV testing and vaccination acceptability: Results from a population-representative sample of British women. *J. Med. Screen.* **2008**, *15*, 91–96. [CrossRef] [PubMed]
32. Marlow, L.A.V.; Wardle, J.; Forster, A.S.; Waller, J. Ethnic differences in human papillomavirus awareness and vaccine acceptability. *J. Epidemiol. Community Health* **2009**, *63*, 1010–1015. [CrossRef] [PubMed]
33. Marlow, L.A.V.; Wardle, J.; Waller, J. Attitudes to HPV vaccination among ethnic minority mothers in the UK: An exploratory qualitative study. *Hum. Vaccin.* **2009**, *5*, 105–110. [CrossRef] [PubMed]
34. Rockliffe, L.; Waller, J.; Marlow, L.A.V.; Forster, A.S. Role of ethnicity in human papillomavirus vaccination uptake: A cross-sectional study of girls from ethnic minority groups attending London schools. *BMJ Open* **2017**, *7*, e014527. [CrossRef] [PubMed]
35. Spencer, A.M.; Roberts, S.A.; Brabin, L.; Patnick, J.; Verma, A. Sociodemographic factors predicting mother's cervical screening and daughter's HPV vaccination uptake. *J. Epidemiol. Community Health* **2014**, *68*, 571–577. [CrossRef] [PubMed]
36. Stearns, S.; Quaife, S.L.; Forster, A. Examining Facilitators of HPV Vaccination Uptake in Men Who Have Sex with Men: A Cross-Sectional Survey Design. *Int. J. Environ. Res. Public Health* **2020**, *17*, 7713. [CrossRef] [PubMed]
37. Craciun, C.; Baban, A. Who will take the blame?': Understanding the reasons why Romanian mothers decline HPV vaccination for their daughters. *Vaccine* **2012**, *30*, 6789–6793. [CrossRef] [PubMed]
38. Miko, D.; Costache, C.; Colosi, H.A.; Neculicioiu, V.; Colosi, I.A. Qualitative Assessment of Vaccine Hesitancy in Romania. *Medicina (Kaunas)* **2019**, *55*, 282. [CrossRef] [PubMed]
39. Pop, C.A. Locating Purity within Corruption Rumors: Narratives of HPV Vaccination Refusal in a Peri-urban Community of Southern Romania. *Med. Anthropol. Q.* **2016**, *30*, 563–581. [CrossRef] [PubMed]
40. Alberts, C.J.; van der Loeff, M.F.S.; Hazeveld, Y.; de Melker, H.E.; van der Wal, M.F.; Nielen, A.; el Fakiri, F.; Prins, M.; Paulussen, T.G.W.M. A longitudinal study on determinants of HPV vaccination uptake in parents/guardians from different ethnic backgrounds in Amsterdam, the Netherlands. *BMC Public Health* **2017**, *17*, 220. [CrossRef] [PubMed]
41. Mollers, M.; Lubbers, K.; Spoelstra, S.K.; Weijmar-Schultz, W.C.M.; Daemen, T.; Westra, T.A.; van der Sande, M.A.B.; Nijman, H.W.; de Melker, H.E.; Tami, A. Equity in human papilloma virus vaccination uptake?: Sexual behaviour, knowledge and demographics in a cross-sectional study in (un)vaccinated girls in the Netherlands. *BMC Public Health* **2014**, *14*, 288. [CrossRef] [PubMed]
42. Salad, J.; Verdonk, P.; de Boer, F.; Abma, T.A. A Somali girl is Muslim and does not have premarital sex. Is vaccination really necessary?' A qualitative study into the perceptions of Somali women in the Netherlands about the prevention of cervical cancer. *Int. J. Equity Health* **2015**, *14*, 68. [CrossRef] [PubMed]
43. Grandahl, M.; Oscarsson, M.; Stenhammar, C.; Nevéus, T.; Westerling, R.; Tydén, T. Not the right time: Why parents refuse to let their daughters have the human papillomavirus vaccination. *Acta Paediatr.* **2014**, *103*, 436–441. [CrossRef] [PubMed]
44. Grandahl, M.; Larsson, M.; Dalianis, T.; Stenhammar, C.; Tydén, T.; Westerling, R.; Nevéus, T. Catch-up HPV vaccination status of adolescents in relation to socioeconomic factors, individual beliefs and sexual behaviour. *PLoS ONE* **2017**, *12*, e0187193. [CrossRef] [PubMed]
45. Wang, J.; Ploner, A.; Sparén, P.; Lepp, T.; Roth, A.; Arnheim-Dahlström, L.; Sundström, K. Mode of HPV vaccination delivery and equity in vaccine uptake: A nationwide cohort study. *Prev. Med. (Baltim)* **2019**, *120*, 26–33. [CrossRef]
46. Amdisen, L.; Kristensen, M.L.; Rytter, D.; Mølbak, K.; Valentiner-Branth, P. Identification of determinants associated with uptake of the first dose of the human papillomavirus vaccine in Denmark. *Vaccine* **2018**, *36*, 5747–5753. [CrossRef] [PubMed]
47. Møller, S.P.; Kristiansen, M.; Norredam, M. Human papillomavirus immunization uptake among girls with a refugee background compared with Danish-born girls: A national register-based cohort study. *Eur. J. Cancer Prev. Off. J. Eur. Cancer Prev. Organ.* **2018**, *27*, 42–45. [CrossRef] [PubMed]
48. Schreiber, S.M.S.; Juul, K.E.; Dehlendorff, C.; Kjær, S.K. Socioeconomic predictors of human papillomavirus vaccination among girls in the Danish childhood immunization program. *J. Adolesc. Health Off. Publ. Soc. Adolesc. Med.* **2015**, *56*, 402–407. [CrossRef] [PubMed]

49. Riza, E.; Karakosta, A.; Tsiampalis, T.; Lazarou, D.; Karachaliou, A.; Ntelis, S.; Karageorgiou, V.; Psaltopoulou, T. Knowledge, Attitudes and Perceptions about Cervical Cancer Risk, Prevention and Human Papilloma Virus (HPV) in Vulnerable Women in Greece. *Int. J. Environ. Res. Public Health* **2020**, *17*, 6892. [CrossRef] [PubMed]
50. Reszka, K.; Moskal, Ł.; Remiorz, A.; Walas, A.; Szewczyk, K.; Staszek-Szewczyk, U. Should men be exempted from vaccination against human papillomavirus? Health disparities regarding HPV: The example of sexual mi-norities in Poland. *J. Prev. Med. Hyg.* **2021**, *62*, E386–E391. [CrossRef] [PubMed]
51. Hansen, B.T.; Campbell, S.; Burger, E.; Nygård, M. Correlates of HPV vaccine uptake in school-based routine vaccination of preadolescent girls in Norway: A register-based study of 90,000 girls and their parents. *Prev. Med. (Baltim)* **2015**, *77*, 4–10. [CrossRef] [PubMed]
52. Navarro-Illana, P.; Navarro-Illana, E.; Vila-Candel, R.; Díez-Domingo, J. Drivers for human papillomavirus vaccination in Valencia (Spain). *Gac. Sanit.* **2018**, *32*, 454–458. [CrossRef] [PubMed]
53. Restivo, V.; Costantino, C.; Fazio, T.F.; Casuccio, N.; D'Angelo, C.; Vitale, F.; Casuccio, A. Factors Associated with HPV Vaccine Refusal among Young Adult Women after Ten Years of Vaccine Implementation. *Int. J. Environ. Res. Public Health* **2018**, *15*, 770. [CrossRef] [PubMed]
54. Nguyen-Huu, N.; Thilly, N.; Derrough, T.; Sdona, E.; Claudot, F.; Pulcini, C.; Agrinier, N. Human papillomavirus vaccination coverage, policies, and practical implementation across Europe. *Vaccine* **2020**, *38*, 1315–1331. [CrossRef] [PubMed]
55. Bonanni, P.; Faivre, P.; Lopalco, P.L.; Joura, E.A.; Bergroth, T.; Varga, S.; Gemayel, N.; Drury, R. The status of human papillomavirus vaccination recommendation, funding, and coverage in WHO Europe countries (2018–2019). *Expert Rev. Vaccines* **2020**, *19*, 1073–1083. [CrossRef]
56. Boyce, T.; Holmes, A.H. Persistence and partnerships: School nurses, inequalities and the HPV vaccination programme. *Br. J. Sch. Nurs.* **2013**, *8*, 71–77. [CrossRef]
57. Fournet, N.; Mollema, L.; Ruijs, W.L.; Harmsen, I.A.; Keck, F.; Durand, J.Y.; Cunha, M.P.; Wamsiedel, M.; Reis, R.; French, J.; et al. Under-vaccinated groups in Europe and their beliefs, attitudes and reasons for non-vaccination; two systematic reviews. *BMC Public Health* **2018**, *18*, 196. [CrossRef]
58. Thornton, C.; Reich, J.A. Black Mothers and Vaccine Refusal: Gendered Racism, Healthcare, and the State. *Gend. Soc.* **2022**, *36*, 525–551. [CrossRef]
59. Colzani, E.; Johansen, K.; Johnson, H.; Celentano, L.P. Human papillomavirus vaccination in the European Union/European Economic Area and globally: A moral dilemma. *Euro Surveill. Bull. Eur. Sur Les Mal. Transm. Eur. Commun. Dis. Bull.* **2021**, *26*, 2001659. [CrossRef]

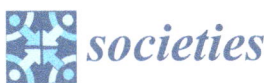

Concept Paper

Medicalization of Sexuality and Trans Situations: Evolutions and Transformations

Alain Giami

INSERM–CESP–Hôpital de Villejuif, 94807 Villejuif Cedex, France; alain.giami@inserm.fr

Abstract: This article explores the evolution of the definition and the process of medicalization of sexuality during the second half of the 20th century. After a review and discussion of the notion of medicalization, the application of this notion to a few examples is discussed, including the emergence of sexuality, the demedicalization of homosexuality, the treatment of "sexual disorders", the prevention of HIV infection, and the gender-affirmation pathways for transgender and gender diverse (TGD) people. The analysis of these situations—in the light of the notion of medicalization—allows us to better understand the multiple facets of this notion. In particular, we observe processes of medicalization and demedicalization, depathologization, and pharmacologization. The notion of medicalization of sexuality appears here as a useful concept for understanding the conceptualization and treatment of diversities in the field of sexuality and gender.

Keywords: medicalization; sexuality; social control; pharmacologization

Citation: Giami, A. Medicalization of Sexuality and Trans Situations: Evolutions and Transformations. *Societies* **2023**, *13*, 3. https://doi.org/10.3390/soc13010003

Academic Editors: Violeta Alarcão, Sónia Cardoso Pintassilgo and Dwai Banerjee

Received: 5 July 2022
Revised: 22 November 2022
Accepted: 6 December 2022
Published: 22 December 2022

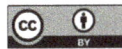

Copyright: © 2022 by the author. Licensee MDPI, Basel, Switzerland. This article is an open access article distributed under the terms and conditions of the Creative Commons Attribution (CC BY) license (https:// creativecommons.org/licenses/by/ 4.0/).

1. Introduction

Since the release in 1998 of new pharmacological treatments for male erectile dysfunction, and, more recently, the release of some pharmacological treatments for women's sexual problems and disorders, there has been a renewal and reformulation of the issues and controversies regarding the medicalization of sexuality. The questions raised by the "medicalization of sexuality" lead to a renewal of the general questions about the medicalization of society in general, which has already been conceptualized in the work of Conrad [1] and others who have developed other notions, such as "biomedicalization" [2]. As historian Olivier Faure has already noted, "the term medicalization refers to multiple realities, has different origins and gives rise to opposing interpretations. Much more than an object of consensus, the notion of medicalization is an inexhaustible source of debate among historians, which makes it rich, but also ambiguous" [3]. The situation observed by Faure with regard to historians applies perfectly to sociology, anthropology, and science and technology studies (STS) in which this work is situated.

Attitudes towards the issue of the so-called medicalization of sexuality are not univocal. Depending on the professional position, the personal conceptions, and the professional interests that one defends and tries to promote, the question of medicalization is not approached in the same way. Everyone may consider the legitimacy of the use of this concept differently, the positive aspects or, conversely, the negative or problematic aspects. The different evaluations of the dimensions and values associated with the processes of medicalization vary also according to the objects under study: male and female 'sexual disorders', HIV prevention techniques, and treatments aimed at facilitating the gender affirmation process for transgender and gender diverse (TGD) people. These different evaluations and their possible designation as forms of "medicalization" of sexuality or gender issues vary according to the historical moments and the actors involved in these processes. In the examples that will be discussed in this work, violent controversies that opposed actors involved at different levels were observed, either, on the one hand, between different professional groups involved in a given situation, or, on the other, an opposition between differently positioned groups regarding a specific condition, i.e., medical doctors and groups of patients, users of care, and consumers. It is, therefore, the understanding and discussion of the fundamentally controversial nature of medicalization processes that makes them interesting and that will be the central focus of the present work.

2. Materials and Methods

The reflection carried out in this article on the question of the medicalization of sexuality has its origins works carried out by the author on the use of drugs to treat "sexual disorders" in men [4] and women [5], on the evolution of HIV prevention with the arrival of effective retroviral drugs [6], and on the questions of medicalization and depathologization of medical treatments concerning gender affirmation pathways [7]. This article proposes a theoretical and political reflection on the qualification of different situations as medicalization and the consequences that this designation entails on a practical and political level. It is based on research performed in Europe, North America, and Brazil.

3. State of the Art

The problem of the "medicalization of sexuality" is the subject of several controversies that oppose health professionals and health care users, sometimes organized into patient and consumer associations that play an increasingly important role in health and health care issues. The question concerns different objects and gives rise to contradictory views concerning the evolution of sexuality, the transformations that are undergoing under the influence of the pharmaceutical industry and medicine, the coherence and even the ethics of professional interventions, and, last but not least, the participation of consumers' and patients' associations.

The use of the term "medicalization" in current debates and controversies about sexuality is, thus, embedded in the social world, and these debates are embedded on the different representations of sexuality and gender held by different groups with different professional and ideological views and objectives. The examples discussed in this paper demonstrate that the actors currently involved in social and political debates about sexuality use the same term "medicalization" with different meanings and representations. The use of this term in the social world is, therefore, different from that observed in the academic world, particularly in sociology and history. However, health professionals use some kind of common sense meaning of the term medicalization which may be somewhat different from its academic definitions. We can, therefore, speak of a "common sense" of the professionals. If there is a plurality of understandings of the professional common sense of medicalization, this is because it is (1) based on different representations of sexuality that refer to a plurality of professional or ideological objectives, as well as to personal subjective positions, and (2) related to the implications of medical and pharmacological treatments for the conditions that fall under the jurisdiction of these professions. Psychologists dealing with "sexual problems" and "impotence" will not have the same representation compared to urologists dealing with "erectile dysfunction" and will not use the same approaches, tools, techniques, and pharmaceutical products.

Thus, not only do these different representations of sexuality conveyed by professionals allow us to understand the dividing lines that have emerged in the debates on the medicalization of sexuality, but they also reveal the blind spots in each of these conceptions of medicalization. For example, there is rarely mention of the "medicalization of sexuality" in the context of HIV prevention, even though this field of activity involves both changes in sexual behavior and medicalized interventions of various kinds (prevention, recommendations, treatment, etc.) that are grounded on medical and public health knowledge, whereas the field of the disorders of sexual function is saturated with controversies around the medicalization of sexuality, including pros and cons. The field of treatment for gender affirmation is more often described and discussed as a process of "pathologization" and "de-pathologization" which excludes a critique of the concept of medicalization.

The study of "medicalization of sexuality", as a system of polarized representations, must be based on a socio-historical analysis of the field of sexuality and the care of which it is the object in the Western world. "Sexuality" is being understood here as the field of words and concepts that define and represent it. This is why, in the present work, even if our initial reflection on the medicalization of sexuality started in the field of 'sexual disorders', we considered it fundamental to test the ideas developed in this field in other areas that were not immediately analyzed from the angle of medicalization. The approach developed in this article is based on the work by the French sociologist Robert Castel (1933–2013) in which he considered that, in order to understand the contemporary mental health system, it was necessary to include "the whole range of practices and theories", starting from the practices of prison psychiatric hospitalization, to the prescription of psychotropic drugs, to the different psychotherapies, and to the practices of personal development and psycho-corporal approaches, which were very much in vogue at the beginning of the 1980s and were carried by an ideology of contestation of the "psy" system [8]. Castel demonstrated that a unifying logic was underlying all of these apparently opposed practices and discourses. The ambition and the aim of this paper are to describe the underlying and unifying logic of medicalization in those situations that are analyzed beyond apparent controversies. In this perspective, this work is different from the work published by Ortega and Zorzanelli, in which these authors discuss the fluidity and potential inaccuracy of this concept [9].

4. The Medicalization of Sexuality: Conceptual Approaches

The expression "medicalization of sexuality" tends to give some substance to the idea that there is an essence of sexuality outside the field of medicalization, and that medicalization would have distorted the very essence of "sexuality". However, an analysis of the history of sexuality since the middle of the 19th century shows that the destiny of sexuality has been inseparably linked to developments in science and medicine and to different medical and psychological approaches. In this perspective, to speak of "medicalization of sexuality" would almost be a pleonasm, insofar as the concept of sexuality appears in the register of physiology and medicine (outside of medicine, there is no "sexuality"). It would be also to ignore that the term "sexuality" is already in itself a historically dated representation of a set of phenomena designated under other terms in the course of history [10]. Michel Foucault has clearly shown how the term "flesh" was used in early Christian pastoral care to address the phenomena currently designated under the definition of sexuality, while referring to a different "experience" and *episteme* [11]. Medicalization then unfolded from the different "foci" of the medical disciplines, each one responsible in its own way for dealing with one of the problems posed by sexual conduct, whether conjugal or non-reproductive and "perverse". More recently, the French historian Alain Corbin has analyzed the phenomena of "sexual life" in the period between the middle of the eighteenth and the nineteenth centuries before the term "sexuality" appeared in the language of physiology and medicine in English and French languages. Corbin, thus, highlights another form of medical understanding of sexuality in which medicine appears to be responsible for a "just measure of pleasure", set aside from questions of procreation, and supports the idea of the necessity of a "moderate" sexual pleasure for the "harmony of couples" and the good health and well-being of individuals [12].

However, if we should take for granted that modern sexuality has indeed developed in a scientific and medical context, the term medicalization, as used by sociologists and historians who have been interested in this question, allows us to understand the genesis and the social, political, and psychological implications that have presided over the elaboration of medical representations of sexuality. Georges Lanteri Laura has approached this question from the angle of "the medical appropriation of sexuality", highlighting that the implantation of sexuality in the field of medicine is the result of a historical process based on the pre-constructions operated by the dominant ideology and the penalization of certain behavior (male homosexuality constituted the paradigm of these approaches) [13]. Thomas Szasz has shown, from the example of masturbation, how the medicalization of sexuality has consisted in a progressive appropriation by medicine of behavior and personalities previously treated by religion or by justice [14]. Arnold Davidson has developed the notion of a "style of reasoning" applied to psychiatry and medicine. The development of different and divergent representations of sexuality, elaborated according to the division of tasks between somatic medicine (such as urology and venereology) and psychiatry, makes it possible to explain how the question of sex inscribed in the body has been transferred to that of the personality and subjectivity of the perpetrators of deviant behavior [10].

Other sociologists, within the framework of sociology of deviance, have understood the process of medicalization in a dynamic form by situating the institution of medicine in relation to other institutions that play a central role in the social world and in the management of the body and behavior: the religious institution and the legal institution. In this perspective, the process of medicalization appears as the object and the result of a conflict between the medical institution and these other institutions, which has as its goal the designation of phenomena and the definition of legitimate response to them. Thinking about medicalization within the framework of sociology of deviance implies a decentering of the conceptions of medicine and its social role, of the conceptions of illness, and of the role and social status attributed to those living with an illness.

In this context, Peter Conrad has defined "medicalization as a process by which everyday life problems come to be defined as medical problems, most often in terms of diseases or disorders" [15]. From a sociohistorical perspective, Conrad and Schneider introduce the idea that medicalization is a form of designation that historically replaces other forms of designation of deviance established by other institutions of social regulation and control. They explain the processes by which Western society has transformed a number of conditions and behaviors "negatively condemned by society" into forms of disease [16]. The "unnatural acts" initially treated as sins in the religious context were transformed into crimes or offences in the judicial context, and then, more recently, into diseases to be treated in the medical register, before leaving the field of pathology and being constructed as a form of social identity and participation in a "community" [17]. Conrad and Schneider, thus, highlight a form of circulation, historically determined, of the processes of designation of deviance, which makes it possible to change the representations and meanings attributed to "deviant" behaviors, as well as the forms of social treatment that are intended for them. A profound transformation of the ideology and functioning of modern society has driven the way in which social behaviors are interpreted. Thomas Szasz has described the following in his work: "With the transformation of the religious conception of man into a scientific one—particularly through psychiatry—which developed systematically during the 19th century, there was a radical shift from the view of man as a responsible agent acting in and on the world to a reactive organism that is acted upon by biological and social 'forces'" [18].

The work of the North American sexologist Leonore Tiefer occupies a singular place insofar as she attempts to situate herself on a double slope as a conceptualizer of the notion of medicalization of sexuality and by engaging in critical debates from a position opposed to what she considers as an inappropriate form of medicalization of sexuality. Tiefer makes a double distinction. First, she analyzes the "medicalization of sexuality" and the "medicalized construction of sexuality" separately. "The first implies that there is an *a priori* field of behavior and problems—sexuality—that is placed in the register of medicine during the historical and social process of medicalization. The second implies that modern medical cosmology (what Foucault has called the *archaeology of the clinic*) has invented a sexuality in its own image" [19]. Second, on the basis of this conceptual distinction, Tiefer also differentiates the analysis of appropriate forms of medicalization of sexuality from that of the excessive medicalization of sexuality. The medicalization of sexuality then concerns the understanding and management of patients with erectile dysfunction, low desire disorders, premature ejaculation, and sexual pain, whereas the over-medicalization of sexuality is defined as an excess of medical diagnosis, recourse to medical or surgical treatments, and the search for exclusive medical causes of sexual problems. Tiefer takes the perspective of a clinical sexologist who defends a specific approach to "sexual disorders" by contrasting "good" and "bad" forms of medicalization of sexuality and by privileging the psycho-social dimensions of sexuality that constitute her own professional object. Gori and Del Volgo follow the same perspective by denouncing the "medicalization of existence" or the "bio-medicalization of the human being" from the point of view of psychoanalysis, thus *de facto* excluding psychoanalysis from the field of medicalization and from the field of questionable medicalization [20].

Overall, the medicalization of sexuality is, thus, thought to be the result of a relatively complex historical and sociological process that does not consist in the simple medical appropriation of the natural phenomenon of sexuality. It consists much more in the reinterpretation of previously existing modes of representation and designation of deviance, such as the religious and the legal by the medical-scientific apparatus.

The study of the medicalization of sexuality, thus, lies first and foremost in the deciphering of the way in which sexuality is constructed and represented in a context marked by the emergence of modern medicine, the development of biological and medical sciences, the organization of the medical profession and health professions, and the development of public health. The medical representation of sexuality has been developed in relation to other ways of designating phenomena related to reproduction, eroticism, marital relations, and social deviance, which are situated in the moral, religious, and legal registers. It consists of, above all, the definition of a set of norms opposing the "normal" functioning of sexual function and activity to its less frequent forms, thus transforming them into pathological forms. The pathologization of behavior and subjectivity is one of the central forms of medicalization. This model of medicalization is based on a binary opposition between the normal and the abnormal, the legal and the illegal, and the common and the uncommon, which rejects conceptions based on the idea of a continuum of behavior, activities, thoughts, fantasies, and emotions.

Secondly, the study of medicalization lies in the analysis of the transformations of representations of sexuality under the effect of the neurological, physiological, hormonal, and pharmaceutical research developed since the end of the 20th century and that calls into question the primacy of psycho-social explanations of sexuality. This new focus on the pharmacological treatment of "sexual disorders" and the emergence of sexual medicine [21,22] have the effect of obscuring situations in which it is rather a lack of medical development that is at stake. Interventions developed in the field of HIV-AIDS prevention are not often represented as a form of "medicalization of sexuality", whereas patients' associations demand the development of effective treatments and vaccines and greater accessibility to the populations concerned in a situation of extremely limited access to these treatments in many regions of the world. In this case, what is criticized is the lack of available medical treatments and the difficulties of access to these treatments, whereas in the field of "sexual disorders", it is the process of over-medicalization or the non-necessary use of pharmacological products that is at stake. The multiplicity of these ways of assessing the "medicalization of sexuality" confirms that these phenomena are the subject of very different and even opposing representations.

5. Male and Female "Sexual Disorders": The Arrival of Pharmacological Treatments

5.1. Medicalization and Over-Medicalization

In the field of sexology and sexual medicine, the expression "medicalization of sexuality" is currently used and claimed in various ways. Medical doctors and researchers who, often in association with the pharmaceutical industry, develop and promote new drugs and treatments, use it in a positive sense. In this posture, medicalization is seen as an important advance of scientific medicine (evidence-based medicine) in a field that is still insufficiently explored and, in full development, that of sexual medicine. In this first sense, the term medicalization of sexuality is, therefore, synonymous with progress [23]. The term is used by others, notably sexologists, sex therapists, and psychotherapists who are not part of the medical profession, in a critical and pejorative sense, and consists of criticism of the transformations of representations of sexuality and of the medical, psychological, and sexological practices that are caused in this context. They perceive a transformation of the characteristics of female sexuality, mainly [19], and, secondarily, a reduction of male sexuality to the sole sexual function (erection, ejaculation, and orgasm) under the influence of the strategic orientations of the pharmaceutical industry. In this second sense, the medicalization of sexuality is considered more as a process that is highly problematic. A distinction can be made between the proponents of this second view. Some denounce medicalization in itself, as well as the domination of medicine and the imposition of a biologistic representation of sexuality that takes little account of the elements of social and psychological context that are consubstantial to the idea of sexuality which emerged at the beginning of the 20th century [4]. Others, while not questioning the legitimacy of medicalization (as a medical approach to these problems), criticize the phenomena of *over-medicalization* of sexuality that is occurring with the bio-medical management of women's sexual difficulties and disorders [24]. They consider it inappropriate or excessive to treat these problems through the exclusive use of pharmacological products.

5.2. Pharmacological Treatments for Male Impotence

The medicalization of male impotence is a phenomenon that dates back to the dawn of sexual medicine [21]. This contemporary form of medicalization of male impotence is based on a process that began in the early 1980s with scientific discoveries and, in particular, the discovery of the effects of Papaverine on erection by the French urologist Ronald Virag. Then, a group of urologists from Boston University undertook to reconceptualize male impotence in the field of organic medicine, away from the psychological and psychoanalytic conceptions that had prevailed during the previous decades, and distanced themselves from the surgical approach (applied to the insertion of penile prostheses), which was then central in urology. Armed with the new concepts (*erectile dysfunction* instead of *impotence*) and new criteria of severity and frequency of occurrence of the condition, these same urologists occupied the field of epidemiology and established data showing a much higher prevalence than that which was commonly accepted until then. The development of the sildenafil molecule, for which Pfizer pharmaceutical company filed a patent in 1993, opened up perspectives and possibilities for research funding that led to the development of an instrument for evaluating the effects of treatment and aiding diagnosis and the conduct of clinical trials demonstrating the tolerance and efficacy of the drug. The development of evaluation questionnaires and clinical trials marked the entry of the pharmaceutical industry into the field of impotence and its association with researchers and physicians who had been working on impotence for many years. The process of organicist reconceptualization of male impotence was not, however, to be total. In their initial ambition, these urologists would have willingly abandoned the psychogenic hypothesis to impose the organic theory, as evidenced by the publications in the early 1990s, which placed strong emphasis on organic etiologies and related risk factors. Their own clinical trials led them to requalify their statement and to recognize the presence of an irreducible form of psychogenic etiology "in most men", which remained accessible to the new treatment. The presence of psychosocial etiological risk factors was finally recognized, as a way of not cutting itself off from a large part of the market [4]. Is erectile dysfunction different from impotence? The term impotence is now considered pejorative and potentially offensive. It is also considered inappropriate in that it can encompass the entire cycle of a man's sexual response, whereas the term "erectile dysfunction" takes into account only the erectile mechanism, as only one part of this cycle and the only target of treatment. Furthermore, impotence, as a pathology, only concerns the severe forms, i.e., "primary"; episodes of secondary, transient, or situational impotence are considered "the limit of normal sexual functioning". The new concepts of erectile dysfunction innovate by establishing a continuum of degrees of severity (from the mildest to the most severe) and by including all men with a lesser degree of this dysfunction in the field of pathology. The etiology of impotence is considered to be mainly psychogenic, whereas that of erectile dysfunction is mainly organic. Erectile dysfunction is, thus, distinguished from impotence by a reduction of its domain to erection and organic etiology and by an increase of the total prevalence by including the mildest forms alongside its moderate and severe forms [4].

If scientists and physicians (and mainly urologists) have played a fundamental role in this conceptual evolution of male impotence, the pharmaceutical industry has very quickly set up a drug and new treatments for this new clinical entity. The pharmaceutical industry then contributed to the diffusion of these ideas and their transformation. By choosing to designate the whole situation as an "effective and well-tolerated treatment for a duly listed disease", the pharmaceutical industry was facing the regulatory bodies of drug distribution, which further contributed to the evolution of ideas and located the problem of 'sexual disorders' on a public health level.

The introduction of Viagra in 1998 led to intense media campaigns in the developed world. Viagra—Viagra is understood here as a discursive device, a "Viagra culture" [24] and not only as a drug—was constructed as a symbol of a new sexual revolution, which countered the sexual pessimism developed all along the early years of the epidemics of HIV infection. Viagra represents a sexual world much different from the world that was constructed in the rhetoric of AIDS [25], in which it is a matter of "restoring a natural and normal sexuality" instead of trying to reduce anal sexual practices, promiscuity, and multiple partnership considered as risk factors. From this perspective, the Viagra discourse is aimed at a different segment of the population, men over forty in a stable heterosexual relationship and practicing penile—vaginal penetration, and is aimed at the "restauration" of this practice within the context of the married heterosexual couple. Generally speaking, it is a rediscovery of the sexuality of older heterosexual people and marital sexuality, a sexuality that had been forgotten in the context of the fight against the HIV infection because it was perceived as not being at risk of contamination. Viagra is constructed as a drug that must be prescribed by a doctor to treat a disease: erectile dysfunction. It is the clinical model of communication between the doctor and the patient that predominates, even if Viagra is the subject of an intense media campaign that occupies the public space. Here, the pharmaceutical industry addresses consumers directly, at the same time as it addresses doctors through the channels of professional communication. Advertising propaganda, thus, functions on both sides. The public dimension of Viagra's advertising communication suggests that its influence goes far beyond the strict framework of the population; it is supposed to address and opens up possibilities of use to other groups of the population who are more engaged in "recreational" sexual activities than are concerned with restoring a "natural sexuality".

6. Homosexuality: Medicalization and de-Medicalization

Homosexuality is also part of an evolution that has consisted in recognizing the legitimacy and normality of non-reproductive sexual practices and non-marital activities. Homosexuality began as a form of "unnatural" sexuality, and, until recently, was considered a crime or at least an offence in a number of European countries and a mental disorder. Within each of these categorizations, the status of homosexuality has followed particular destinies, taking on specific meanings according to the times and contexts and becoming subject to different punishments or penalties [26]. More recently, the medical fate of homosexuality has undergone important changes. Homosexuality, considered as a mental disorder, was excluded from the *Diagnostic and Statistical Manual of Mental Disorders* (DSM) in 1973 following discussions between gay organizations and representatives of the different trends of American psychiatry: "By deciding to exclude homosexuality from the nomenclature, the American Psychiatric Association not only placed itself in opposition to the systematic models of formal and informal exclusion that prevented the complete integration of homosexuals into social life, but also deprived civil society of an ideological justification for a certain number of its discriminatory practices" [16]. The exclusion of homosexuality from the field of mental disorders testifies to the anchoring and political function of this medical discipline, its submission to ideological influences and the *zeitgeist*, and its function of legitimizing social norms and prejudices. A few years after leaving the field of psychiatry and mental illness, homosexuality entered the field of medicalization again through the HIV-AIDS epidemic, becoming the first visible figure of this disease [27] in the form of a "lifestyle" that could cause a serious illness: the so-called "gay cancer". The "lifestyle" hypothesis was the first attempt to explain HIV-AIDS in the early 1980s before the discovery of the acquired immune deficiency virus [28]. But beyond the representation of AIDS in the guise of male homosexuality, it is the entire so-called "recreational" non-reproductive sexual life, "promiscuity", and "multi-partnering" that have fallen into the net of medicalized pathologization.

7. Public Health Responses to the HIV Epidemic: The Pathologization of "Deviant" Behavior

The HIV social and political responses, including HIV prevention, grew out of the first responses to the epidemic among gay men and is one of the most important forms of medicalization of sexuality that has taken place in the 20th century on a global scale. The main objective of the fight against HIV-AIDS has been (and still is) to "change sexual behavior" and to develop "protected" sexual practices, i.e., to avoid transmission of the virus by using condoms during sexual relations (anal, genital, and oral). It is, therefore, a behavioral change effort based on scientific and medical rationality and public health lessons. The *AIDS system* [29] has become part of the public health field, working with "risk groups" and deploying methods of social communication, education, and counseling. Sexual behaviors began to be assessed in terms of their potential risk of infection, distinguishing between high-risk, low-risk, and very high-risk behaviors. A hierarchy of behaviors was established, distinguishing between genital, oral, and anal sex according to risk exposure, and between monogamy and multi-partnership according to the same criteria. As a result, the meanings of sexual activity and sexual relationships have changed and love has come to be seen as "a risk factor" insofar as one does not feel the need to protect oneself from someone one loves [30].

In the past, multi-partnership was seen as a moral issue related to infidelity, whereas at the times of HIV-AIDS multi-partnering has become a "risk factor". Much attention had been paid to gay men and not at all to lesbians, as they were assumed not to be at risk of HIV infection. In this perspective, there was a sustained interest in anal practices (insertive and receptive) considered as "higher-risk" sexual practices. This stigmatization of anal sexual behavior and the attempt to reduce them are parallel to the decriminalization of sodomy by the United States Supreme Court in 2003. While attempts were made to reduce anal practices in the name of health, legal and criminal prosecution of those who were alleged to engage in them had been stopped.

Minority behaviors considered deviant, such as sex work and group sex, have become public health issues [31]. The logic of public health does not overlap with that of legality, nor with that of morality. Moral issues are translated into health problems. The fight against HIV infection has focused on young people and multi-partners and has neglected the elderly and married heterosexual and monogamous couples who are considered less exposed to risk. From this perspective, the "fight against AIDS" has taken less account of issues of contraception and procreation and has often failed to consider the links and contradictions between the various forms of "protection" for sexual relations, especially heterosexual relations. There was a strong contrast between the Global North and its focus on Gay and Bisexual men and Intravenous Drug Users (IVDU) and the high prevalence of HIV infection among heterosexual women and men in countries from the Global South, such as Brazil for example [32]. We can, thus, see how the contours of risky sexuality and its health framework have been redrawn by implicitly excluding the most common form of sexual behavior from the field of risky sexuality and from public health interventions and recommendations [33]. However, the history of the medicalization of sexuality from the perspective of AIDS is not yet complete. Current developments in HIV prevention policies, which fall within the paradigm of risk reduction, reflect a shift in this medicalization with the use of pre-exposure and post-exposure antiretroviral pharmacological treatments and male circumcision [34].

8. HIV Prevention as a Form of Biomedicalization of Sexual Activity

The introduction of new efficient drugs available for HIV prevention and treatment has created a situation in which the potential exposure to the risk of HIV infection becomes a medical condition in itself, which can be treated medically with these new drugs. The exposure to the risk of HIV infection—whether situational or behavioral—becomes itself available to chemotherapy in replacement of (or in "combination" with) behavioral approaches. There is a shift from a situation in which behavioral modifications were the only possibility to prevent the occurrence of HIV infection towards a situation in which these behavioral modifications will no longer be necessary thanks to the use of pharmacological medication. This kind of transformation of therapeutic devices into prevention tools is not unique and specific to HIV-AIDS. Based on her work in the field of breast cancer prevention, Fosket has developed the notion of "chemoprevention" in which the risk of breast cancer is treated as a disease: "Chemoprevention is based on the concept that biologically active compounds can be administered not only as tumor-destroying chemotherapy but also as tumor-preventing chemotherapy. (. . .) Drugs developed as treatments for health problems given instead to healthy populations as a way to stay healthy highlight the intense biomedicalization of society such that technoscientific biomedical interventions are increasingly normalized as part of everyday life" [35]. Fosket demonstrates how chemoprevention, which remains controversial, is developed in combination with and/or in replacement of other more traditional preventive approaches, such as surveillance, self-examination, and early response, which are behavioral practices.

The approach developed in the field of cancer treatment and prevention presents a strong analogy to understand the important changes occurring in the field of HIV-AIDS prevention. The concept of Pre-exposure Prophylaxis (PrEP), which refers to the act of using a drug designed for the treatment of HIV infection to prevent the occurrence of the infection, reflects this evolution. Risk exposure and risk behavior become conditions that can be—and need to be—treated biomedically, using the same drugs that are used to treat patients who are already infected to HIV. However, these drugs do not have the function to treat these behaviors; they prevent the occurrence of some adverse potential consequences of such behaviors without the possibility to reduce or suppress their occurrence [36]. The treatment becomes prevention: "Treatment as Prevention" (TasP) replaces the obligation to engage in sexual behavior change among those who have already been infected by HIV, which is now considered to have been a failure by most of the advocates of the biomedicalization of HIV prevention [37].

The discovery of the relative protective effect of biomedical (pharmaceutical) and surgical approaches (ART and male circumcision) is now a motivation for the adoption of new health behavior and adherence to medical prescriptions, and for a reduction in the effort expended on education on sexual behavior change, which is now considered less necessary. This relative reduction in educational efforts, with the increased emphasis on awareness of risk situations, is associated with the use of bio-medical methods. In any event, the promoters of this new pharmacological HIV prevention strategy consider that biomedical recommendations are easier to adopt rather than the long-term modification of sexual behavior, and that adherence to biomedical prescriptions will provoke a reduction of the social and individual control exerted on sexual conducts, thanks to the shift to adherence to pharmacological prescriptions.

The situation that is currently developing around responses to HIV infection is part of a long history of the medicalization of sexuality in the twentieth century that has seen the setting of the behavioral approaches and their progressive abandonment, be they psychosocial, psychotherapeutic, or sexological, in favor of methods based on the use of medication. For example, the development of hormonal oral contraception, considered to be highly effective, has, in most industrialized countries, replaced behavioral methods, such as *coitus interruptus* and male condom, which are located at the very moment of the actual sexual interaction. The widespread use of hormonal contraception, presented as a 'magic bullet' and endowed with total efficacy in the prevention of unplanned pregnancies, is actually disconnected from the moment of the sexual interaction and placed under the control of women. It has been proven over time to have important limitations. Undesirable side effects linked to the regular ingestion of hormones were reported and provoked controversy. Recent surveys demonstrated that the use of hormonal contraception did not eradicate the occurrence of unplanned pregnancies and, consequently, abortion [38]. In the domain of "sexual disorders", there has been an extensive movement pertaining to the pharmacologization of sexuality since the introduction of Viagra, building on the idea of the abandonment of the psychogenesis of "sexual disorders" and the potential for their psychotherapeutic treatment. As in the domain of contraception, after the euphoria of the possibility of completely restoring male sexual function, there was a redeployment of psychotherapeutic responses complementary to, or independent of, the use of these drugs [39]. It can, therefore, be seen that psychosocial and behavioral approaches were initially put in place as a first step towards achieving certain health goals, with the objective of changing people's behaviors and cognition. These treatments and approaches had limitations, as much in the prevention of HIV as in the domains of contraception and the prevention of abortion and sexual dysfunction. One must also note that the development of biomedicalized measures and tools remain constructed on the ground of disciplinary conducts. The major change in this regard is the shift from the discipline related to sexual behavior to a discipline related to health behavior (use of medication and circumcision). Biomedicalization and the development of biopolitics cannot be effective without the sustained use of some disciplinary approaches, be they focused on sexual behavior or on health-oriented behavior.

The case of HIV prevention illustrates the migrations of the medicalization of sexuality, initially between the use of educational and preventive methods based on risk awareness and the application of complex body techniques and, in a second phase, a return to approaches rooted in the bio-medical model based on the persuasion and adherence of individuals in the perspective of population management.

9. "Trans" Situations: Between Medicalization and Depathologization

The question of the coverage and reimbursement of gender affirmation pathways in health insurance systems is central to the conceptual thinking and policy development of user associations, health professionals, and international organizations. The WHO's ICD-10, the major international classification of diseases, was used as a reference by the majority of the world's states [40]. This issue is taken into account in the work of the groups responsible for revising the ICD-10 and, in particular, chapter F 64, which includes "gender identity disorders" and "transsexualism", and to the same extent by the international "Task Force" responsible for revising the DSM-IV into the DSM-5 [41]. Finally, it should be noted that almost the same experts have been appointed to address gender identity disorders in both groups. They are the US psychiatrist Jack Drescher and the Dutch clinical psychologist Peggy Cohen-Kettenis, whose legitimacy in dealing with these issues is unquestionable both in terms of their clinical practice and in view of their impressive lists of publications on the subject. Both of these authors have already published extensive reviews of their work on the DSM-5 Task Force [42,43] and ICD-11 revision process, and it can be assumed that they draw on this prior work for their interventions in the WHO working group.

From the outset, these two experts stated that the main challenge of the revision of ICD 10 was to be able to reconcile the avoidance of stigmatization while protecting the modalities of access to care, insofar as this access is dependent, in the majority of WHO member states, on the existence of a recognized and codified condition. It was, therefore, necessary to maintain a nosographic category allowing access to care and health insurance systems while limiting the effects of stigmatization and the consequences on the mental health of trans people, such as internalized transphobia. The definition and maintenance of such a nosographic category are, thus, the result of decisions that go beyond the simple medical or psychiatric space to take into account in a decisive way the psycho-social consequences of the very establishment of the diagnosis and to allow access to care and its coverage by health insurance systems. Thus, the definition of a nosographic category depends as much, if not more, on the responses that societies provide to conditions than on the strictly medical dimensions of the problems and disorders in question. Since the ICD is a classification of somatic and psychiatric disorders, it would have been possible to classify "gender identity disorders" and "transsexualism" outside of psychiatric mental disorders and, for example, among endocrine disorders or neurological disorders. One could also redefine "gender identity disorders" along the lines of sleep disorders or in the pregnancy register [44]. Furthermore, the ICD has a "Z" category that would have allowed "gender identity disorders" to be coded as "factors influencing health status and reasons for seeking health services," which would make it possible to avoid specifying these disorders in a pathological register while maintaining the possibility of their management and coverage in the health care systems.

The logic of the ICD-10, thus, allows for more room for maneuver than the DSM-5. If the WHO would have decided in the last instance not to exclude "gender identity disorders" from the register of diseases, the possibilities offered would have been numerous to maintain the place of "transsexualism" in the register of conditions without maintaining its definition as a general pathology on the one hand, or even psychiatric on the other.

The potential demedicalization of the trans situations and "gender identity disorders"—if it is desirable for some—appears, however, difficult to achieve at the general level. The first demand is for the depsychiatrization of these conditions, but apparently in the discussions that have taken place in the framework of the DSM-IV Task Force, this possibility has not been put on the agenda. The experts are moving towards a definition of these disorders under the term "gender dysphoria" (after a first proposal made in 2010 to use the term "gender incongruence"). However, Heino Meyer-Balhburg warns policy makers that any new definition of these disorders cannot be based on scientific grounds alone and must be in compromise with the claims and needs of people with gender identity variants [45]. The ICD offers broader possibilities for the depsychiatrization of "transsexualism" and reclassification of this condition under a new name, but the experts, concerned with reducing the harmful effects of stigmatization, did not envisage removing this category completely from the field of pathologies, which would have the effect of depriving the persons concerned of quality care and of coverage by health insurance systems.

In the discussions that developed around the development of erectile dysfunction drugs, it was hypothesized that the medicalization of 'sexual disorders' had come under the control of the pharmaceutical industry and was, thus, a result of the pharmacologization of "sexual disorders" [46]. With transgenderism and diverse expressions of gender identifications, it is much more the economics of health and health insurance systems that contribute to the maintenance of minority identities in the register of medicalization. The total depathologization of "transsexualism" does not seem possible for the moment insofar as it would imply an exclusion of the assumed responsibility of health insurance systems, which is wished neither by the doctors nor by the representatives of the trans associations. Non-medical factors, thus, contribute to keeping the trans situations within the bounds of medicalization. The situation of transsexualism, thus, opens up a renewal of the questioning of medicalization by revealing the non-medical factors that are at work in the construction of medical categories and definitions. Finally, the WHO working group proposed the creation of a new category "problems related to sexual health" in which "gender incongruence" would be included as a way of excluding the trans situations from the realm of a psychiatric (mental disorder) category and the subcategory of paraphilic disorders. The creation of this new category is a half-way process toward depathologization. It is certainly a way of excluding the trans situations from the field of psychiatric disorders while maintaining these situations in the field of registered response to a medical condition, allowing its full or partial coverage by local insurance companies and social security systems. Ironically, at a time in history where transgender and gender diverse situations are moving away from any reference to a sexual etiology and paraphilia (as it was the case in previous medical and psychiatric classifications), the WHO created a new category of "conditions related to sexual health" in order to depathologize these situations. The sexual dimension of transgender identities and situations makes a kind of unexpected comeback. Including transgender and gender diverse situations in the realm of sexual health helps to remove these situations from the field of psychiatry and, at the same time, brings them back in the extended field of sexuality [47].

10. Conclusions

The various forms of the medicalization of sexuality and gender that have been discussed in this article (responses to the HIV-AIDS epidemic, conceptions of homosexuality, treatments for "sexual disorders", and gender affirmative pathways for transgender and gender diverse situations) have appeared at different times in the history of the 20th century. Each of these approaches represents a particular form of medicalization, that is, a form of medicalized representation of sexuality or gender identity issues which has social, political, economic, medical, and subjective implications. Some of these situations are denounced by groups of actors involved in these issues (feminist organizations, gay organizations, and transgender and gender diverse organizations), others are considered acceptable and even sometimes necessary (HIV prevention), and some are not considered to fall within the scope of the medicalization of sexuality and therefore exempt from criticism.

The medicalization of sexuality takes the form of interventions, planned within the medical framework, on situations qualified as sexual, and on the actors involved in them, which can take the form of clinical and therapeutic interventions, but can also be outside the narrow framework of medical practices and preventive, psychotherapeutic, or educational interventions which are oriented through a medical perspective. These interventions can take place within a medical framework in the strict sense of the word, or in partnership with public health, health education, or criminal justice institutions. The anchoring of these practices in the dichotomy of normality/pathology established by medicine orients the objectives of these practices and interventions in the direction of restoring or enhancing supposedly reduced sexual activities, which are considered as normal, or in the direction of reducing or repressing physical or mental sexual activities considered, either from a strict medical point of view or from a legal and moral point of view, as deviant or excessive.

These analyses demonstrate that medicalization is a very complex process. Moreover, medicalization has numerous ramifications and, primarily, the movement of medicalization/demedicalization has been observed regarding the depsychiatrization of homosexuality. There is also a possibility to try to depathologize a situation, such as the medical pathways of gender affirmation among trans people, and not demedicalize, i.e., not removing medical interventions and participation of members of the medical profession. The medicalization of sexuality was first framed and organized around the distinction and separation between procreative and non-procreative activities, which provided the onset of the concept of sexuality to establish a discourse and a practice [9]. Then, since the beginning of the 20th century, the organizing principle of the medicalized representation of sexuality has gradually changed by recognizing the legitimacy of non-procreative activities. In its contemporary meaning, the terms "sexuality" and sexual no longer necessarily include procreative functions in their normal course. The pathologization of these terms now focuses on the difficulties in developing and maintaining an erotic life, which is a guarantee of satisfactory sexual health and well-being. While medicalization initially consisted of the medical appropriation of a field of human activity, more recent developments show how health has progressively become the foundation and justification of individual and collective moral values [48].

Funding: This research received no external funding.

Conflicts of Interest: The author declares no conflict of interest.

References

1. Conrad, P. *The Medicalization of Society*; The Johns Hopkins University Press: Baltimore, MD, USA, 2007.
2. Clarke, A.E.; Fishman, J.; Fosket, J.; Mamo, L.; Shim, J. Biomedicalization: Technoscientific Transformations of Health, Illness, and U.S. Biomedicine. *Am. Sociol. Rev.* **2003**, *68*, 161–194. [CrossRef]
3. Faure, O. La médicalisation vue par les historiens. In *L'ère de la Médicalisation*; Aïach, P., Delanoe, D., Eds.; Anthropos: Paris, France, 1998.
4. Giami, A. De l'impuissance à la dysfonction érectile. Destins de la médicalisation de la sexualité. In *Le Gouvernement des Corps*; Fassin, D., Memmi, D., Eds.; Editions EHESS: Paris, France, 2004; pp. 77–108.
5. Giami, A. L'invention des médicaments des troubles féminins du désir: Controverses autour de la sexualité feminine. In *Les Sciences du Désir La Sexualité Féminine de la Psychanalyse aux Neurosciences*; Gardey, D., Vuille, M., Eds.; Editions le bord de l'eau: Paris, Franece, 2018.
6. Giami, A.; Perrey, C. Transformations in the Medicalization of Sex: HIV Prevention from Discipline to Biopolitics. *J. Sex Res.* **2012**, *49*, 353–361. [CrossRef] [PubMed]
7. Giami, A. Médicalisation et dépathologisation des identités trans: Le poids des facteurs sociaux et économiques (Commentaire). *Sci. Soc. St.* **2012**, *30*, 59–69. [CrossRef]
8. Castel, R. *La Gestion des Risques. De l'anti-Psychiatrie à l'après-Psychanalyse*; Les éditions de Minuit: Paris, France, 1981.
9. Zorzanelli, R.T.; Ortega, F.; Bezerra Júnior, B. An overview of the variations surrounding the concept of medicalization between 1950 and 2010. *Cien Saude Colet.* **2014**, *19*, 1859–1868. [CrossRef] [PubMed]
10. Davidson, A. Sex and the emergence of sexuality. *Crit. Inq.* **1987**, *14*, 16–48. [CrossRef]
11. Foucault, M. *Les Anormaux—Cours au Collège de France 1974–1975*; Gallimard, Le Seuil, EHESS: Paris, France, 1999.
12. Corbin, A. *L'harmonie des Plaisirs. Les Manières de Jouir du Siècle des Lumières à l'avènement de la Sexologie*; Perrin: Paris, France, 2008.
13. Lanteri Laura, G. *Lecture des Perversions. Histoire de leur Appropriation Médicale*; Masson: Paris, France, 1979.
14. Szasz, T. *Sexe sur Ordonnance*; Hachette: Paris, France, 1981.
15. Conrad, P. Medicalization and social control. *Annu. Rev. Sociol.* **1992**, *18*, 209–232. [CrossRef]
16. Conrad, P.; Schneider, J. *Deviance and Medicalization: From Badness to Sickness*; The C.V. Mosby Company: St. Louis, MO, USA, 1980.
17. Bayer, R. *Homosexuality and American Psychiatry. The Politics of Diagnosis*; Basic Books: New York, NY, USA, 1981.
18. Szasz, T. *Ceremonial Chemistry*; Doubleday & Co, Inc.: New York, NY, USA, 1974.
19. Tiefer, L. The medicalization of sexuality: Conceptual, normative and professional issues. *Annu. Rev. Sex Res.* **1996**, *7*, 252–282.
20. Gori, R.; Del Volgo, M.-J. *La Santé Totalitaire, Essai sur la Médicalisation de L'existence*; Denoël: Paris, France, 2005.
21. Perelman, M. The history of sexual medicine. In *American Psychology Association Handbook of Sexuality and Psychology*; Tolman, D.L., Diamond, L.M., Bauermeister, J.A., George, W.H., Pfaus, J.G., Ward, L.M., Eds.; American Psychological Association: Washington, DC, USA, 2014; Volume 2.
22. Giami, A. La médecine sexuelle: Genèse d'une spécialisation médicale? *Hist. Médecine St.* **2018**, 131–147. [CrossRef]
23. Jardin, A. Le traitement médicamenteux des troubles érectiles: Aspects éthiques. In *Progrès Thérapeutiques: La Médicalisation de la Sexualité en Question*; Jardin, A., Queneau, P., Giuliano, F., Eds.; John Libbey, Eurotext: Paris, France, 2000.
24. Tiefer, L. Doing the Viagra Tango. *Radic. Philos.* **1998**, *92*, 2–5.
25. Gagnon, J. Disease and Desire. *Daedalus* **1989**, *118*, 47–78.
26. Leroy-Forgeot, F. *Histoire Juridique de L'homosexualité en Europe*; PUF: Paris, France, 1997.
27. Fee, E.; Fox, D. (Eds.) In the eye of the storm: The epidemiological construction of Aids. In *Aids, The Burden of History*; University of California Press: Berkeley, CA, USA, 1988; pp. 267–300.
28. Gilman, S. *Disease and Representation. From Madness to Aids*; Cornell University Press: Ithaca, NY, USA, 1988.
29. Grmek, M. *Histoire du Sida*; Payot: Paris, France, 1989.
30. Henriksson, B. *Risk Factor Love: Homosexuality, Sexual Interaction and HIV Prevention*; Goteborgs Universitets Skriftserien: Goteborg, Sweden, 1995.
31. Frank, K. Rethinking Risk, Culture, and Intervention in Collective Sex Environments. *Arch. Sex. Behav.* **2019**, *48*, 3–30. [CrossRef] [PubMed]
32. da Silva Campany, L.N.; Murta Amaral, D.; de Oliveira Lemos dos Santos, R.N. HIV/aids no Brasil: Feminização da epidemia em análise. *Rev. Bioét.* **2021**, *29*. [CrossRef]
33. Gagnon, J. Theorizing risky sex. In *The Role of Theory in Sex Research*; Bancroft, J., Ed.; Indiana University Press: Bloomington, IN, USA, 2000; pp. 149–176.
34. Giami, A.; Perrey, C.; de Oliveira Mendonça, A.; Rochel de Camargo, K. Hybrid forum or network? The social and political construction of an international 'technical consultation': Male circumcision and HIV-prevention. *Glob. Public Health Int. J. Res. Policy Pract.* **2015**, *10*, 589–606. [CrossRef] [PubMed]
35. Fosket, J.R. Breast Cancer risk as disease/Biomedicalzing risk. In *Biomedicalization Technoscience, Health and Illness in the US*; Clarke, A.E., Mamo, L., Fosket, J.R., Fishman, J.R., Shim, J.K., Eds.; Duke University Press: Durham & London, UK, 2010; pp. 331–352.
36. Nguyen, V.K.; Bajos, N.; Dubois-Arber, F.; O'Malley, J.; Pirkle, C.M. Remedicalizing an epidemic: From HIV treatment as prevention to HIV treatment is prevention. *AIDS* **2011**, *25*, 291–293. [CrossRef]

37. Cohen, M.S. HIV Treatment as Prevention: To be or not to be? *JAIDS J. Acquir. Immune Defic. Syndr.* **2010**, *55*, 137–138. [CrossRef]
38. Moreau, C.; Trussell, J.; Desfreres, J.; Bajos, N. Patterns of contraceptive use before and after an abortion: Results from a nationally representative survey of women undergoing an abortion in France. *Contraception* **2010**, *82*, 337–344. [CrossRef]
39. Giami, A.; Chevret-Méasson, M.; Bonierbale, M. Recent evolution to the profession of sexologist in France. *First results of a 2009 survey in France. Sexol. Eur. J. Sexol. Sex. Health* **2009**, *18*, 238–242.
40. Bowker, G.; Leigh Star, S. Sorting things out. In *Classification and Its Consequences*; MIT Press: Cambridge, MA, USA, 1999.
41. Zucker, K. Editorial: Reports from the DSM-V Work Group on Sexual and Gender Identity Disorders. *Arch. Sex. Behav.* **2010**, *39*, 217–220. [CrossRef]
42. Drescher, J. Queer diagnoses: Parallels and contrasts in the history of homosexuality, gender variance, and the Diagnostic and Statistical Manual. *Arch. Sex. Behav.* **2010**, *39*, 427–460. [CrossRef]
43. Drescher, J. Personal Communication, 2012.
44. Cohen-Kettenis, P.T.; Pfäfflin, F. The DSM diagnostic criteria for gender identity disorder in adolescents and adults. *Arch. Sex. Behav.* **2010**, *39*, 499–513. [CrossRef]
45. Meyer-Bahlburg, H. From Mental Disorder to Iatrogenic Hypogonadism: Dilemmas in Conceptualizing Gender Identity Variants as Psychiatric Conditions. *Arch. Sex. Behav.* **2010**, *39*, 461–476. [CrossRef] [PubMed]
46. Tiefer, L. Sexology and the Pharmaceutical Industry: The Threat of Co-optation. *J. Sex Res.* **2000**, *37*, 273–283. [CrossRef]
47. Drescher, J.; Cohen-Kettenis, P.T.; Winter, S. Minding the body: Situating gender identity diagnoses in the ICD-11. *Int. Rev. Psychiatry* **2012**, *24*, 568–577. [CrossRef] [PubMed]
48. Epstein, S. *The Quest for Sexual Health. How an Elusive Ideal Has Transformed Science, Politics, and Everyday Life*; University of Chicago Press: Chicago, IL, USA, 2022.

Disclaimer/Publisher's Note: The statements, opinions and data contained in all publications are solely those of the individual author(s) and contributor(s) and not of MDPI and/or the editor(s). MDPI and/or the editor(s) disclaim responsibility for any injury to people or property resulting from any ideas, methods, instructions or products referred to in the content.

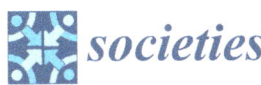

Concept Paper

A New Time of Reckoning, a Time for New Reckoning: Views on Health and Society, Tensions between Medicine and the Social Sciences, and the Process of Medicalization

Diogo Silva da Cunha [1],* and Hélder Raposo [2,3]

1. Institute of Social Sciences, University of Lisbon, Av. Prof. Aníbal Bettencourt 9, 1600-189 Lisbon, Portugal
2. Lisbon School of Health Technology, Polytechnic Institute of Lisbon, Av. D. João II, Lote 4.69.01, 1990-096 Lisboa, Portugal
3. CIES-IUL—Centre for Research and Studies in Sociology, ISCTE-IUL, Avenida das Forças Armadas, 1649-026 Lisbon, Portugal
* Correspondence: cunha.diogo@ics.ulisboa.pt

Abstract: This article seeks to capture variations and tensions in the relationships between the health–illness–medicine complex and society. It presents several theoretical reconstructions, established theses and arguments are reassessed and criticized, known perspectives are realigned according to a new theorizing narrative, and some new notions are proposed. In the first part, we argue that relations between the medical complex and society are neither formal–abstract nor historically necessary. In the second part, we take the concept of medicalization and the development of medicalization critique as an important example of the difficult coalescence between health and society, but also as an alternative to guide the treatment of these relationships. Returning to the medicalization studies, we suggest a new synthesis, reconceptualizing it as a set of modalities, including medical imperialism. In the third part, we endorse replacing a profession-based approach to medicalization with a knowledge-based approach. However, we argue that such an approach should include varieties of sociological knowledge. In this context, we propose an enlarged knowledge-based orientation for standardizing the relationships between the health–illness–medicine complex and society.

Keywords: medicalization; knowledge-based approach; medical dogmatism; medical skepticism; medical imperialism; sociological imperialism; sociological objectivism; sociological subjectivism; pharmaceuticalization; therapeuticalization

Citation: da Cunha, D.S.; Raposo, H. A New Time of Reckoning, a Time for New Reckoning: Views on Health and Society, Tensions between Medicine and the Social Sciences, and the Process of Medicalization. *Societies* **2022**, *12*, 119. https://doi.org/10.3390/soc12040119

Academic Editors: Violeta Alarcão and Sónia Cardoso Pintassilgo

Received: 14 June 2022
Accepted: 4 August 2022
Published: 13 August 2022

Publisher's Note: MDPI stays neutral with regard to jurisdictional claims in published maps and institutional affiliations.

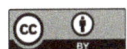

Copyright: © 2022 by the authors. Licensee MDPI, Basel, Switzerland. This article is an open access article distributed under the terms and conditions of the Creative Commons Attribution (CC BY) license (https://creativecommons.org/licenses/by/4.0/).

1. Introduction

Since the mid-20th century, strong fluctuations have been identified in the discourse on the 'health–illness–medicine complex' (HIMC), to use Renée C. Fox's accurate formulation [1] (p. 10). The renowned social historian of medicine Roy Porter opens his proposal of a medical history of humanity by saying, "these are strange times, when we are healthier than ever but more anxious about our health" [2] (p. 3). In the last chapter of his book, he repeats this idea, writing that "the irony is that the healthier Western society becomes, the more medicine it craves" [2] (p. 717). There are many factors to consider in the oscillations in the discourse on the HIMC and several available theoretical perspectives and analytical models to explain them. The medical journalist James Le Fanu treated Porter's irony as a paradox composed of four growing layers: physicians' own disillusionment with medicine, general public's concern with health, the resort to the so-called alternative medicines, and the costs of health care [3]. According to Le Fanu, each of these layers can be seen as a facet of the pattern of the historical development of modern medicine.

Le Fanu's central argument is that this development followed the standardized up and down narrative that serves as the title of his book, *The Rise and Fall of Modern Medicine*. In the post-war years, roughly from the mid-1940s to the late 1970s, the development of clinical research as applied science, drug discovery, and technological innovation would spark the rising movement. From the late 1970s onwards, there would be exhaustion of these forces and a break in optimism surrounding modern medicine. This rupture would have produced, in turn, an empty space to be filled in the early 1980s by two emergent projects.

On the one hand, 'The New Genetics' is a project based on molecular biology and comprises the application areas of biotechnology or genetic engineering, genetic screening, and gene therapy. On the other hand, what the author calls 'The Social Theory', basically epidemiological studies, considers cultural, social, and economic conditions of health and works through statistical inference. These two projects supposedly brought a new notion of the etiology of disease, the first guided by a naturalistic and reductionist perspective, focused on genes, and the second guided by environmental and social conditioning. Solutions based on genetic manipulation and social engineering followed these notions, namely technological treatments and social prevention, respectively. For Le Fanu, these projects failed mainly because their etiology was wrong. According to him, the causes of diseases are not genetic nor social, but biological, determined by age, or simply and above all, unknown. The lack of this perception would have represented the downfall of modern medicine.

As with other interpretive generalizations, this narrative is not entirely false, but it simplifies a much more nuanced reality. Although Le Fanu's work contains pertinent criticisms of the geneticist enterprise, his perspective seems to be deeply conditioned by the very model of clinical medicine that he seeks to defend, which mainly skews his understanding of social theory but also limits the very conception of medicine. We are undoubtedly facing a transition in the discourse on the HIMC. Nevertheless, to understand what is specific in this transition and in a new discourse on the HIMC, it is mandatory to start by questioning not only what is new in our objects of study but also the limits of our old perspectives and methods of analysis. This is not equivalent to accepting the anti-realist and even nominalist theses that are still present and dominant in some sectors of the social sciences. "The key task for medicine is not to diminish the role of the biological sciences in the theory and practice of medicine", as Leon Eisenberg and Arthur Kleinman wrote, "but to supplement it with an equal application of the social sciences" [4] (p. 11). "The problem is not 'too much science', but too narrow a view of the sciences relevant to medicine", they add [4] (p. 11).

From our point of view, it will be necessary to begin by realizing that the relations between the HIMC and society are not strictly formal. They are inscribed in multilevel conditions and variations and are crossed by several agonal tendencies, as the COVID-19 pandemic crisis has recently shown. Those conditions and variations and these tensions do not allow the idea of a social theory to be reduced to epidemiology and a quantitative approach, nor to the medical fields of public health or social medicine. If, on the one hand, there is no systematic, coherent, and, above all, consensual theory that relates the HIMC to society, on the other hand, concepts, hypotheses, and theses, implicit or explicit, about this relationship are abundant.

More specifically, the social components of the discourse on the HIMC seem to find expression in, or at least are consistent with, some of the constitutive assumptions of the various subdisciplines of the social sciences dealing with research on health and medicine. As can be seen by the efforts of synthesis undertaken in authoritative works such as Deborah Lupton's *Medicine as Culture* [5] or Marc Berg and Annemarie Mol's *Differences in Medicine* [6], there are among these subdisciplines, including medical anthropology, history of medicine, sociology of health, political economy of medicine, or even strict domains of STS, cultural studies, and media studies, a discipline-oriented division of work, the construction of peculiar research traditions, but also remarkable convergences of contemporary epistemological transformations.

In this article, we are interested in considering those conditions, variations, and tendencies and these transformations. Beyond the excessive analytical segmentation resulting from any division of labor, which produces approaches that are not only distinctive but tend to be captive to an insularity that makes reciprocal understanding difficult, we believe that it is possible to demonstrate that the new discourse on the HIMC follows, and is followed by, epistemological transformations transversal to the diverse social sciences, or to social theory in a broad sense. Some of these transformations escalate disputes on the meaning of health and illness, the limits of medical authority and the autonomy of patients, or even on broader aspects of the entire social structure. For some social scientists, as in the case of Vicente Navarro, it is the very flux of social and economic transformation, namely the accumulation crisis of capital, that produces crisis in the field of medicine [7].

In the face of specificities of this type, we must take into account that, as Graça Carapinheiro points out, the meeting between sociology (but perhaps we can generalize it to other social sciences) and health is presided over by the idea that health problems cannot be treated exclusively from the perspective of medicine, by the hypothesis that these problems require a collaborative effort that challenges the organization of knowledge and the division of professional work, and by the need to develop a critical epistemology that opens the causal nexus of pathological facts [8].

In this paper, we will sustain as a central argument that the concept of medicalization and the development of a theoretical, empirical, and critical movement called 'medicalization critique' constitute a paradigmatic illustration of the problematic coalescence of perspectives between the HIMC and society. We also believe this occurs in accordance with the previously mentioned epistemological transformations, as that concept and this movement incorporate problems inherited from fundamental tensions inscribed in the relational variability characterizing the relationship between the HIMC and society.

Let us summarize our argument according to the structure of the present paper. It is constituted of three main parts. Along them, we carry out several theoretical reconstructions, reassess and criticize established theses and arguments, realign known points of view according to a new theorizing narrative, and also propose, as necessary, some new notions.

In the first part, Sections 2 and 3, we will analyze epistemological problems transversal to the development of the history of ancient science, modern medicine, public health, medical anthropology, history of medicine, sociology of health, philosophy of medicine, and STS. We will argue that relations between the HIMC and society are not formal–abstract, or historically necessary but material and conceptual, developed at various levels, inscribed in cognitive, historical, cultural, and socio-structural variations and values. We will demonstrate the antiquity and diversification of the tensions between what is understood by the HIMC and society, showing that they are part of the Western medical tradition.

In the second part of our text, from Section 4 to Section 8, we recapture medicalization critiques following the problems and the epistemological transition exposed. We will show that this movement faces problems inherited from fundamental tensions inscribed in the relational variability mentioned above. However, at the same time, it follows and stimulates the transformation in the discourse on the HIMC, providing features that allow new heuristics in this regard. Our aim is not to reshape the concept of medicalization but to suggest a new synthesis of medicalization critique, reconceptualizing it as an already established but poorly defined set of modalities of the same process. The first will be the negative modality of medicalization, based on the concept of social control and characterized by repressive realism. Exploring the discussions around imperialism, we will argue, on the one hand, that medical imperialism corresponds to the professional variant of this first modality, and that, on the other hand, by reformulating the critique impetus and considering sociological analysis as an extension of professional imperialism, it renews and deepens the variations and tensions represented by medicalization critique. A positive modality of medicalization, still supported by the notion of social control, will be thematized from the convergence between social constructivism and the social and historical interpretations of Michel Foucault's works. This modality implies a shift from professional analysis to the analysis of power relations and forms of knowledge, which implies the recognition of the productivity of these forms and the adoption of a corresponding anti-realist point of view, which contrasts with the natural–scientific force of Western medicine. The expansion of medicalization studies will imply reassessing new critical scrutiny, and analytical contributions, namely the accusation of biophobia, and including new structures, new agents, new behaviors, and new dynamics also explored not only by the concepts of moralization and misinformation but by concepts such as biomedicalization, pharmaceuticalization, therapeuticalization, or complementary and alternative medicalization (camization).

Finally, we will consider the proposal of replacing a profession-based approach with a knowledge-based approach, excluding the concept of social control from the semantic field of medicalization. However, we consider that a knowledge-based approach should not be sustained only in recognizing the variability of medical knowledge but also include the variability of sociological knowledge. Thus, in the third part, consisting of Sections 9 and 10, we make a case for what we can call an 'enlarged knowledge-based approach'. Such broadening involves questioning the intersection of commonplaces between medicine and the social sciences and increasing the dose of sociological reflexivity. This reflexivity will not, however, be merely professional but relative to sociological knowledge in its own variations. In this context, we can finally propose an orientation for standardizing the problematic relationships between the HIMC and society according to parameters related to the possibility of medical knowledge (skepticism and dogmatism) and related to the perspective on societies (objectivism and subjectivism).

This proposal does not exhaust the diversity of theoretical approaches but organizes them through a correlative conceptual scheme. We are not just living in the new time of reckoning Eliot Freidson alluded to, referring to the need to respond to the reckoning being made of health institutions, educational institutions, and welfare services, overlooked by commercial enterprises [9], but in a time for new reckoning, an epoch that simultaneously demands comprehensive empirical knowledge, but also profound theoretical redefinition, and sophisticated critical sensitivity.

2. The Health–Illness–Medicine Complex and Society

Nothing general can be said about phenomena as general as those of health and illness. This limitation does not arise from endorsing a relativist epistemological point of view—this is not even our case. Instead, it is an epistemological consequence resulting from the very structure of reality. On the one hand, these words, 'health' and 'illness', seem to describe universal conditions of human existence: all human beings are potentially subject not only to what we call illness but also to related circumstances such as malnutrition, aging, pain, suffering, or even death. Additionally, every human being is also, we must add, a potential subject of therapies. Nevertheless, we do not relate only empirically to these aspects, as, on the other hand, we have peculiar representations of them. We select, organize, and frame them according to different value systems and carry out diverse correlative practices. However different our conceptions may be, each of us, at each time, under each cultural bond, within each social formation, within the framework of different political regimes and forms of economic organization, has ideas about what a body is, perceptions, representations, beliefs, and even knowledge about what it is to be healthy or sick, practices and values about how to nourish, care, and cure, and how to deal with aging and death.

Thus, the space described by the terms 'health' and 'illness' is unavoidable and presumably warranted but, at the same time, highly fluctuating. As Gary L. Albrecht, Ray Fitzpatrick, and Susan C. Scrimshaw say in the introduction to the *Handbook of Social Studies in Health and Medicine*, "Health is one of the most vital but taken-for-granted qualities of everyday life" [10]. In the new edition of this book, published 20 years later as *The SAGE Handbook of Social Studies in Health and Medicine*, Scrimshaw, along with Sandra D. Lane, Robert A. Rubinstein, and Julian Fisher, wrote that "Disease, illness, and conceptions of health are complex, interrelated phenomena", whereby "simple explanations of these phenomena give only partial insights into them", leading to "inadequate and poorly fitting policies or interventions" [11] (p. 7). Faced with the COVID-19 pandemic, the authors emphasize "the need to shift from seeing problems to be solved in an insular way to accepting that these are complex and evolving challenges" [11] (p. 11).

According to Bryan S. Turner, precisely because they express vital assumptions, notions such as those of health and illness are linked to the structure of power relations and the set of values of a society, aligned with moral and theological concerns [12]. We might add that these concerns are followed by fantasies, aesthetic sensibilities, cultural codes, and metaphorical resources [13]. Nevertheless, more than being systematically developed, the idea of value-ladenness finds expression in different theoretical frameworks of reference, study hypotheses, and particular concepts.

For instance, as the theme of the social regulation of the body theorized and investigated by Friedrich Nietzsche, Sigmund Freud, Marcel Mauss, Charles H. Cooley, Norbert Elias, and Erving Goffman and recovered by Thomas Scheff and Turner himself within the scope of medical sociology demonstrates, we are not only in the field of representations, but in a context of mediation between the biological, the psychic and the social, all this mixed with culture, morality, and religion [14–17]. In this sense, we could understand the notions of health and illness in the light of Marcel Mauss' Durkheimian concept of 'total social fact', as complex transversal realities subject to multiple approaches, including biomedicine, without exhausting the very understanding of those notions [18]. It will thus be very difficult, as Turner argues, retrieving Walter B. Gallie's concept of 'essentially contested concepts', to establish a cross-cultural consensus between what is meant by 'health' and 'illness', or to define a corresponding rigorous history [12].

Just as nothing general can be said about health and illness, it is also difficult to speak of medicine in general terms. Medicine, being associated with human vital and existential problems, also seems to be inscribed in the variability of such notions and to be conditioned by its resulting tensions. Bearing in mind that, alongside a widespread structure of health beliefs, as the medical anthropologist Arthur Kleinman suggests, there is also a widespread "institutionalization of decisive therapeutic practices", the institutionalization of care processes and systems of healing, it would be possible to think about medicine itself as a "universal in human organizations" [19] (p. 15). Kleinman considers that, regardless of cultural differences, there are similarities between these systems, namely disease diagnosis categories, forms of symbolic interpretation of disease, pathology, and therapeutic practices (including idioms, metaphors, and narrative structures), healing roles, discursive strategies, or symbolic and practical operations to control symptoms.

Nonetheless, the substantive differences between conceptions, practices, and values seem to be more severe than those structural similarities. This is certainly a legacy of the variability of the very notions of health and illness, both fundamental in the scope of diverse aspects of medicine. In this sense, it can be said that, like the former notions, medicine will also involve social totality, being crossed by significant cultural and historical variability, and undergoing generalized conceptual contestation. In fact, the concept of total social fact has already been evoked to describe the COVID-19 pandemic [20].

The recognition of socio-cultural conditions of health and illness is not entirely new. There is an abundance of relevant works from various disciplinary areas that seek to elaborate historical reconstructions of particular disciplines or subdisciplines related to health and medicine, showing us a common set of variations in the respective representations, practices, and values. Among other circumstances, such works demonstrate the transhistorical awareness of socio-cultural aspects as factors that positively or negatively condition, or even determine, health and illness. This notion was already partially conscious, at least since classical antiquity. Furthermore, it has developed and integrated more social and academic groups over the centuries, according to a particular set of transformations. Among these, we must count the threats posed by communicable diseases, namely from epidemic and pandemic events, and the respective structural control responses, scientific and technological changes, developments in religion, morality and manners, the regionally differentiated processes of modern state formation, economic metamorphosis and the corresponding organization of power relations and class struggle, and correlative changes in the supply and quality of food and water, housing, sanitation, and medical care.

Theoretically systematic, empirically grounded, well-argued, and now profusely studied examples are George Rosen's *A History of Public Health* and Samuel W. Bloom's *The Word as Scalpel: A History of Medical Sociology* [21,22]. Rosen begins his book by exploring ancient worldwide sanitary ideas and practices, including those within the framework of ancient Eastern civilizations. However, as Bloom will argue, based on a long ballast of historical evidence, there will be for centuries, inside or outside the Western world, the absence of an "effort to develop a systematic theoretical basis for the administrative program of public health" [22] (p. 22), "the systematic investigation of these relationships and the institutionalized expression of such ideas in public policy" [22] (p. 14). Both authors demonstrate that awareness of social and economic conditions of health is very old, that the problems of community life highlighted facets that today fit within the framework of the notion of public health, but that only from the Renaissance onwards did the conscience about these conditions expand.

Particularly important is the thesis advanced by Rosen, endorsed by Bloom, according to which from the 16th to the 18th centuries, the political and economic doctrines of mercantilism, or cameralism in Germany, and its respective conception of society, were structuring the formation and development of the state and the concomitant centralization of the national government. Seeking to place social and economic life at the service of the state, it was understood that it was necessary to protect the health of individuals and groups, making health a fundamental topic of public policy. Both authors also emphasize the importance of the struggle for recognition of the constraints caused by economic and technological developments in the health of the poorest and working classes. It is a struggle that dates back at least to the 15th century, being deepened after the Industrial Revolution, with increasing morbidity and mortality among the poor, a problem, as Bloom argues, that economic liberalism was not able to resolve because poverty was considered as part of the natural and moral order. According to Bloom, it is only the report to the Poor Law Commission prepared in 1842 by Edwin Chadwick that breaks with this perspective. In this regard, one cannot ignore, in our view, the contribution of Karl Marx himself in formulating his critique of political economy and his economic theory in the first book of *Das Kapital*, namely in the chapter dedicated to the discussion of the working day [23].

During the 19th century, according to Bloom, social medicine or public health began to emerge as a branch of medicine that identified the need to understand medical problems from the idea of a reformist social science, under the name of Chadwick in England, but also Rudolph Virchow or Salomon Neumann in Germany. However, the institutionalization of this area would have regional variations and would be generically deferred to the turn of the century. Even so, according to Bloom, the absence of systematic effort and its institutionalized expression would only be overcome with the emergence of medical sociology.

We must add, despite the relevance of these disciplinary areas that, in the wake of the recognition of the importance of cultural, economic, and social factors in the etiology of the disease by physicians and epidemiologists in the early part of the 20th century, the study of what can be called the binomial 'health and culture' has become common among certain empirical trends of social research. In line with some substantive issues within foundational anthropological works and with the practical orientation of ethnographic fieldwork and participant observation, medical anthropology became the main disciplinary formation responsible for comparative, cross-cultural studies on health, health behavior, practices, systems, and medical care [24]. Especially important in this regard was, through unavoidable works such as those of Kleinmann and Charles Leslie, the definition of 'medical systems' and 'ethnomedicine' as the basic units of anthropological analysis, the approach to the various representations of illness as 'explanatory models', as the concomitant composite understanding through the concept of 'medical pluralism' [25–28].

From an early age, medical historians also understood that, both in terms of theorization and analysis, the history of medicine would necessarily have to integrate cultural, social, and economic conditions. The biography and intellectual and institutional work of Henry E. Sigerist demonstrate this. He wrote, "medicine is the most closely linked to the whole of culture, every transformation in medical conceptions being conditioned by transformations in the ideas of the epoch" [29] (p. 103). This aspect is particularly distinctive and created specific tensions with the historiographical orientations prevailing in other areas, namely in the history and philosophy of science, which has produced a direct controversy between Sigerist and George Sarton, the founder of this area [30–32].

There seems to be, in a way, an epistemological anomaly here since, while serving as foundational concepts for medical science, health and illness are also more general representations; they are notions endowed with values and closely related to certain practices. However, this is not an anomaly but a constitutive tension. At least since ancient Greece, medical vocation deals with the recognition of difference but also of peculiar fusion, to use Stephen Toulmin's terms, between the theoretical and the practical, the general and the particular, the universal and the existential [33]. While aiming at the great scale of the universal, medicine is linked to the mundane world, to the problems of human existence. That is why, even if we do not subscribe to a relativistic frame of reference, we must recognize the relativistic lesson that many of the non-scientific notions available in the field of health are not even properly pre-scientific, having different relationships with scientific theories. They can even be, to use a concept elaborated by Ludwik Fleck, 'proto-ideas', that is, not only ideas that further turn scientific but also a kind of ideas that remain in scientific substance as guiding principles, let alone subconsciously [34].

The constitutive distinction between the universal and the particular in medicine structured the humanist medical tradition [35,36] and, following medical humanism against technicism, maintains a great philosophical relevance in the face of the hegemonic threat of Western mercantile technoscience, namely in particularly sensitive cases of the transformation of nature and the human condition, where there is no need for intervention to preserve life, such as cosmetic surgery, human experimentation, some cases of genetic engineering, liberal eugenics, certain situations of human enhancement, some clinical scenarios of decision making, or even in some cases of normative, prescriptive, or regulatory health frameworks, whose critiques sometimes coincide with those of the critique of medicalization that we will explore later [37–47].

There are several grounds where we find the transposition of this foundational opposition. The scope of the analytical philosophy of health and medicine has been marked by a strong opposition that, in its own way, has transposed that distinction into a debate on the values associated with the medical and social conceptions of health and illness. This focus on values results from several developments in the natural sciences, in technologies for medical use and in medical practice, transformations in the fields of philosophy of science and philosophy of biology, and applications of the orientations known as analytic philosophy and phenomenology.

In particular, the debate was somewhat launched by the works of Christopher Boorse and was largely built around the commentary on Boorse's article "Health as a Theoretical Concept", published in 1977 [48,49]. In confrontation are, on the one hand, value-excluding naturalists, or neutralists, who, as in the case of Boorse's analytical approach and biostatistical theory of health, argue that the concept of health is determined by biology and is, therefore, a value-free notion. On the other hand, the value-entailing descriptivists, or normativists, for whom, as in the case of Lennart Nordenfelt's action-theoretic approach and holistic theory of health, health depends on elements of human agency, for whom assessing whether the sick subject can reach his vital goals is, therefore, a value-laden or value-relative notion [50,51]. Although the arguments on each side of the dispute remain the same, intermediate positions have been defended. It is worth mentioning K.W.M. Fulford's proposal of a bridge theory of illness, an advocate of values-based practice, for whom concepts of disease and social conceptions of health are structurally interdependent, as demonstrated by the fact that Boorse's theory implies evaluations, not being value-free, and Nordenfelt's theory implies biological criteria, not breaking with a certain dimension of scientific objectivity [52,53].

The same ground has also been plowed by physicians, philosophers, and social scientists who, independently but with numerous conceptual points of contact, have advocated a conceptual distinction between disease, on the one hand, as an objective abnormal condition based on the analysis of biological structures, functions, and changes, and illness as a subjective, or intersubjective, experience, whose analysis depends on psychological and social factors (e.g., [54,55]). In the context of the debate on values, the former would be value-free, while the latter would be value-laden.

At no point does the recognition of the value-ladenness or the contested nature of the notions of health and illness imply the rejection of the theoretical content of a natural-scientific point of view on these notions, nor the acceptance of a contrary approach, holistic, which links these concepts to all human life, paradoxically strengthening the processes of medicalization considered below. This discussion on values is crucial here, as it signals that the conflict generated around the HIMC does not reside only in ideas or representations but also in values, including the values that govern the selection of certain ideas or certain representations, to the detriment of others. This has been a subject insufficiently appreciated by social scientists. Despite those philosophical discussions, in the framework of the diverse social sciences, the idea of value-ladenness of health is mainly consensual but is broadly taken for granted. What is needed, for now, is to frame and organize the perspectives we have in more general frames.

For example, for Turner, following Mary Douglas, all these kinds of complexity seem to be able to be controlled by grasping the development of historical and cultural schemes around these categories and the respective phenomena, processes, or experiences they designate [12]. The reflexive transformation of these notions into systematic concepts implies a process of secularization, framing in scientific theories, the differentiation of several levels of conceptual application (such as physical health and psychological health), and the mutation of corresponding treatment practices among other aspects. This scheme helps to reduce the complexity of the contested concepts of health and illness (or even disease), but as soon as medicine is considered, one is again faced with a great increase in complexity.

These relatively introductory remarks allow us to understand that the relationships between the HIMC and society are complex, but they are not ideal formal relationships. They are not purely abstract nor historically necessary, but contingent-dependent material and conceptual relationships. The notions now mobilized also allow us to state that the multilevel conditions, variabilities, and tensions that characterize the relationship between the HIMC and society are not recent, nor can they be circumscribed only within a sphere of lay beliefs or rationalities. They are part of multiple views on health and medicine. For all these reasons, we can never take for granted the relationships between the HIMC and society. Anachronism and ethnocentrism are traps that we must avoid, at the cost of jeopardizing the understanding of our subject matter. We must make an effort to look at health–society relations independently, or only partially depending on, of the current medical configuration based on biology, the 'medical model' or 'biomedical model'. A less obvious effort, but one that we will also have to undertake, concerns the independence, or partial dependence, of these relations in terms of our understanding of society and, by extension, the ways in which the social sciences perceive, represent, and describe social life. In this sense, we must be suspicious of the excess offered by the biomedical model, as well as that given to us by an opposite 'social model'.

3. On the Acknowledged Internal Heterogeneity of Western Medicine

It is important to emphasize that Western medical theory, history, and practice are not homogeneous, which has long been known within the Western medical tradition and outside its borders. However, contrary to what today's dominant discourses conveyed by supposed experts in health care may imply, more through the media than in background inquiries, the release of doubts about medicine is neither just a product of contemporaneity, nor only reactive and inorganic conspiratorial action. The doubt about medicine, not of a question about a particular medical intervention but of a broader questioning horizon, is also an important part of Western philosophical, scientific, and artistic traditions and of the Western medical tradition itself. Notwithstanding their analytical relevance and substantive contribution, from a historical–critical point of view, it is not necessary to turn to the comparative studies of health and medicine, nor to the application of the ethnographic method to Western medicine itself to assert its diversity against a supposed unity. In other words, it is not necessary to come from the outside. Not least because, from within Western medicine, the acknowledged diversity is not limited to the circumscription of conceptual or practical variations, pointing to deep and multilevel re-articulations of that founding tension between the theoretical and the practical, the general and the particular, the universal and the existential.

We can recall different analytical topics that run through the very foundations of Western medical heterogeneity. In particular, the historical transformations of medicine have been widely considered. For instance, among the various dimensions that Scrimshaw, Lane, Rubinstein, and Fisher underline in the set of methodological and epistemological complexity referring to the chapters published in the book they edited is "the importance of historical depth" [11] (p. 7). However, besides this general call for attention, the discipline of medical history has specifically established its validity, legitimacy, and practice around the historical variation of several medical topics. Considering studies on medical history, but also the history of ancient science and public health history, we can indeed discover widespread recognition of historical variabilities of the concepts of health and illness, the ontological status of the body, the etiology of disease, medical theories, clinical practice, the role of the physician, hygiene and nutrition, lay attitudes towards medicine, and the human relation to death, among other similar subjects (e.g., [56–65]).

In addition to considering cultural variations in health, illness, and different therapeutic systems, in light of these areas of study, and also taking into account medical literature and works on the philosophy of medicine, we will be able to perceive how different modes of thought coexist in a single culture. First, we can mention the historical variants of the very organization of medical knowledge, such as anatomical tradition, microscopical tradition, physiological tradition, biochemical tradition, pathological tradition, and immunological tradition [66].

Second, structural variants of the organization of medical practice and activity can be mentioned. For instance, the great historian of Hellenistic and early Roman medicine Vivian Nutton forged the concept of a 'medical market-place' to refer to the fact that medical practice in the period of classical antiquity is characterized by a logic of marketplace trade [67,68]. Contrary to what the anachronistic application of contemporary notions of public health or social medicine to ancient medicine would suggest, medicine and physicians have not always, nor in the West, been linked to public good or function. In classical antiquity, the physician had an ambivalent social status, highly dependent on his patients and patrons. With ancient medicine being a science, contact with the patient's individuality forces us to speak of a 'science of the individual' [69]. There was no formal medical education nor regulation of medical practice. In fact, medical knowledge was widely accessible, being available according to individual literacy and socio-economic conditions. Moreover, there were lay people who could dispute without barriers the opinions of physicians, and also a bunch of healers of all kinds competing for the same type of opportunities. So, the doctor had to, in Nutton's economic language, know how to sell his knowledge.

Erwin H. Ackerknecht was responsible for periodizing the development of Western medicine in a classic phase of 'library medicine', later replaced by 'bedside medicine', and in turn, changed in the early 19th century in France to 'hospital medicine', having later been succeeded by 'laboratory medicine' [70]. This distinction and the central role of French hospitals, and specifically the Paris Clinical School, in this development remains a valid working hypothesis [71–75].

More recently, N. D. Jewson reformulated this distinction in a way that intersects the organization of medical knowledge and the organization of medical practice and activity [76]. Based on the notion of medical cosmology and the concept of the mode of production of medical knowledge, Jewson developed a correlation between the patron, the occupational role of the medical investigator, the source of patronage, the perception of the sick man, the occupational task of the medical investigator, and the conceptualization of illness. This type of conceptual proposal took on some prominence in the sociological approach, so the idea of medical cosmology shaped other analyses committed to capturing new distinctive characteristics both at the level of discourse, practices, and forms of medical knowledge. This is certainly what explains the existence of analytical proposals that, although emphasizing and problematizing different aspects of modern medicine, converge in the objective of trying to identify the dimensions that appear to be more structural in the way of thinking and doing medicine, such as 'surveillance medicine' [77], 'precision medicine' [78], and now 'digital medicine' [79], or 'translational medicine' [80]. It is the same unifying assumption that presides over those exercises.

Third, one can speak of the existence of internal ontological, epistemological, and practical variants of medical theory or, in other words, refer to the various branches of medicine in a broad sense, as for example, Hippocratic and Galenic humoralism or Louis Pasteur and Robert Koch's germ theory of disease. The range of the clusters in this regard can be highly variable, depending on the systems of classification of nature, body, disease, etc. A suitable designation to integrate these variants without disregarding them from the criteria of contemporary science lies in the expression 'medical pluralism'. As the great historian G.E.R. Lloyd recently argued from the study of Egyptian, Chinese, Greek, and Roman sources (in fact, in the explicit wake of Nutton), in the ancient medical marketplace, we find nothing but medical pluralism in the sense of complexity, diversity, and heterogeneity of practitioners and practices [81].

Different metaphysical and ethical conceptions of medicine can, fourthly, also be mentioned as one of those specific analytical topics that signal the internal heterogeneity of Western medicine. In classical antiquity, medicine, as Hans Jonas states in his great work *Das Prinzip Verantwortung*, would be the only domain of *techne* that was non-ethically neutral [45]. Given the unitary nature of the Hellenic way of life, several of these conceptions have played a structuring role in the history of medicine since antiquity. A clear example lies in the secular distinction between two dimensions of medicine, or two entirely different conceptualizations of it: medicine as a science and medicine as an art, *scientia medica* and *ars medica* [37,82].

However, this is not the only important issue in this context. As health and illness engender moral and theological bonds, metaphysical and ethical medical conceptions integrate the vast scopes of culture, morality, and politics. In this regard, it is worth bearing in mind that there is a notion of philosophy as a form of therapy being appreciated from classical antiquity to contemporary philosophy [83] and that, in the same context, especially in the frame of the *Corpus Hippocraticum*, medicine was established as what came to be understood not only as a form of humanism but also as a proper human science [22,36]. A similar meaning was accommodated by the contemporary conceptualization of medicine itself as a social science. This understanding of medicine as an art, as a human science, as a social science, or the very conception of medicine from a humanist point of view has been mainly mobilized to respond to conceptions not only more scientific but above all, more technological of medicine, having a non-negligible role in the organization of hospital services and in the articulation of, or resistance to, new movements within institutionalized medicine, such as evidence-based medicine or personalized medicine [84–87]. In turn, it is not alien to this nexus the correspondence of the idea of social science itself, especially that of sociology, with a form of medicine, a very common correspondence in the American sociological literature of the 20th century [88].

Fifthly, it will be very worthwhile to consider that doubts about medical knowledge, practices, values, and institutions and the effectiveness of the medical act are very old. In his fascinating book *The Word as Scalpel: A History of Medical Sociology*, Samuel W. Bloom places the genesis of medical sociology within the scope of a pattern of social change that includes conceptual and institutional transformations and writes that the different aspects of physicianhood "always evoked ambivalent response in society" [22] (p. 13). Of course, for the reasons outlined above, these doubts inhabit lay attitudes toward medicine from an early age to modern industrial societies. However, it is crucial to underline that there is an affinity between skepticism and medicine and that the latter is very ancient. Whatever the answer to the debates about the theoretical priority and the reciprocal influence between ancient philosophy and ancient medicine, as shown by John Christian Laursen in a recent text, "the practice of medicine and philosophical skepticism have gone hand in hand at several points in history", including authors such as Sextus Empiricus, the physician who is also the major source for ancient skepticism, or Francisco Sanches, Ernst Platner, or Martin Martinez [89] (p. 305). The most important thing to glean from this legacy seems to be not so much a closed sense of skepticism as a doctrine of radical uncertainty, but, as Maurice Raynaud points out, following Claude Bernard, the universal doubt and critical attitude that is characteristic of it, that is extended by the modern scientific spirit, and should also be present in medicine [90]. Without taking this into account, it is difficult to understand some contemporary views on health and how they articulate with, say, the self-criticism of Western medicine.

Even from a less skeptical point of view, but not less critical, there is no doubt that the results of medical interventions can be effectively ambivalent, carry error, and be followed by malpractice, which means, as abundantly documented (e.g., [91–93]), that they are not harmless or unproblematic in their effects and implications. There are, therefore, several substantive arguments for not slipping into a simple salvific exacerbation of medicine's successes or into a reified view of medicine's technical superiority. On the one hand, in the exercise of its practice, medicine is confronted with areas of indeterminacy, complexity, and contingency that signal the constitutive character of uncertainty and, thus, the always limited scope of its interventions [94]. Because the measurement of the effectiveness of this intervention is demonstrably lower than what is believed, Jacob Stegenga's recent research into medical skepticism, or even, in his own phrase, 'medical nihilism' in Western philosophical, scientific, artistic, and medical thought reinforces the importance of taking these doubts into account on a rational and argumentative level [95–97] (see also [98]).

On the other hand, despite many innovations and objective gains in health, multiple inequalities persist, reflecting structural tensions between economy, health, and politics, which means that the distribution of positive impacts in terms of health indicators is differentiated according to the hierarchical divisions of social stratification. This idea was famously presented, perhaps for the first time and within the scope of Western medicine, by Thomas McKeown, who argued that health improvement stems more from social change than from medical interventions [99–101]. Several government efforts have extended this point of view, which has crystallized in the publication of several important technical reports, such as the so-called 'Black Report' on Inequalities in Health of 1980, authored by the Department of Health and Social Security of the United Kingdom [102], and more recently in the creation of the Commission on Social Determinants of Health by the World Health Organization, with a specific research agenda (see [103]).

It is important to note that this agenda has been challenged by the explicit criticism of some of its socio-political assumptions and the search for a redefinition of the relations between the HIMC and society attentive to health structural inequalities and injustices from the individual and community recognition of the right to health [104–106]. This is happening in a macroeconomic environment with long-term growth of the gross domestic product rates of Global South nations and their statehoods, now accelerated and impacting healthcare spending [107–110]. Accordingly, the Low and Middle-Income Countries (LMICs), the South Eastern European countries (SEE), the leading emerging markets of

Brazil, Russia, India, China, and South Africa (BRICS), or the Emerging Markets Seven (EM7), the MIST nations (Mexico, Indonesia, South Korea, and Turkey), the Central Asian Republics Information Network (CARINFONET), or the Association of Southeast Asian Nations (ASEAN), have been recognized as an economic and social driving force, despite facing specific epidemiological difficulties.

4. Social Control and the Realist-Negative Modality of Medicalization

One of the classic and most consolidated currents of the social study of health, illness, and medicine explicitly expresses the variabilities and conflicts just alluded around the HIMC and society and the respective tensions between medicine and the social sciences. Early on, a substantial part of the theoretical heritage that was being developed in the context of sociology regarding the role and action of medicine followed a critical vision of the growing power and permanent expansion of the medical profession, conceived as a form of regulatory action whose more tangible effects were translated into effective mechanisms for social control of deviant behavior. One of the concepts that, in this context, gained prominence and widespread acceptance was that of medicalization. It ended up giving rise to an abundant theoretical–empirical streak. This concept takes us from the domain of the variations in the concepts of health, illness, and medicine and throws us into the field of medical feedback from society.

We believe that it is possible to sustain the thesis that medicalization critique, as a very heterogeneous movement, constitutes a paradigmatic illustration of the difficult coalescence of the perspectives between the HIMC and society and, simultaneously, the perspectives between the social sciences and medicine. It was, and maybe still is, a potential source of extraordinary theoretical inventiveness in the field of the social sciences in dialogue with medicine and an excellent base of thematic issues for thinking about the new pandemic age.

Medicalization critique today has vast intellectual patrimony. We know in our days that several authors developed the concept of medicalization, that it was inscribed in different disciplinary areas and theoretical–empirical approaches, that it integrated different political families, that it was thus still supported by different assumptions and starting hypotheses, but also that it served purposes and was developed in different contexts, that it was focused on a wide range of historical periods, empirical areas and objects, cut according to the most diverse sampling processes and interpretative horizons. This rich heritage ended up being translated into the accumulation of semantic layers around its meaning, the very definition of the term 'medicalization'.

Joseph E. Davis argues that from the 1990s onward, medicalization theorists tried to give the concept greater generalizability, but the result was excessive, causing the concept to become "a complete muddle" and lose "its way" [111] (p. 51). As Rafaela Teixeira Zorzanelli, Francisco Ortega, and Benilton Bezerra Júnior argue in a more recent article, this generalization created disagreements and great conceptual confusion [112]. Based on an excellent analysis of the uses of the term 'medicalization' by different authors and in various contexts between 1950 and 2010, Zorzanelli, Ortega, and Júnior reject the possibility of a definitive definition of the concept of medicalization, suggesting a set of possible and not necessarily excluding specific meanings of the term. Due to the need for theoretical attention and precision, without neglecting the conceptual complexity of medicalization and its cultural, historical, and local boundaries, those authors also stand for 'transitivity' as a necessary principle for the use of this concept, that is, that such use should be followed by the specification of the particular meaning of the term and the respective object under analysis.

Here, we look for what Zorzanelli, Ortega, and Júnior call the "common conceptual ground" of medicalization critique [112] (p. 1860). However, unlike these authors, we do not do so directly through the definitions established by Peter Conrad, the contemporary author who would become the main reference in the field of medicalization critique. In this text, we do not have a particular interest in the exegesis of the work of this or that author but in the critique of medicalization understood as a whole. For this, it is perhaps not necessary to admit the transitivity of the concept of medicalization as a determining principle of the critique of medicalization, but rather to understand this critique as a historically situated movement and to ascertain to what extent the previous principle emerges, or not, from the process of conceptual formation itself.

In a chapter discussing Michel Foucault's contributions to the understanding of medical knowledge, practice, and encounter, Deborah Lupton establishes a comprehensive framework that fits the diversity of perspectives on the concept of medicalization [113]. It is from Lupton that we retain the expression 'the medicalization critique', or more especially 'the orthodox medicalization critique'. The transversal and general reading evoked by these designations allow us to capture the arguments of the original proponents, but it also enables the reassessment of new critical scrutiny and analytical contributions and the incorporation of new actors and new dynamics in the reconfiguration of what is understood as the very process of medicalization.

Following Uta Gerhardt, Lupton's genealogy of medicalization critique begins with the Marxist and liberal humanist perspectives underlying social movements emerging in Europe in the 1960s and 1970s. As justice and inequality acquired legitimacy in academic research, several authors began to underline the relevance of "individual freedom, human rights and social change" and at the same time criticize "the ways that society is structured", including the scrutiny of the "social role played by members of powerful and high-status occupational groups such as the legal and medical professions" [113] (p. 95). According to Lupton, medicalization critique would become one of the most dominant sociological perspectives in the 1970s and the 1980s, remaining largely dominant in the 1990s in Marxist, feminist, and consumerist-based works. This development implied accusing Talcott Parsons' structural functionalism, which commanded medical sociology in the previous decades, of political conservatism, namely of reproducing medical authority. As we will see, the break with the structural functionalism view of social order in general and the sick role in particular is supported by an even more general epistemological transition in sociology, mainly guided by the development of symbolic interactionism, labeling theory, phenomenological sociology, ethnomethodology, and the dialogue with the anti-psychiatric movement and several political movements [88], but it did not dispense the sociological analysis of the Parsonian account of illness as deviance.

The term 'medicalization' was coined by the American sociologist Jesse Pitts in 1968 in an *International Encyclopedia of Social Sciences* entry on the concept of social control [114] (pp. 390–392). The set of works consensually considered classic in medicalization literature includes articles, chapters, and books authored by Eliot Freidson, Irving Zola, Ivan Illich, Thomas Szasz, Michel Foucault, Catherine Kohler Riessman, Howard Waitzkin, and Peter Conrad, although some of these authors did not regularly use the term 'medicalization'. Other works of reference will be considered later in our paper, such as those of Renée C. Fox and Philip M. Strong [1,115]. However, it is important to emphasize that, in addition to the classics, different authors can be pointed out as pioneers of the movement, according to the subscribed definition of medicalization and the effective field of its application. In a brief period prior to the 1960s, even before the concept of medicalization was coined, systematized, and disseminated, some of the understanding of the process described by this concept was established within the scope of the study of the development of psychiatry and around the idea of mental illness. Some specific works of Barbara Wootton, Thomas Szasz, and Thomas J. Scheff from the 1950s and 1960s are, in this sense, identified as pioneers in the critique of medicalization [116–121]. Some of those works are cited by the classics themselves. In this sense, it can already be advanced that psychiatrization can be understood as an internal variant of medicalization and, at the same time, the 'critique of psychiatrization' as an internal variant of the critique of medicalization.

Proponents of the medicalization critique, as Lupton demonstrates, will argue in different ways that, with this process, medicine, medical discourses and practices, and also medicine allied professions and care structures become increasingly powerful, influential, and dominant. The central thesis shared by those authors is that, following the scientificization and professionalization of medicine, there was an extension of the monopoly of the field of medical practices, medical jurisdiction, and its expert authority to more and more aspects of life. Medical intervention in the management of human life has increased; its scope is indefinite and potentially ubiquitous. This idea would correspond, in conceptual terms, to the reduction of a growing set of social and political problems to medical problems, treatable according to the practices of professional medicine, namely through drug therapies.

According to each author, the focus of theorization, analysis, and criticism had been placed on different segments of this process, such as, continuing to follow Lupton, the medical error, the putative lack of effectiveness of medical treatments, or the side-effects of medical intervention, the reproduction of all sorts of social and economic inequalities in the medical encounter and in the medical definitions of illness and disease, the identification of the medical profession as a patriarchal institution, or the increase in dependence of lay people or, on the contrary, the loss of their autonomy. According to June S. Lowenberg and Fred Davis, the conceptualizations of medicalization bring together three main components: causality conceptions and locus of causality, the purview of the pathogenic sphere, and professionalized unequal status relationships between providers and clients [122].

Although we are not interested in a detailed exegesis, it is important to understand the aspects that each main orthodox author added to the concept. In Pitts' foundational text, the concept of medicalization manifests itself with transitive character; that is, it is not formulated as a general process, as medicalization as such, but specifically as 'medicalization of deviance'. This formulation resulted, on the one hand, from the analysis of social control arising primarily from the American sociological tradition and, on the other hand, from the consideration of the influence of Freudian thought since the 1920s upon the social organization of stigma and penal sanctions. Looking at illness as a pattern of deviance, Parsons' approach is one of the main sources for Pitts to correlate illness, deviance, and social control. In this context, the term 'medicalization' designates the process of "redefining certain aspects of deviance as illness rather than crime" [114] (p. 390). In the same framework, this process implies reassessing individual responsibility and assessing unconscious psychological motivation in understanding illness, followed by the respective therapeutic practice.

Therefore, in Pitts' paper, the concept of medicalization was also linked to a psychological and social dimension of illness, namely the control of people classified as mentally ill. Another crucial aspect of this first formulation is found in its critical but not entirely negative sense. Pitts accepts that there may be some decrease in individual autonomy through the medicalization process, including political castration of the deviant and threat of their civil liberties. Nevertheless, he believes that medicalization can be a more humanized method of controlling deviance than imprisonment. In his words, "social control becomes more humane and forgiving, but perhaps also more relentless and pervasive" [114] (p. 391). Pitts considers that medicalization may also be more effective than the judicial method, as the medical and paramedical professions will resist corruption and political pressure more than the judicial and parajudicial professions.

The point of view introduced by Freidson is unavoidable. As Fredric D. Wolinsky underlines, in this author's work, it is not only the issue of the emergence (and organization) of the medical profession that arises but also, as part of his theory of professions, a perspective on professional dominance [123]. Freidson, in fact, rarely uses the term 'medicalization', and when he does, implicitly or explicitly, it is framed by his theory of professions, by his empirical evaluation of the dominant autonomous professions, and fits his idea of dominance as can be seen in his book *Professional Dominance: The Social Structure of Medical Care* [124]. We cannot fail to say that in his best-known work, his book on the profession of medicine, Freidson does not even use the word 'medicalization'. It appears only in the recourse to the citation of Pitts' foundational text in the chapter "The Professional Construction of Concepts of Illness" [125]. In Wolinsky's concise and accurate words, it can be said that the essence of the professional dominance perspective developed by Freidson has to do with two crucial aspects: the definition of the medical profession as an occupation that has achieved 'organized autonomy' or 'self- direction' and that this autonomy is structurally guaranteed, namely through formal institutions, in such a way that the profession can be self-regulating. According to Wolinsky, this perspective was addressed by the observation of a progressive erosion of the autonomy of the medical profession. The notions of deprofessionalization, mainly developed by Marie Haug, and that of proletarianization, mobilized, for example, by John McKinlay, have served to criticize the point of view of domination and thus question medical power as a professional power.

Here, we are facing an important disciplinary and epistemological event. A disciplinary event is before us; it is profoundly known but seldom recognized and rarely noted: there is an agreement between the sociology of professions and the sociology of medicine—the first is dependent on the high relevance of the medical profession in the system of professions, while the former needs a theory of professions and methods to explain and understand health care systems. Eliot Freidson's life and work, in its entirety, are the perfect example of the intersection between the sociology of professions and the sociology of health [126–128]. However, it should be noted that this relationship does not occur only in the professional domination version of the medicalization critique but in the entire scope of the orthodox understanding of this critique and the respective repressive–negative modality of medicalization. A clear example of this lies in republishing Irving Kenneth Zola's main text on medicalization in a collective anthological volume that did not include Freidson's participation, which was organized around Ivan Illich's notion of 'disabling professions' [129].

As it began to structure itself based on the experimental sciences, medicine acquired greater disciplinary coherence and a new scientific identity that was fundamental to its growing institutional power and the cultural legitimacy of the profession [130]. From the perspective of some of the authors responsible for the sociological approach to the power of professions, medicine is precisely a paradigmatic case of a profession whose institutionalization has historically translated into the ability to convert its specific and professional knowledge into organized forms of power, which proved to be fundamental for the defense of its jurisdiction [131], as it ensures a space of expertise protected from external interference from other groups and actors [125,132,133].

The emergent conventional narrative of medical sociology as a subdiscipline repeatedly associated with Parsons wrongly assumes that the theorizing heritage of the classic founders of sociology would denote an alleged alienation regarding health and illness [134,135]. Now, not only is this postulate debatable, but this whitening is particularly illuminating for the sociological project itself in terms of disciplinary institutionalization. Since its emergence as a subdiscipline, there has been a well-established division of labor between sociology and medicine. In the case of the sociological approach, specialization resulting from this division influences criticism directed at the biophysical approach of medicine, building, from there, the study of the dimensions that are excluded from the medical perspective.

The analysis privileges the social interpretation of reality, condensed, for example, in the distinction between illness and disease, fundamental in Parsons' foundations of the sociology of medicine, subscribed by Freidson and crucial as a basis for the conception of the analysis of the emergence and professional dominance of medicine [136]. It supports the assumption that medicine has the exclusive right to approach the biological body and its pathologies, while sociology strictly focuses on the social. This relegation of classical approaches has made us forget not only some sociological theories about disease, health, and mortality but also, and especially, the content of various critical approaches to the emerging biologism, vitalism, the new physiology, or pathological anatomy [137], which resulted in the gradual uncritical incorporation of the idea that the medical notion of illness constitutes a stabilized biological and physiological fact. The suppression of illness in sociological analysis can thus be understood as an illustrative indicator of the dynamics of disciplinary differentiation and professionalization since it seeks to base itself on a focus on the social as explanatory nexus.

A crucial article for the systematic development of the concept of medicalization was published by Irving Kenneth Zola in 1972 [138]. It had an expressive title: "Medicine as an Institution of Social Control". This document resulted from a residency at the Netherlands Institute for Preventive Medicine in Leiden and a subsequent presentation at the Medical Sociology Conference of the British Sociological Association in Weston-Super-Mare, in November 1971. In this article, there is significant generalization of the concept of medicalization. The transitive character of this concept seems to be relatively dissipated by this generalization. Zola no longer speaks of the medicalization of deviance but, in his terms, of the 'medicalizing of society'.

According to Zola, the practice of medicine has always been "inextricably interwoven into society" [138] (p. 488). Additionally, this relationship is not only *de facto* but also *de jure*; that is, medicine has always had a normative role. In historical terms, Zola finds in psychiatry the main scope for dealing with social deviance and in public health a fundamental field for the transformation of diverse aspects of social life. However, the author argues that the critique of medicalization cannot be reduced to a critique of psychiatrization since the psychiatric profession "by no means distorted the mandate of medicine" and, at most, carried out this mandate at a faster pace [138] (p. 487). Zola also rejects the thesis that medical involvement in social problems removes them from religious and legal spheres, demoralizing them. On the contrary, recovering the link between the concepts of medicalization and social control, he believes medicine "is becoming a major institution of social control, nudging aside, if not incorporating, the more traditional institutions of religion and law" [138] (p. 487). Explicitly relying on Freidson, Zola highlights the relevance of the correlation between the medical profession and the jurisdiction over the label 'illness'. Nevertheless, he moves away from a reading that reduces medicalization or its causes to 'professional imperialism', understood as an intentional action by medical professionals. For Zola, medicalization is not, nor does it result from, an intentional process.

Furthermore, Zola thinks it also does not come from the medical class' political influence or political power, nor does it consist only of an expansion of medical jurisdiction. For Zola, there is indeed an extension of medical jurisdiction and an extension of the physician's power, but he understands medicalization as a more insidious issue, reaching beyond the medical profession itself. It resides precisely in "medicalizing much of daily living, by making medicine and the labels 'healthy' and 'ill' relevant to an ever-increasing part of human existence" [138] (p. 487). Zola proposes to categorize medicalization in four concrete ways. First, following the change from a specific to a multi-causal etiological model of disease, medicalization takes place through the expansion of what in life is deemed relevant to the understanding, prevention, and treatment of disease, followed by the emergence of forms of social control. Finding roots for medicalization in the "increasingly complex technological and bureaucratic system" [138] (p. 487), which fosters extreme confidence in the figure of experts, Zola cannot fail to note, secondly, that medicalization is also carried out through the expansion of the use of medical devices, medical evidence, and medical rhetoric to explain what is good in individual, social, political, and economic life. Medical judgment is not based on virtue or legitimacy but on the label 'health'. Thirdly, the same process of medicalization lies in the retention of access to taboo in areas of mental and social life, including in the medical field natural processes such as aging and pregnancy and social issues such as drug addiction and alcoholism. Medicalization thus goes far beyond organic disease; the question becomes what can be labeled as an 'illness' or 'medical problem'. We are facing a growing list of human conditions and daily activities. Many other cases of cultural, social, and political situations are mentioned by Zola, such as male circumcision, abortion, child abuse, sterilization, sex change operations, homosexuality, drug use, or dieting. Eventually, lay people themselves attribute organic problems to some of these conditions. Nevertheless, medicalization is also made, fourthly, of the retention of control over some procedures, namely the right to carry out surgery and prescribe drugs, not only placing the body and mental life under medical care but also doing it under criteria that go beyond organic repair and include moral and aesthetic standards. Therefore, medicalization, as conceptualized by Zola, is followed by processes of moralization. The danger, for Zola, lies not only in masking these processes as strictly scientific and technical but also in being for 'our own good'.

Illich reformulated the critique of medicalization through the concept of iatrogenesis and with a frame of reference inspired by the critique of the political economy of industrialization. Other authors, namely Vicente Navarro and Howard Waitzkin [7,139], also focused on the criticism of medicalization from issues of the political economy. However, Illich's vision stands out because he is usually pointed out as the most radical critic of medicalization. He was recently appointed, together with Zola, as responsible for an 'extreme Medicalisation thesis' [140] (see also [141,142]), which we will see makes little sense when we look at the Foucauldian point of view.

In *Medical Nemesis. The Expropriation of Health*, Illich hypothesizes that there are three levels of iatrogenesis: first, clinical iatrogenesis, which concerns the undesirable effects of the medical system; second, social iatrogenesis, which concerns the sponsorship of disease by medical practice, encouraging diverse forms of preventive medicine; third, cultural or structural iatrogenesis, which is related to the inculcation of health improvement with a current value, as a commodity [143]. For Illich, iatrogenesis has become medically irreversible at each of its three levels. Illich also considers that whenever an attempt is made to avoid harm to the patient, a loop of negative institutional feedback is created, which he calls 'medical nemesis'. Illich seeks to recover the figure of Nemesis from Greek mythology. According to the author, for the Greeks, Nemesis represented divine revenge on mortals who went beyond the limits of the human, looking for what the gods kept for themselves. Nemesis was the inevitable punishment for attempts to be a hero instead of a human. As a deity, it represented nature's response to arrogance, to the individual's presumption in seeking to acquire the attributes of a god. By invoking ancestral myths and gods, Illich sought to clarify that his framework for analyzing the collapse of medicine is alien to industrially determined logic and ethos. Therefore, he rejects the use of bureaucratic, therapeutic, or ideological language.

What can be conceived as this initial vision or as the more general or orthodox perspective of the medicalization critique began with the identification of medicalization as the social–cultural and political–economic process through which the function or role of social regulation traditionally exercised by religion and law is now being carried out by medicine. It can accordingly be argued that there is a continuity between the broader processes of Western secularization and modernization and the understanding of medicalization [144]. If we consider that this process, so understood, inaugurates a new era in social development, 'the medicalization era', recovering the title of the book directed by Pierre Aïach and Daniel Delanoe, we can, at the same time, as the subtitle of the same book points out, speculate about the emergence of a new type of human, or a social specification of the species, the *Homo sanitas* [145].

Despite all the differences, the group of authors that can be considered orthodox share not only the previously mentioned thesis but also an ontological, epistemological, and normative orientation. The view subscribed by these authors is realist and negative. For them, medicalization is a real but undesirable process. As Lupton writes, "the term 'medicalisation' is generally used in the sociological literature in a pejorative manner", "to be 'medicalised' is never a desirable state of being" [113] (p. 96), "Medicalization is typically represented as negative, a repressive and coercive process" [113] (p. 106). This perspective is based on a notion of power as "a property of social groups" and in a respective concept of social control [113] (p. 106). In this context, the concept of medicalization points out the limitation of the field of freedom, thought, and action of the individual and the community to which he belongs by a dominant social, cultural, economic, and political structure. This perspective can be extended directly into a "negative view of members of the medical profession", concerning power relations, in the sense of "seeing doctors as attempting to enhance their position by presenting themselves as possessing the exclusive right to define and treat illness" [113] (p. 96).

When we look at the previously mentioned group of authors as a whole, we see that, despite textual variations here and there, they share a set of assumptions that allow us to speak not only of a semantic sense of medicalization but of a whole modality of this process. We prefer to speak of modalities of medicalization, and corresponding versions of the critique of medicalization insofar as the expression 'modality' allows us to underline a process of a specific type as a counterpoint to a perspective on certain processes of this or another type. Talking about different modalities implies recognizing some degree of existence, which may have been discovered through specific discussions, but which is not reduced to the discursive layer that puts them in evidence.

In this case, in epistemological terms, their vision is supported by a realistic epistemological conception, followed by an explicitly critical normative conception, directly dependent on the negative evaluation of this process which is called medicalization as real. For authors who subscribe to a version of the repressive–negative critique of medicalization, such conceptions translate into the understanding of certain phenomena of the social and political order as medicalizable, while others would be of a natural, biological order—illnesses, let us say, truly acceptable as illnesses. As Thomas Szasz mentions within the opening of his book *The Medicalization of Everyday Life*, the concept of medicalization "rests on the assumption that some phenomena belong in the domain of medicine, and some do not" [146] (p. xiii). That is, for this author, there are, in fact, some phenomena that belong to this domain. The question is truly about 'over-medicalization' (see [147,148]). The example he offers us is crystal clear: "we speak of the medicalization of homosexuality and racism, but do not speak of the medicalization of malaria or melanoma" [146] (p. xiii).

In the context of such an understanding, according to Lupton, orthodox critics of medicalization end up considering that medicalization is a two-way process, being possible and desirable to diminish medical power and restore some power to lay people through demedicalization strategies. Lupton mentions challenging medical rights, knowledge, and decisions, empowering patients, promoting engagement in preventive health activities, patient advocacy groups, or even seeking the attention of alternative practitioners, and encouraging greater state regulation over the actions of the medical profession to limit its expansion or even to deprofessionalize it. Through these demedicalization strategies, lay people could 'take back control' over their own health. In this respect, critics of medicalization are very close to the bioethical discourse on patient autonomy (see [149]).

5. Medicalization and Varieties of Imperialism

We can recognize a focus of tension in the relationship between medicalization and imperialism that deserves further clarification in the critical reactions to the discourse on medicalization found in the sociological literature. In the 1970s, some sociologists began to critically limit the critical perspective on medicalization itself, addressing a specific internal tension. The best-known cases are the article "The Medicalization and Demedicalization of American Society", published in 1977 by Renée C. Fox [1], and Philip M. Strong's article "Sociological Imperialism and the Profession of Medicine—A Critical Examination of the Thesis of Medical Imperialism", published in 1979 [115].

The semantic field of imperialism is quite vast, which forces us to establish that there is a whole genealogy of imperialism that goes beyond the content of these texts and the work of these authors. According to *The Cambridge Dictionary of Sociology*, the term 'imperialism' refers to the indefinite expansion of the territorial sovereignty of a political unit [150]. Furthermore, it articulates diverse sociological and political notions, such as capitalism and colonialism. In both cases, concomitant forces are at play with imperialist ambitions of territorial acquisition and multilevel forms of control and domination. In turn, the plasticity of this type of force allows us to think about different varieties of imperialism. There is little doubt that various contemporary processes of globalization have made the cultural variety of imperialism, the so-called 'cultural imperialism', one of the most discussed.

The specific variety of what is designated by the expression 'medical imperialism' is used more sparingly, almost always going back to Strong's text, but the introduction of this formulation has been traced back to a letter by the physicians Herbert A. Schreier and Lawrence Berger, published in 1974 in *The Lancet* [151] and which Strong does not cite. In its foundational usage, the term is used widely as a synonym for colonialism, economic, and cultural imperialism. For Schreier and Berger, the term 'medical imperialism' designates "the use of foreign populations, for example, by American corporations, Federal agencies, and private foundations, for American ends" [151] (p. 1161). Starting by talking about the economic exploitation of the antibiotic drug chloramphenicol, then also referring to the tobacco industry and the use of cyclamates, those authors argue that giant multinational corporations based in the US, despite international regulation, promote sales abroad and earn billions of dollars in foreign sales of products whose internal consumption is at least scientifically contextualized or even limited.

The concept of medical imperialism was later used by several authors, including some critics of medicalization or connoisseurs of medicalization critique. Nevertheless, not all retained the same meaning. In his book, *Medicine Out of Control. The Anatomy of a Malignant Technology*, also published in 1979, the same year as Strong's article, Richard Taylor directly addressed and developed the concept as forged by Schreier and Berger [152]. Illich, in turn, understands medicalization as a form of medical colonization and refers to the letter of these authors but does not mobilize the concept of imperialism in these terms [143].

Most researchers associate this notion with another variety of imperialism, 'professional imperialism'. This variety is perfectly harmonized with the Parsonian association between social control undertaken by physicians and their belonging to a professional complex. In fact, it seems to have been from there, even if not accepting the structural-functionalist program, extended by the sociology of professions through the approach of professional analysis of medicine. This intersection in the critique of medicalization already occurred, paradoxically, after Zola argued that medicalization did not result from any professional imperialism. Such a variety may have been first formulated by Howard B. Waitzkin and Barbara Waterman, also in 1974, when they considered the international, institutional, and interpersonal levels of medical imperialism [153]. As mentioned, Freidson's life and work exemplify the intersection between the sociology of professions and the sociology of health, but the author rarely mobilized the concept of medical imperialism, having preferred to speak of professional domination.

In Fox's and Strong's works, the intersection is more corpulent, critical, and directly related to medicalization critique. We can find here an analytical autonomization of the tension between medicine and the social sciences, specifically sociology, an approximation with greater consistency than usual.

Fox puts us in front of one of the first critiques of the medicalization critique. Since this is a sociological work that does not entirely deny the medicalization critique, we are not dealing with an external critique but with what can be understood as an internal critique or a meta-sociological critique. According to Fox, the complexity of the medicalization process and its putative inconsistency, widely understood by the author in terms of the realist–negative medicalization modality, make its analysis difficult. The vast extension of the implied notion of illness does not allow defining illness itself in a strict sense, either as "objective reality", "a subjective state", or "a societal construct" [1] (p. 11). However, the author considers that the main difficulties in the analysis of the medicalization process stem from two sorts of assumptions made by critics of medicalization in America. The first is that "the central and pervasive position of health, illness, and medicine in present-day American society is historically and culturally unique" [1] (p. 13). The second is that "it is primarily a result of the self-interested maneuvers of the medical profession" [1] (p. 13). Fox believes that neither of these assumptions can be taken to be true without further clarification.

Throughout his text, he seeks to defend that younger health professionals, political activists, and also some social scientists, reacting to what they consider to be "over medicalization" with a discursive and practical countertrend process of demedicalization, contended the historical and cultural transience of medical categories [1] (p. 17) (see also [147,148]). The very concept of illness, for example, and there is no doubt about that, is considered to vary between cultures and over time. Fox also argues that the HIMC designates a broad nexus, which involves several structures (biological, social, psychological, cultural) and institutions (economic, magic, religious, scientific), in such a way that the current process of medicalization in American society could not result exclusively from the privileged action of physicians.

Additionally, focusing on the criticism of medicalization and the advocacy of demedicalization, Fox argues that there are apparently opposite transformation movements. On the one hand, the gradual emergence of a conception of health as a right would entail major conceptual rather than structural shifts, while, on the other hand, particular effective processes of demedicalization would concern a transformation of structures and values.

Strong's text seems more relevant to us. His critique can also be considered within the framework of a meta-sociological critique of the perspective of medicalization critique. Nevertheless, it operates from a reformulation of this perspective. In this sense, it is also, shall we say, a sociological meta-critique. Strong's starting point is to reformulate not the process of medicalization in any applied sense or directed to any particular condition, but in a very vast sense, also here coincident with the realist–negative modality. This generality constitutes a focus of attention and interest for the author. According to Strong, it is the generality encompassed by medicalization that attracted several researchers, including himself, to the study of this process. This occurred because the conceptualization of this process would make it possible to frame in an overall picture smaller problems in scale, concrete research findings, and even looser ideas arising from readings and everyday experiences.

Based on his generalist perspective, Strong proposed to reformulate medicalization as a form of imperialism, which the author specifically calls the 'thesis of medical imperialism'. The critique of medicalization is thus understood in terms of a critique of medical imperialism. However, as can be seen from the title of his article, Strong's purpose is the critical introduction of a sociological kind of imperialism. That is why he presents his essay as controversial. According to Strong, the thesis of medical imperialism arose from the general sociological analysis of professional ambition and constituted influential developments in the sociologies of deviance and medicine. Strong does not neglect the merits of this thesis of medical imperialism, nor does he abandon the reflection upon the conditions for successful medicalization. However, he considers this thesis, this critique, "both exaggerated and self-serving" [115] (p. 199).

For Strong, the same type of analysis that underlies this thesis could be applied to sociology, providing, in its own programmatic synthesis,

> "a more satisfactory theory of professional change, one which explains the appeal of both conservatism and radicalism at different points in a profession's trajectory. Applying this to medical sociology, it is argued that current critiques of medical expansion, although containing much that is of value, are in some places misleading or exaggerated, for this young discipline and its ally, public health, have a vested interest in the diminution of the present form of the medical empire. Moreover, the social model of health which they themselves prefer is in some ways a better vehicle for medical imperialism than the much abused 'medical model'" [115] (p. 199).

This constitutes the reason why it can be said that Strong's perspective is, at the same time, a meta-sociological critique and a sociological meta-critique. In our view, his reformulation of the critique of medicalization as anti-imperialism, as a variety of imperialism critique, a kind of mirror effect of the critique of medicalization, is perhaps the highest point that the tension between medicine and the social sciences has reached. Furthermore, we believe that understanding the reformulation of the critique of medicalization as anti-imperialism is a *conditio sine qua non* so that, in further research, we can make intelligible how this tension reaches a critical situation an even more critical point, in the present pandemic context.

Some authors believe that this reformulation is, in itself, greatly exaggerated. In the commentary tradition that has established itself around Strong's work, Peter Conrad will be largely responsible for recovering the idea first advanced by Zola in the frame of reference of the medicalization critique that medicalization cannot be explanatorily reduced to the thesis of professional imperialism.

Seeking to support this critique of critical criticism, Conrad and Joseph W. Schneider published a commentary on "Strong's Critique of the Thesis of Medical Imperialism" as early as 1980, in the same journal in which Strong had published his text one year before [154]. The theme was recovered in several texts by the same authors [155,156]. Conrad and Schneider recognize the value of Strong's positionings. Overall, they positively evaluate the idea of Strong's proposal of a reflexive analysis of medical sociology. They think, for instance, that the author rightly corrects oversimplified conceptions and exaggerated claims about medical imperialism. They also consider that Strong is quite right to point out that sociology is a profession and that, as such, it maintains its own interests. Conrad and Schneider believe, in particular, that the growing professional interest of sociologists in the medical field may well represent "the appeal of the social attractions and rewards" in this domain [154] (p. 76).

Despite this, Conrad and Schneider feel that Strong's approach has several serious shortcomings. Essentially, the authors argue that Strong has a narrow view of medicalization, missing the complexity of the concept and the perception of the various contexts of occurrence and study of the respective process. For both, the understanding of medicalization as imperialism is reductive and normative, and its sociological corollary is inconsistent. Such an understanding does not correspond to the concept of medicalization employed by several critics, such as Zola, thus blurring the diverse argumentative distinctions that follow the debates on medicalization. This is a reductive understanding because, resulting from Strong's own ethnographic field research on doctor–patient interaction, medicalization is thought of by this author only at the level of these interactions, leaving aside the conceptual and institutional levels and the political and definitional character of medicalization. This understanding is normative since it imputes to the concept of medicalization motives, a load of intentionality, which is not only not defended by critics such as Zola but which is very difficult to verify empirically, not seeming to be verified in Conrad and Schneider's own historical research on the medicalization of deviance. In this context, these authors suggest "to conceptualize the expansion of medical jurisdiction as *medicalization*, which is a more descriptive term" [154] (p. 75).

Considering the sociological corollary of the understanding of medicalization as imperialism also involves unverified intentionality, since the sociological profession cannot expand its potential jurisdiction in the same way as the medical profession, since it has no individual clients, has no direct prescriptions, nor can it provide the satisfaction of such a direct intervention, Conrad and Schneider further consider this corollary to be inconsistent because, while the analysis of medical imperialism focuses on the level of doctor-patient interaction, the analysis of sociological imperialism is only dealt with at the conceptual level. Ultimately, Conrad and Schneider consider this corollary irrelevant to medicalization thought. In our view, it is the opposite: the idea of sociological imperialism represents a step forward in the tensions between health and society to which we cannot be indifferent.

Despite the pertinence of Conrad and Schneider's critical response observations, a good part of the evaluation of Strong's arguments presented by these authors, provided with a comprehensive source of case studies in the context of medicalization critique, is nothing more than a corrective of short range. In addition to the major foci of criticism, Conrad and Schneider accuse Strong of grossly simplifying the attended difficulties and respective perspectives on them, of having been selective in his examples, of ignoring the then-recent literature on medicalization, of inventing problems that can be considered false, of underestimating modern medicine's technical achievements and overstating some constraining forces, namely that of the modern capitalist state. However, all these accusations are followed by notes of argumentative agreement. The variation is not of substance but of degree. Therefore, in our opinion, Conrad's and Schneider's statements, taken together, demonstrate Strong's creativity rather than the imminent failure of his argument.

Notwithstanding the recognition achieved in the meantime by Strong's formulation of the thesis of medical imperialism, and although several of the criticisms pointed out by Conrad and Schneider are legitimate, perfectly acceptable, and accurate, the substance of some of them were previously considered within the framework of the limitations presented by the author himself. The question will eventually be to ponder the extent to which Strong was coherent in recognizing his limitations; that is, if and when he overstepped the limits he recognized in his own work. For the sake of our argument, we must then rehearse his view once again.

6. The Professional Variety of the Negative Modality of Medicalization

The thesis of medical imperialism is expounded by Strong as a segment of a broader thesis of 'professional imperialism'. In Strong's view, this is a general thesis, applicable to all professions, revealed by the "general debunking of professional pretensions", particularly by the "general sociological analysis of professional ambition", and revealing special danger in the case of professions that accumulate more power [115] (p. 199).

The thesis of professional imperialism is summarized by the author through the exposition of a set of basic assumptions. There is an elementary tendency for handling social problems to be assigned to full-time professions and professionals. Certain professions monopolize the provision of certain solutions or services. This provisioning tends to control that service's nature and normative criteria. Such control tends, in turn, to expand beyond its original remit, redefining problems in other areas and discovering new problems whose solutions can only be provided by its professionals. This expansion is potentially indefinite. Moreover, any profession can give rise to such a process. This expansion will be articulated with the tendency to understand the etiology of social problems in individualistic terms, which obscures causality and depoliticizes social processes. In conjunction with the modern relevance of science, the professions most called for expansion are those that deal scientifically with the properties of individuals. The expansion of the domain of such professions will also be stimulated by the increase in demand from clients who have become addicted to prevention and treatment products. Ultimately, all problems identified, even when it comes to bodily harm, can be considered products of social forces, so disease prevention and treatment imply social change.

Strong argues that critics of medical imperialism share "a rough consensus" about its shape [115] (p. 200). However, he acknowledges and assumes several limitations of his study. First, he finds that his synthesis does not do justice to the diversity of views on imperialism. He admits Zola's criticism of intentionalism in the case of medical imperialism but considers that the very notion of imperialism does not embrace an intentionalist perspective. Furthermore, he finds that the notion of imperialism correctly captures the professional expansionary potential and the associated professional political threat. Second, Strong also believes that critics of medical imperialism do not agree on the nature of society. This implies that the notion of imperialism is inscribed in different causal and axiological schemes, examples being the studies of Vicente Navarro and those of Illich. Third, Strong clarifies that he will only address one segment of the medical imperialism thesis: the part Conrad and Schneider will understand as the medicalization level of doctor-patient interaction.

After clarification, Strong proceeded to the exposition of his 'sociological imperialism thesis' as a sociological version of the professional imperialism thesis and, in this condition, in his reading, rival of the medical imperialism thesis. As Strong says, "the thesis of professional imperialism cuts two ways" [115] (p. 205). He begins by arguing that most sociologists have been unreflexive about professional imperialism. Perhaps we can speak of a deficit of reflexivity in the sociological analysis of the medical profession: sociologists accuse doctors of conditions that they themselves suffer without realizing it. In order to increase reflexivity, it would be necessary, in Strong's view, for the discipline to fold in on itself based on the analysis of the professions. The author applied the same perspective sociologists mobilize to study the medical profession to the sociological scope itself. He used the method of professional analysis in the theoretical framework of what he manages to be a theory of professional change. However, he considered that the thesis that sociology is a practicing profession in a narrow sense is not acceptable. It is, first and foremost, an academic discipline insofar as it has no individual clients and has resisted the usual processes of professionalization. Despite this, Strong defends that sociology may be seen as a profession in the sense that it does possess "most of the crucial traits by which we normally identify professional occupations" [115] (p. 202), namely, it seeks to serve humanity, it is supported by an academic body of knowledge, it maintains concerns regarding the practical application of such knowledge, it has clients although they are not individuals, but groups, such as governments, bureaucratic organizations, or representatives of less powerful groups, such as trade unions. It is in these terms that Strong understands sociology as a profession and 'practicing sociologists' as professionals.

He frames the application of the thesis of professional imperialism to sociology in the broader context of Alvin Gouldner's critical characterization of the history, social position, and ideological functions of modern sociology (also referring to the Marxist critiques of Martin Shaw and Martin Nicolaus). Gouldner considered sociology a product of the bourgeois social order, of modern interventionist capitalism, of the welfare state, and a means of legitimizing and maintaining it. In this context, sociology is a form of "mindless empiricism" and "atheoretical managerial" social science [115] (p. 201). Nevertheless, Strong believes that Gouldner and his fellow-critics analysis exaggerated the interdependence between capitalism and sociology.

From Strong's point of view, it is necessary to take into account, in general, some conditions of production of bourgeois sociology and, in particular, associated factors of analytical distortion specifically related to the sociological analysis of the medical profession. Strong talks about those conditions and these factors separately, but they are deeply articulated, so it is worth considering them in an integrated and conjoint way.

First, contemporary sociology lacks historical sensitivity, which contributes to devaluing and exaggerating present trends. Second, sociologists suffer from professional skepticism in the sense that there is great proximity between analysis and critical devaluation. Based on the ideas of Paul Halmos, Strong considers that this skepticism, in addition to conveying the idea that sociologists are incorruptible, supposedly generates the paradox that sociological criticism of the way society is organized allows sociologists to progress within this society. Third, the intellectual freedom that sociologists enjoy is superior to that of other academics. The articulation between the second and third elements allows us to perceive that, in this way, sociologists can more easily become great critics of the societies in which they live. Fourth, sociologists' professional status is neither passive nor disinterested; sociologists are part of the professional schema of ideological and technical competition. They are, to use Strong's quite liberal tone, "in the market-place" [115] (p. 202).

Strong argues that, like any other profession within bourgeois society, sociologists thus have imperial ambitions. In particular, they are not passive commentators on the medical profession, and sociological commentaries are not disinterested. While he recognizes that medicine now has a power that sociology does not have, Strong does think that sociology seeks to rival medicine. Note that, for the author, the point is not just what we call the deficit of reflexivity. The point is again a paradox: by criticizing the imperialism of other professions, sociologists advance their own empire. The lack of reflexivity of sociologists on professional imperialism turns into a danger of "unreflexive radicalism" [115] (p. 204).

Fifth, sociology has a sales appeal of its own, which leads sociologists to become involved in ambivalence. In a society where individualism is heavy, by not having individual clients, sociology is socially weakened because it depends on group clientele and, in addition, this clientele is divided between more powerful groups, such as rulers of countries, and less powerful groups, such as the working class. This situation is inherently tense. Yet, sixth, sociology is never compromised by committing to the less powerful, given that sociologists belong to an elite class and occupy an advantageous structural position. Seventh, Strong does not let us forget that sociologists will never simply be medical students, for sociologists too will, in a certain context, be the patients of doctors (while, let us add, doctors will hardly be clients of sociologists).

Only after looking at the sociological discipline and profession in general, trying to show how it can represent the rival to medicine, did Strong consider the thesis of sociological imperialism in the context of the specific situation of medical sociology. He argues that medical sociology had a managerial role until the 1970s, but that since then, this has been changed thanks to the study of the history of the subdiscipline, attacks on empiricism, and criticism of administrative abuses and their political connotations, following the general sociological self-awareness that characterized the previous decade. However, Strong considers that these transformations only altered the phase of sociological imperialism, not having provided the necessary reflexivity. By critically understanding their establishment and constantly emphasizing the social and political nature of medicine, sociologists ask for more attention. However, they do it without giving up their subservience to the medical order. We may perhaps add that other sociologists, generally and independently, have referred reflexively and critically to some form of sociological imperialism [157].

Notwithstanding all the above conditions, Strong defends the validity of sociological ambitions and productions and that even the analysis of the medical profession is not mere hypocrisy, but that these ambitions and the thoughtless naivety on which they are based have made this analysis exaggerated. For Strong, this exaggeration constitutes a source of empirical selectivity and distortion, leading sociologists to ignore or distort evidence, especially if the evidence contradicts established views on medicine.

The author speaks of six particular kinds of distortion. The first distortion common among medical sociologists is the tendency for critiques of medical imperialism to be based on what Strong calls "the benefit of hindsight", and the second for these critiques to suffer from a lack of historical or anthropological awareness [115] (p. 205). The fourth distortion is a tendency to underestimate the success of modern medicine in technical terms. The fifth is the putative misrepresentation of capitalist control over medical imperialism. The sixth distortion is the trend to overstate patient addiction to medicine. Strong detects, commenting on this tendency, an assumption that deserves to be mentioned: as medicine is important to physicians and scholars, they assume that medicine should be equally important to others. This assumption can be particularly harmful in questioning patients in empirical sociological research, namely structuring interviews. "By focusing on what patients make of medical services", writes Strong, "they fail to set their comments in the wider context of patients' lives and thus often ascribe to them an unwarranted importance" [115] (p. 298). We purposely skip the third kind of distortion mentioned by Strong, leaving it for the end because it more directly concerns the argument of our article. This is the "tendency for sociologists to perceive the dispute as one *between* sociology and medicine itself" [115] (p. 205). The point that Strong seeks to underline in this case is that the generality that medicalization criticizes homogenizes a universe of disciplinary and sub-disciplinary diversity, forgetting that the expansion of medicine may vary in terms of interest, expertise, and ideology of medical specialties.

In addition to these distortions, Strong identifies factors embedded in the very position of medicine within the modern bourgeois society which serve to limit or restrict the threat of medical imperialism but which sociological exaggeration has obscured. The author mentions four factors: the capitalist financial system is not limited to positively financing the medical profession, it also constrains it; the medical community has limited the number of people entering the profession, which limits professional expansion; medicine, as understood by Strong, is an "applied science, a fundamentally pragmatic discipline" [115] (p. 209), so its professionalization is followed by scientific, technical and practical concerns, and doctors themselves have skeptical attitudes towards the medicalization of social conditions such as alcoholism (see [158]); finally, the state granted doctors a monopoly of practice, but patients' behavior is protected by bourgeois freedoms.

As can be seen from the observations of Conrad and Schneider, an enterprise as creative and critical as Strong's naturally lends itself to much criticism. We could undoubtedly add a few more to the list. From the outset, we could speak of the weak argumentative foundation to support the idea of a sociological profession, which is essential for the rest of his analysis. In this context, when his entire perspective is so dependent on defending the professional character of a given activity and despite having Everett Hughes or Terence J. Johnson in his bibliographic references, the absence of a clear distinction within the sociological theory of professions of degrees of professionalization or concepts such as 'occupation' and 'profession' is quite questionable, either to undertake a social history or a historical sociology of medicine, or to adopt an analytical conception of sociology. This absence, among others, is due to a significant elemental flaw in Strong's approach. In our view, his mistake in the reconfiguration of the critique of medicalization as a critique of medical imperialism does not seem to be found in its substantive content. Instead, it lies in the profession-based approach dominant in the sociological study of health, illness, and medicine and with which Strong does not break but which develops to the limit of sociological contradiction. In this sense, Strong's mistake is also Conrad's mistake, but also Parsons's and Freidson's. The lack of understanding of imperialism in the field of health and sociology is not, in our view, found in the argumentative dispute between the authors but in the fact that sociological analysis is reduced in this context to the analysis of professions. This kind of reflexivity is not dispensable, but it is not enough.

7. Foucault, Social Constructivism, and the Anti-Realist-Positive Modality of Medicalization

Although Illich's work typifies for many authors a critical and skeptical approach to medicine, it is essential to underline that, on the one hand, as we have seen, criticism and skepticism regarding medicine are not new, nor is it restricted to the outside eyes of the medical tradition. It is also important to emphasize that, on the other hand, concepts such as professional dominance or iatrogenesis do not fully cover the innovation that skepticism has to deal with in our time. That is, the problems of medicine no longer concern the errors of the medical profession but the very scientific transformation and scientific specificity of medicine.

The scientific mutation, or scientificization process, of medicine has been perceived, analyzed, and scrutinized by researchers from different research subfields dedicated to the study of the HIMC. It has been articulated with other macro, sub, or complementary processes alongside the development processes of various sciences, laboratories, and industries, such as the molecularization of biology and the progressive formalization of medical decisions [159–164]. However, at the same time that in the scope of the study of the dynamics of professionalization, an erosion of the autonomy of the medical profession has been evidenced, mainly thanks to managerial policies and the corresponding quantitative reorganization of medical work and knowledge [165–171], on the side of the social sciences, there has been a generalized and profound change in the scale of analytical values. What, as we said initially, referring to the works of Lupton [5] and Berg and Mol [6], can be understood as remarkable convergences of contemporary epistemological transformations concerns, above all, convergence in an increasingly radical perspective of critique of the biomedical model.

It is a convergence between poststructuralism, phenomenology, sociology of knowledge, and sociology of science with a constructivist bent, especially from the relationship established between knowledge and power in Michel Foucault's work [5,16,17,172–178]. A number of authors in the post-war period found in this convergence a way to overcome the absence of a broad theory in the social study of health and medicine, and from there, they also defined their research topics. The more classical approaches of medical sociology and sociology of health, such as that of Freidson, had already absorbed elements of constructivism; they accepted without any exception the existence of social factors in the scope of health, illness, and medicine. However, as M. R. Bury highlights [178], the causal effect of these factors was restricted to the social sphere, and the distinction between illness and disease was accepted.

What is happening now is that the limit has been breached. There is, therefore, no constructivist turn but a constructivist radicalization. The theoretical centrality of these approaches reflects the epistemological centrality of social constructivism in diverse areas of the social sciences (see [179]). Such approaches allowed us to think about illness and disease beyond their supposed status as fixed physical realities, which is essential for social scientists. The ideas about illness and disease categories came to be seen as phenomena shaped by social experiences, shared cultural traditions, and changing frameworks of knowledge. However, instead of illness and disease being understood as invariable natural objects, what has alternatively been maintained is that they correspond to socially constructed evaluative concepts insofar as they can assume a plurality of social and cultural meanings, meanings that can be (and often are) variable in time and space. The scope of this constructivist approach was not limited to understanding the socio-cultural meanings underlying illness and the analysis of the variation of disease experiences. This type of analysis was also extended to scientific knowledge itself as it was developing in a specific political, economic, and technological context (see [180]). On the one hand, professional conceptions and categories of medical knowledge began to be equated as socially situated symbolic systems. On the other hand, it became increasingly challenging to disarticulate these two dimensions (disease experience and medical knowledge) since the way of managing and giving meaning to the disease is carried out within the framework of biomedical understandings that, by giving existence to certain conditions, organize experiences into specific diagnose categories [181,182].

These approaches allowed many areas to question the conceptual limits of the disciplines that study health and medicine. What remains to be seen is that the progressive approach of medicine in relation to the natural sciences has homogenized culturally, socially, and politically what we understand by health, illness, and medicine and, with that, also how we relate to medical knowledge, erasing a series of tensions inherent to the intrinsic diversity of health-related and medical phenomena. There were, in particular, internal disciplinary breaks. For example, in the case of medical anthropology, the application of the concept of ethnomedicine to biomedicine [183] and a move away from the notions of medical systems and medical pluralism in the name of the notion of syncretism [184]. In the context of the history of medicine and the sociology of health, an attempt is made, for example, to understand the type of historical orientation that has governed the reconstruction of the biomedical model [185].

The recognition of these achievements becomes more debatable and paradoxical when the development of such questions, based on a relativist epistemological orientation and an ontological orientation of an anti-realist type, translates into frameworks that reiterate reductive interpretations of medical knowledge, actively committed to rejecting any idea of autonomy from the natural world. What tends to prevail is the denial of the ontological reality of the natural world, which results in the basic postulate, when applied to medical knowledge, that illness and disease categories do not necessarily correspond to natural phenomena. These are, on the contrary, conceived either as the result of scientific consensuses essential to produce legitimate knowledge or (in their most relativistic version) as the expression of fabrications and discursive constructs oriented towards the dissemination of a disciplinary power structurally rooted in the modern world. In the sociological field, following the previously mentioned thematic specialization around the social dimensions of illness, there is a constructivist worsening that is well captured by the idea of a medicalization nominalist orientation [186] and by the expression 'biophobia' [187,188]. We can capture this idea well if we look at Foucault's influence.

In Lupton's chapter previously mentioned, the author introduces and develops the interpretative thesis that there is no explicit and systematic Foucauldian adherence to the critique of medicalization but that it is possible to add from the study of medicine in a Foucauldian perspective a specific perspective on medicalization. Lupton even considers that Foucault and his readers agree with the idea that "medicine is a dominant institution that in Western societies has come to play an increasingly important role in everyday life, shaping the ways that we think about and live our bodies" [113] (p. 106). However, in his words, "the Foucauldian perspective articulates a more complex notion of the role played by medicine in contemporary Western societies" [113] (p. 94).

The interpretation that Foucault did not define his own version of the critique of medicalization should not –let us underline carefully – equate to the interpretation that the author did not address this concept. In fact, the distinction between his understanding of the medicalization process and that of the repressive-negative version, namely that of Illich, was very well captured by Foucault himself in a series of conferences held in 1974 as part of the Social Medicine course at the Instituto de Medicina Social at the Biomedical Center of the State University of Rio de Janeiro and later published, between 1974 and 1978, in article form in the journal *Educación Médica y Salud*, under the responsibility of the Pan American Health Organization [159].

We know since *Naissance de la clinique: une archéologie du regard médical*, published in 1963, that there were several areas of disease distribution in addition to the one that concerns the human body and several corresponding epistemological configurations of medicine [75]. One of Foucault's fundamental theses is that the emergence of pathological anatomy and its development at the end of the 18th century, particularly with Marie F. X. Bichat and his disciples, led to a reconfiguration of medical perception; clinical experience came to concern an anatomo-clinical gaze. The body, with its tissues and organs, becomes the space of clinical experience, symptomatic medicine recedes, and the analysis of the body becomes crucial in the pathological process. Foucault also did not forget that this transformation follows a process of secularization, in which medical intervention replaces the religious figure of salvation insofar as it confronts humanity with its finitude. We find this notion in several passages of *Naissance de la clinique*.

The important aspect that Foucault adds and clarifies in the 1974 conferences is that the critique of medicine itself is not new, that the novelty is, with the scientificization of medicine, it leaves the regime of error. According to Foucault, it was not necessary to wait for the critics of medicine in the 20th century to know that medicine has negative effects. What has changed is the configuration of these effects due to its development as a science:

"It was not necessary to wait for Illich or for the anti-medical agents to know that one of the properties and one of the capabilities of medicine is to kill. Medicine kills, it has always killed, and we have always been aware of that. The important thing is that until recent times the negative effects of medicine have been registered in the register of medical ignorance. Medicine killed because of the physician's ignorance or because medicine itself was ignorant; it was not a true science but just a rhapsody of ill-founded, ill-established, and verified knowledge. The harmfulness of medicine was evaluated in proportion to its unscientificity. However, what has emerged since the beginning of the 20th century is the fact that medicine can be dangerous, not insofar as it is ignorant and false, but insofar as it constitutes a science" [159] (pp. 21–22).

Let us return, once again, to Lupton's unlimited text to observe the synthesis she makes of a Foucauldian perspective on medicalization from the comparison between what she understands as the orthodox medicalization critique and the Foucauldian commentaries on scientific medicine. We have already mentioned the brief similarity. Now it is time to look at the significant differences. According to Lupton, Foucault's work challenges the prevailing conception among critics of medicalization on power and medical knowledge.

This challenge can be understood from three points. The first concerns his conception of power, which is more complex than in the case of repressive-negative critics. The Foucauldian conception of power has, in turn, three basic characteristics. Power, in Foucault, is relational, dispersed, productive, or positive. That it is relational means that it "is not a possession of particular social groups", it is "a strategy which is invested in and transmitted through all social groups", it is a relation [113] (p. 99). The physician is not a figure of dominance but, as Lupton writes, quoting Foucault, 'links in a set of power relations'. Therefore, contrary to what the other critics propose, Foucauldians consider that it is not possible to take power away from doctors and pass it on to patients. The demedicalization strategy would thus be contradictory.

Power is dispersed in the sense that it is unintentional, lacking a central political rationale. In this way, although they recognize a margin for medical dominance and a role for the state in the regulation of medical activity, from the point of view of Foucault and his followers, the intentional load of the notion of medicine is so small that it reaches such heterogeneity that physician's exercise is placed far beyond the clinic and the hospital, including workplaces, schools, supermarkets. This perspective is profoundly incompatible with the idea of medicalization as professional dominance.

Finally, power is productive or positive; it is not negative, it is not repressive. According to Lupton, from the Foucauldian perspective, in the medical encounter, disciplinary power is exercised not through direct coercion or violence but through knowledge. According to Lupton, Foucault is very close in this respect to social constructivism. From both points of view, medical knowledge is not seen as simply factual but as a belief system shaped by power relations. From this, as Lupton rightly points out, the other critics of medicalization would not disagree. The point is that Foucault and his followers go further in that, as already said, they adopt an anti-realist ontological and relativist epistemological point of view. Furthermore, this is the most distinctive aspect of this second modality of medicalization. For Foucault and his followers, the body does not exist outside of power relations and forms of knowledge. The body is, in a strict sense that annihilates biology, a socio-discursive construction. Medical knowledge and practice are not representations of the body but agents that actively participate in its construction. Once again, the orthodox solution of demedicalization could only sound paradoxical, as it would imply more involvement in medical knowledge and thus more medicalization. Therefore, the concept of demedicalization is incompatible with this modality of medicalization.

Lupton presents several criticisms of the Foucauldian perspective, but her presentation largely boils down to difficulties created either by internal inconsistencies in Foucault's work or the effects of the reception of his work, with greater attention given to early works than to later ones. The way that Lupton solves these problems lies in a phenomenological reorientation of Foucault's latest works. This does not seem to us to be the most pertinent point.

The most pertinent point seems to be to understand this change in the context of the epistemological transformation that, from one end to the other, the social sciences of health have been going through. In one of the last revisits to the thesis of sociological imperialism as formulated by Strong, Simon J. Williams sought to understand which aspects of this thesis can be retained, taking into account the criticism it was subjected to and in the light of the most recent developments in medicine, of medicalization and beyond the very scope of the sociology of health [189]. Williams' text interests us because it underlines the problematic epistemological and ontological duplicity that follows the radicalization of constructivism.

Williams accepts that medicine is not homogeneous and that the expansion of the medical empire cannot be an undisputed assumption. Echoing Strong directly, he then suggests that the central issue has to do with limits and comes to defend the limits of medicalization and the limits of sociological critique. Looking at the over-medicalization and demedicalization debates, Williams follows up on Conrad by emphasizing the bidirectional character of the medicalization process and the levels and degrees of medicalization – a theme that we will approach in the following section. However, he promotes an update of Strong's critique within the framework of the debates on the social construction of medical knowledge undertaken by Michael Bury, Malcolm Nicolson, and Cathleen McLaughlin and the development of the Foucauldian scholarship critiques of medicine, the body, and disease.

Following the perspective of Andrew Sayer, Williams considers that the social constructivism extended by Foucault does not solve the fundamental problem that constructivism initially proposed in the scope of the study of the body, health, and illness: the problem of strong essentialism, biological reductionism, and determinism. What it does is invert the solution: instead of being strictly biophysical entities, body, health, and illness become mere social fabrications, specifically discursive entities. Following Ian Craib, Williams declares that this reversal is a paradoxical form of sociologism, as it ends up reducing sociological explanation itself to discursive determination. Without abandoning the limitation of a strictly medical vision, which gains relevance with the development of the new genetics and evolutionary psychology, Williams then suggests that the limits suggested by Strong also encompass the limitation of social constructivism and Foucauldian scholarship.

For Williams, all these limitations must converge to accept the partiality of all forms of knowledge, to recognize the importance of the diverse contributions of knowledge according to the intellectual division of labor, to understand an ontologically and epistemologically complex world, to recognize the heterogeneity of medical and sociological perspectives, and not to reject the relevance of medicine to our quality of life. In short, as we have been defending from the study of tensions between the HIMC and society, it is necessary to redirect our gaze, clinical or not, to the diversity of forms of knowledge.

8. Reassessing the Concept of Medicalization in a Technoscientific Society and Therapy Culture

As we already stated, the concept of medicalization was addressed and developed by several authors in a wide range of contexts. Since the emergence of the concept and its subsequent theoretical developments, many conceptual debates have taken place, and much empirical research has been developed, which has contributed to the level of sophistication of the social analyses built upon this concept. From them, we obtain important heuristic devices for the clarification of several dynamics regarding the way medical perspectives have become constitutive of the ways of thinking and knowing health, as well as in the way of organizing experiences and complaints according to diagnostic categories. Therefore, while the effective processes of medicalization have been covering more areas of life, the critique of medicalization has also been widening. There are undoubtedly deep theoretical nuances in the authors' perspectives. However, there are other changes that should be considered. As Zorzanelli, Ortega, and Bezerra Júnior say, "the relevance and actuality of the concept of medicalization is demonstrated by the reach that the theme has been acquiring in publications in the field of human and social sciences in the last decades" [112] (p. 1860).

In the case of the line of argument that we seek to develop here, the effort of theoretical discussion does not imply that the analytical merits of a concept that has been systematically mobilized and operationalized over practically five decades are not recognized. The census exercises already carried out, or the critical reassessment carried out by some of its main promoters, are indicative not only of the multiple contributions that have been developed but also of the very mutations that the concept has known, which is in itself denoting its elasticity, as well as the adaptive nature of the processes that this concept seeks to cover. A characteristic that has always been notorious is how this critical view has been branching out into different problem areas, forming a well-defined diatribe regarding the role of medicine. Within the framework of this development, many authors and positions were deepening the scope of the concept by means of new lines of exploration, which contributed to the gradual consolidation of discussions aimed at clarifying the complex, plural, adaptive, and contested character of medicalization processes, but also noticing that they started to assume new facets and configurations.

Gradually, it has become necessary to recognize that medicalization can have multiple dimensions and levels of analysis (see [190]). First of all, one must recognize the drastic expansion of the segments of life that were medicalized and turned into a terrain or object, an empirical field. Abortion, political activism, AIDS, alcoholism, child abuse, hyperactivity, infant death syndrome, aging, poisoning, menopause, premenstrual syndrome, race, pregnancy, masturbation, sexual orientation, sexual gender, obesity, compulsive buying, disability, breastfeeding, drug consumption, childbirth, shyness, sleep, sadness, and even death and normality. These are some topics that have been studied within the scope of medicalization studies.

Conrad, initially in collaboration with Joseph W. Schneider, is one of the main authors responsible for imagining medicalization as a complex process and, especially, for developing the corresponding idea that medicalization processes occur and can be studied in various contexts [154,155]. In their critique of Strong, the authors define for the first time that medicalization can occur on the conceptual, the institutional, and the doctor–patient interaction levels. Precisely in view of some of these main changes, Conrad concedes that medicalization processes are bidirectional and partial. He does not fail to emphasize that despite the existence of 'shifting engines' of medicalization grounded in commercial interests, this dynamic persists rather than contradicts, as multiple possibilities for new medical categories may arise [191].

Moreover, Conrad himself recognizes that medicalization does not necessarily require a professional anchorage but rather an acceptance, on the part of various actors, of medical knowledge [156]. As he himself maintains, "an entity that is regarded as an illness or disease is not ipso facto a medical problem; rather, it needs to become defined as one" [192] (pp. 5–6). Conrad changed his analytical emphasis and shifted it from fundamentally jurisdictional aspects to definitional aspects, the process by which social problems become medical problems. This vision gives a more constructivist content to the concept [193]. Medicalization came to be understood as a process of definition. In other words, a process that results in the conversion of social problems into medical problems, which in practice means that they are defined in medical terms, described in medical language, understood in a medical frame of reference, and treated or managed through medical interventions [156,192].

Additionally, at the same time that the meaning changes, the process starts to welcome more actors and to be comprehended in a sense that no longer fits the professional perspective. "This is a sociocultural process", as Conrad puts it, "that may or may not involve the medical profession, lead to medical social control or medical treatment, or be the result of intentional expansion by the medical profession" [156] (p. 211).

Thus, recognition that there are new actors and new dynamics that play an important role in the reconfiguration of medicalization gains strength. With the end of the assumption of inexorable professional dominance, namely through the expansion of critical and skeptical attitudes towards professional authority (medicine becoming linked to greater public scrutiny), as well as a growing involvement of governments in funding and regulation [191,194], the narrative of medical imperialism, as well as the assumption of the docility of individuals, fails. It is becoming evident that the public is actively searching for medicalization to legitimize existential experiences and problems [195]. This shows that medicalization must be understood as a form of collective action where patients and other lay actors can be active collaborators. They are committed to the medicalization of their problems, especially when they mobilize to exert pressure, or even demand (as with contested diseases), medical categories for their conditions, even when physicians express reluctance to do so [171,196].

Equally relevant is the fact that more than the simple bidirectional nature of these processes, medicalization and demedicalization can, in their articulation, configure continuous processes in the sense of occurring simultaneously [190,197]. It follows that they should not be viewed as rigid categories that are limited to being present or absent in each context. On the contrary, they are processes referring to mutable possibilities of increase or decrease, although it is still significant that the analysis tends to be more systematically inattentive to demedicalization. This can be interpreted, as Drew Halfmann maintains, as a reflection of the conceptual weakness of the literature on medicalization in reifying the idea that one process will be common and the other rare [190] (p. 187).

Other authors attribute meaning to the contestation of medicalization, assuming it as the expression of dynamics strongly articulated to a societal context marked by a more significant critical questioning that takes shape in scrutiny fed by increasing levels of social reflexivity and a keener awareness of the risks and limitations of expert approaches [198].

Thereby, the typical approach of the 1970s of medical power criticism changed, opening space for new approaches and more oriented towards analyzing other dynamics and other actors outside the professional field of medicine. However, the resonances of the agonistic positions that we have been emphasizing are still in the air. Especially when underlying the criticisms of medicine, there still seems to be resonances suggestive of the permanence of a vision that presumes the existence of a professional monopoly with normalizing and regulatory ramifications in the production of health. Even though, in the case of Strong's perspective, it is important to bear in mind the vital point that criticisms of medical expansion have often translated into exaggerated and disproportionate analyzes of medicalization, especially when the emphasis of its conceptualization made it equivalent to a ubiquitous process based on an inexorable expansionist tendency and, as such, denoting the increasing colonization of multiple spheres of human life by medical imperialism.

All the new redefinition was responsible for considerably enlarging and generalizing the concept, but also for the emergence of criticism or reassessment readings. In recent decades, the very concept of medicalization has begun to be viewed with some suspicion, as we have already mentioned. In a recent article, Joan Busfield gathers and organizes the different types of criticism on the concept of medicalization itself and seeks to challenge them [193]. The first type of criticism stemmed from the putative confusion between medicalization and medical imperialism. According to Busfield, reflecting Illich's emphasis on industrialization as the cause of medicalization, Strong and also Simon J. Williams confused the two concepts. Although industrialization can be considered as a preponderant factor of medicalization, the latter, as a process, is not reduced to it as a cause. Thanks to this confusion, the critique of medicalization came to be seen as an exaggerated form of criticism, namely for having a passive conception of the patient and being interested in defense of public health as a branch of interest in medical sociology. Medical imperialism thus gives rise to sociological imperialism.

The second type of critique, again reflecting Illich's perspective, assumes that the critique of medicalization is a total critique of medicine. This is what supposedly happened with Nikolas Rose, who, based on such an assumption, considered that the very concept of medicalization is nothing more than a cliché of social criticism, not recognizing any explanatory power. According to Busfield, there are several formulations and uses of the concept of medicalization. Although in Illich, we can find the insinuation of a generalized attack on medicine, Busfield finds two reasons for not adopting such a comprehensive concept of medicalization, at least as a starting point. First, the criticism of medicalization is usually based on studies of 'specific instances of medicalization', which are not even medical specialties, but particular problems. Second, to the extent that critics of medicalization recognize the potential and benefits of medical action (even in complex fields such as sexual and reproductive health). For Busfield, the central aspect of the value of medicine resides in the ability to articulate description, explanation, and criticism. This assessment is tied to what we call the repressive-negative modality of medicalization since this point would no longer be verified in the case of the other modality.

In fact, in 1985, in consultation at the Pennsylvania State University, Illich argued that, after medicine had monopolized the social construction of the body and, in the 1960s, the medical profession had become prominent in this regard, from the 1970s, the symbolic character of health care changed [199]. Medicine continued to play a role in the sociogenesis of our bodies, but its importance was reduced. According to Illich, a new epistemological matrix emerged in which it is the pursuit of a healthy body that becomes pathogenic and no longer needs medical intervention. Medicine continues to influence the way the body is perceived, but medical theories and concepts are so publicly questioned that the medical system loses the ability—to use Illich's terms—to 'engender a body'. Perhaps we can add that, from a critical but realistic point of view, what is relevant from the 1980s onwards can no longer be the loss of the social agency of medicine but a strong contrast between this loss and the biotechnological conquest of agency in the artificial construction of bodies.

The third criticism of the concept of medicalization, according to Busfield, concerns attempts to replace this concept with others. An example can be found in the defense by Adele E. Clarke, Laura Mamo, Jennifer Ruth Fosket, Jennifer R. Fishman, and Janet K. Shim of the thesis that, in the 1980s, medicalization was replaced by a more complex process of biomedicalization, resulting from major political, economic, and technological changes. In Busfield's view, this new concept's complexity does not imply the rejection of the first but one of the paths for its development. Another attempt at replacement was carried out by John Abraham, who proposed the concept of pharmaceuticalization, emphasizing not only the dimension of drug therapy as a response to medicalization but also the expansion of the pharmaceutical industry. In this case, the author himself, maintaining some doubts, assumes that the concept of medicalization can subsume the other.

Busfield defended that the concept of medicalization retains its relevance. In order to justify it, she exposed two fundamental reasons. The first is that this concept identifies a process that is still taking place, making it possible to explore new factors in the development of known instances of medicalization or even to point out new domains of medicalization. The second reason given by Busfield to justify the relevance of the concept of medicalization is that it refers to the social, political, and economic causes and consequences of the changes considered in direct relation to the transformation of medicine.

What we argue is that the reappraisal of the analytical merits of medicalization needs to be considered within a framework of great articulation with a variety of social processes since the very limited focus around medicine can become reductive or even reify a reality that has become more pulverized in terms of protagonists and bundles of causality. From this point of view, it is important to integrate several other related concepts that denote new and differentiated articulations that constitute medicalization itself. This means that it is necessary to improve reading grids that are porous in the face of different transformative dynamics with an impact on ways of thinking about health and medicine in society. Whether these dynamics go through the recognition of the importance of biotechnological innovations that are at the base of the proliferation of biomedical solutions for the maintenance, improvement, or optimization of health, condensed in the concept of biomedicalization [200]; by considering the role of the pharmaceutical industry in the 'corporate construction of disease' across borders, via marketing, of treatable conditions to sell medical solutions with debatable clinical relevance, condensed in the concept of disease mongering (see, e.g., [201]); by, as the brand new concept of camization points out, subjecting problems that have become medical into perceptible and treatable health problems within the scope of CAM with the respective attempts to encroach upon mainstream healthcare [202]; or by the increasingly significant importance of pharmaceuticalization process, that is, in the transformation of human conditions into pharmacological issues that can be treated or improved [203].

In the latter case, and despite the fact that there are different assessments regarding the analytical importance of this concept, the realization of the relevance of the role of the pharmaceutical industry seems increasingly unavoidable. Not just because the impacts of the growing pharmacological expansion constitute one of the main driving forces (more than medicine itself) of the medicalization of contemporary societies [204], but also because this process is defined and manifested through two aspects of great relevance. First, by the generalization of the use of drugs to an increasingly broad spectrum of aspects outside the field of pathology. Second, by the development of new categories of need for medical and drug consumption, as a result of the pharmacological innovation itself.

More than just a concept derived from medicalization that would always depend on some degree of medical legitimation, pharmaceuticalization can effectively grow without the expansion of medicalization, as it happens in the context of multiple social uses of medicines based on very different investment logics and oriented towards purposes that do not require the precedence of their medicalization as clinical conditions, being, consequently, refractory to the expert supervision of medicine. This is clearly the case, for example, of the pharmaceuticalization of daily life in that medicines, instrumentalized for the realization of a set of personal and social aspirations, are used to improve the quality of life in spheres of bodily hedonism such as sexual and aesthetic self-fulfillment [205], or for the improvement of several other issues related with lifestyle [206,207].

Equally illustrative of these new logics of pharmaceuticalization is the non-medical use of drugs for recreational ends, namely in university contexts by young people [208,209], the use of pharmacological resources to customize or manage sleep [210,211], chronobiological optimization interventions to address circadian disruptions resulting from the diverse impact of life rhythms [212], the use of pharmacological resources for enhancement purposes [213,214], or the consumption of medication for performance management and, therefore, human conditions that are not medicalized [215–219].

In this last case, what the empirical evidence highlights is precisely the autonomy of pharmaceuticalization in relation to the sphere of medical authority since the relationship with therapeutic resources is guided by the logic of the management of the social imperatives of everyday life. By means of a research project on the performance consumption of the young population in Portugal, it was found that therapeutic investments are developed not so much in the logic of overcoming the norm but in achieving this norm more quickly or with less effort [215,216,219]. This means that the imperatives of performativity and the expectations of response to its management are shaped by the pharmacological solutions available on the market, a circumstance that configures what can be called the 'therapeuticization of everyday life' [216]. That is, the use of a technology designed for therapeutic use but which also serves non-therapeutic purposes, replacing or gaining ascendancy over other types of non-drug investments, such as diet, sport, sleep, or meditation [219].

Looking at these examples collected from empirical research, the position of Simon J. Williams, Catherine Coveney, and Jonathan Gabe [220] gains greater consistency regarding the importance of analytical articulations and the variable relationships between these concepts. These interactions introduce a much more productive potential for analysis than if we perpetuate a look strictly focused on medical definitions or their ineluctable expansion. It is clear that the conceptual trajectory of medicalization configures an open narrative, not only for a theoretical reason but also given the heterogeneity and ambiguities of the empirical world.

9. Goodbye, Social Control: The Knowledge-Based Approach to Medicalization

The development of tensions accumulated in the critique of medicalization results from the development of the analysis of the medical profession as it has developed in the sociological literature, slipping towards the analysis of the sociological profession and being followed by the foundational instability of the sociology of health. However, while the object of this analysis is of a professional nature, non-linear developments of medical and sociological concepts emerge from it, including basic notions about what is meant by medicine and social science, especially sociology. This is emphasized by Conrad's and Schneider's distinction between levels of medicalization, especially their consideration of a specifically conceptual level. The same is also partially signaled when Conrad and Schneider accused Strong's version of sociological imperialism of inconsistency. It is inconsistent because it treats the sociological realm in conceptual terms while it treats medical imperialism from the level of doctor–patient interaction. Conrad and Schneider believed that Strong's concern with biology had to do with the author not having gone much beyond the doctor–patient interaction level of medicalization, but it can also be understood as naturalization of medicine resulting from a professional analysis that by default accepts the biomedical model that dominates the present development of the profession of medicine.

The affirmation of the theoretical relevance of the sociology of health remains profoundly current, perhaps more current than ever. However, ironically, we will not be able to understand its true scope if we do not consider the impasses that the sociological theorization of health, illness, and medicine has been going through. One of them is, without a doubt, that the professional perspective has become dominant. The evaluation of the knowledge dimension is not foreign to medicalization studies, but it was largely subsumed in the analysis of the professions. In order to understand the scope of the theoretical relevance of the sociology of health and to understand all this accumulation of tensions and consequent instabilities, it seems necessary to replace, or at least supplement, the profession-based approach. The fundamental reasons for doing so and some of its theoretical–empirical effects deserve careful attention. A recent article in which Tiago Correia proposes his version of the 'knowledge-based approach to medicalization', or 'knowledge-based critique of medicalization', actually coining those expressions, constitutes an important starting point for this [221]. Regarding the concept of medicalization, his perspective involves considering both theoretical and empirical scopes of analysis, giving special attention from the outset and stressing the importance in conclusive terms of the theoretical scope of medicalization.

Correia's perspective is a kind of non-constructivist off-shot of the constructivist development of medicalization studies. It is based on what we might call 'epistemological pluralism of medicine'. This point of view, as we interpret Correia's words, is explored by the author according to different argumentative frameworks throughout his text. It stems from a set of notions we think we can summarize in the following terms. First, the notion of the cognitive and cultural variability of medicine, exposed by the author according to the idea that the problems categorized as medical are not exclusive to Western professionalized medicine. Second, a methodological notion that follows this variability: if this form of medicine does not have this exclusivity, those problems are not, and cannot be understood, on the strictly biological or physiological infrastructure that underlies the medical knowledge of such a form of medicine.

From this rationale derives the broader consideration that a knowledge-based approach must appreciate different branches of medical knowledge. Regarding the concept of medicalization in particular, this means that a framework is needed that expands the medical categorization of problems to include "all forms of medical knowledge in a global society" [221] (p. 1), "irrespective of the political or scientific status of these branches in society" [221] (p. 2).

Correia delved into the field of medical ontology via the hermeneutical philosophy of Hans-Georg Gadamer to assess two underlying features of clinicians' praxis that have remained unchanged in the history of medicine. He did not do so to abandon the legitimacy of medical knowledge but to broaden the scope of its foundation regardless of empirical manifestations and empirical observations on medicine, namely beyond the institutionalized scientific foundation of biomedicine. As a reader of *Über die Verborgenheit der Gesundheit*, Correia refers to the scope of praxis as the first feature, in the sense that medical decisions are intrinsically contingency-dependent, or discretionary, and correspondingly only partially controllable. The second feature mentioned is that, despite the drastic variability in the meaning of the categories of health and disease and health care systems, the aim of medical practice concerns ordered explanations and judgment of what is understood by health and illness and interventions with the purpose of curing or treating. Correia believes that, considering the stability of those two core features of medicine's ontology, it is possible to establish a stable correspondent concept of medicine, which theoretically subsumes a diversity of practices, influences, and disputes among the different branches of knowledge, including non-scientific-natural or even non-scientific (including magical) knowledge and unregulated medical knowledge.

This plural opening enables Correia to question the dominant sociological perspective on medicine and medical knowledge and its expression in the very critique of medicalization. His drawing on hermeneutic philosophy allows us to question the "empirical-based view of medicine and medical boundaries" [221] (p. 6). For Correia, propositions on medicalization, demedicalization, or remedicalization have as their basic condition the clarification of what is meant by medicine. Without necessarily opposing the hypotheses of biomedicalization and camization, it cuts with the underlying definition of medicalization, or, better still, with the definition of medicine underlying this underlying definition of medicalization. As Correia rightly argues, such definitions result from the effects of the profession-based approach dominant in medicalization critique. By focusing on the process of professionalization of medicine at the same time as biomedical knowledge gained relevance in social life, this approach accepted and reproduced the medical boundaries and definitions from the biomedical model. Just as the development of biomedicine excluded other branches of knowledge from the medical domain, so too would medicalization be overlapped by biomedical knowledge. Therefore, the sociological study of health, illness, and medicine would have adopted a reductive notion of medicine and medical knowledge, not only leaving out other forms of knowledge but also forgetting forms that, as Correia emphasizes, can be forces of medicalization. This is how Correia's proposal involves replacing the dominant profession-based approach with a knowledge-based approach.

Added to these notions is the consideration that adherence to medical truth does not depend only on this type of knowledge but on the extension of what Freidson called a 'lay reference' and on the institutionalization of social control itself. The epistemological pluralism of medicine on which Correia's knowledge-based approach is endured was then followed by a fundamental sociological argument around this last question of control. Following the discussions by Joan Busfield, Simon J. Williams, Catherine Coveney, and Jonathan Gabe on Conrad's concern with the definition of medicalization, Correia sought to save the critique of medicalization from the main criticism it has been subject to by establishing a "more analytical neutral [concept] in relation to different players and different forms of medical knowledge" [221] (p. 3), analytical neutral meaning less normative. The author himself recognized that with a knowledge-based approach, considering that medicine comprises different branches of knowledge but maintains ontological traits, it is possible not only upstream to separate the theoretical scope of medicalization from empirical observations but also downstream to operationalize with more accuracy the concept to be applied in the scope of comparative empirical research, allowing to critically explore its variations, namely clarifying the link to medical knowledge of degrees of social control, controlling players and respective procedures. In a way, our attempt to systematize modalities of medicalization is the result of the same type of ideas. Correia's considerations about social control allow us to take a step forward.

Correia reassessed the little-questioned link between medicalization and social control, taking into account, in our view quite correctly, in contrast not only with the tradition of medicalization critique but also with a good part of the naivety that governs current biopolitical critics of medicalization, that there is no a direct link between the two. The author emphasizes that he does not disagree with Conrad's conceptualization of medicalization as making things medical. Going further than Conrad, who had come to accept that medicalization precedes medical social control, Correia argues that, insofar as medicine and social control "stem from analytically independent dimensions" [221] (p. 7), medicalization is independent of the institutionalization of social control, that it does not presuppose social control and that social control may even precede medicalization.

As Correia argues, the branches of medical knowledge are a specific constitutive part of the medical realm. The institutionalization of control over societies is not isolatedly related to this knowledge. Contrary to what a Foucauldian vision implies, this control is not immanent. Drawing on works in the history and sociology of science and medicine, Correia has convincingly tried to argue that it depends on specific social and political contexts in which different players call upon medical knowledge and practitioners themselves engage in disputes over clients and state legitimacy. Finally, medical knowledge does not necessarily create disputes for social control but becomes creatively involved in these disputes.

In the Western social and political context, the link between medicalization and social control is obvious, but it is also there, according to Correia's perspective, that it is most easily inverted. The author argues that, with the process of the professionalization of medicine, thanks to the development of the biomedical field within the framework of the various branches of medical knowledge, it is possible to observe that several forms of medical social control took place before the consolidation of Western medicalization on a large scale. Relying on works such as those of Foucault, Freidson, Porter, David Armstrong, and Deborah Lupton, Correia argues that the first forms of medical-type social control occurred in the late 17th century in the context of state processes of normalization, normativization, and moralization of the human body, whereas disputes among different forms of medical knowledge only had a formal outcome in the 19th and 20th centuries. Reading George Weisz's work on medical specialization, Correia also warns of the cultural variability of these forms according to state integration. In short, in his words:

> "What these arguments highlight is that biological medicine only institutionalized medical social control (the process usually referred to as the medicalization of society) after having successfully monopolized the truths of the medical field, thereby becoming a profession. Therefore, medical social control emerged before the medical profession actually existed as such.
>
> Therefore, what happened in Europe at the turn of the nineteenth to the twentieth century was not the rise of medicalization of society as one can assume by the overlap between medicalization and biological knowledge. Rather, it was the comprehensive institutionalization of medical social control through the professionalization of medicine (Porter, 1999). Medicalized conditions and problems existed before and will continue to exist irrespective of the degree and scope of medical control in societies." [221] (p. 5).

What the knowledge-based approach ends up demonstrating is that there is a wide overlap between the profession-based approach and social control on medicalization discourse. The rupture with the profession-based approach is, accordingly, at the same time, a rupture not only with a dominant mode of knowledge but also a blow to the normative Western and professionalized notion of medicalization. What results from this is the realization that medicine should not be confused with biomedicine since the influence of the former actually precedes the historical context of modernity and the cultural space of the West that made the latter possible. These departures enable us to pluralize the concept of medicalization definitively. There is no 'medicalization of society' but several medicalizations which follow cognitive, historical, cultural, social, and political variability. Correia seeks to demonstrate from this opening that, in the Western context, it will be possible to observe that processes such as biomedicalization and camization are not alternatives to medicalization but different forms of it. Likewise, it can be seen that certain demedicalization processes are not generic but specific in relation to forms of biomedicalization. Outside the framework of the development of biomedicine in Western countries, the same view allows arguing that the link between medicalization and social control is not so direct, with medicalization taking place without the institutionalization of biomedical control.

Correia's attempt to understand the epistemological complexity of medical knowledge, substitute a profession-based approach for a knowledge-based approach, and to correct the issue of social control within the critique of medicalization by broadening the meanings of this concept, seems accurate to us but incomplete. We consider it right because it conceptualizes in an integrated way the target difficulties that seem crucial, in the sense that these are the difficulties that have prevented a better understanding of health, illness, and medicine in society. However, we believe that it is an incomplete adventure for three reasons. The first, and for us the most important, is that it is not based on a typology of knowledge. We do not believe that the focus should be exclusively on medical knowledge but on the relations of this type of knowledge with other forms of knowledge, namely social knowledge and knowledge produced within the social sciences. Second: adopting the hermeneutic perspective of medicine already implies, in the field of theory, accepting a certain image of medicine, which means that Correia's approach may contradict the pluralism on which it seeks to be based. It is necessary, in this respect, to take a step back and look for an approach that, in the name of pluralism, guarantees an even more general image of medicine, such as the one that we have tried to go through in the first part of this article. The third reason derives from the second, concerning the feature mentioned that the aim of medical practice refers to ordered explanations and judgment of what is understood by health and illness, or disease, and interventions with the purpose of curing or treating. This definition of the aim of medical practice, being imbued with the medical image derived from the hermeneutic approach, theoretically subsumes a diversity of practices but precisely given the influence of such an image, it does not allow us to capture, for example, the problems raised by the practice of what Hermínio Martins called 'thanatocratic medicine' [42].

We argue that claims about medicalization and its correlative processes require not only a clear understanding of what medicine is but also of what social science is in its relation to medicine, an understanding that has as a necessary basis the very relationship between society and health, an enlarged knowledge-based approach to medicalization and medicalization critique.

10. Adding Reflexivity: On the Status of Social and Sociological Knowledge Regarding Medicine

Several authors have tried to study in more fundamental terms, following what we may consider knowledge-oriented approaches, the tensions between the HIMC and society as they are mirrored in the relationship between medicine and sociology. Under the old initiative of the Conferences on Social Science and Medicine, several papers of this type were produced, some published in proceedings or in the journal of *Social Science and Medicine*. P.M. Strong addressed related topics in this context. Although his papers are less well known and discussed than his article on the medical imperialism thesis, they contain important contributions to the theoretical and empirical evaluation of the above-mentioned relationships. We think notably of his text "Natural Science and Medicine: Social Science and Medicine: Some Methodological Controversies", co-authored with K. McPherson, originally prepared as a Joint Background Paper for the Seventh International Conference on Social Science and Medicine, Leeuwenhorst, The Netherlands, and reprinted in Strong's volume *Sociology and Medicine. Selected Essays* [158]. They frame medicine among the methodologies of the natural sciences and the social sciences, addressing issues that were left up in the air by the philosophy of science of the 1960s and 1970s and received by several sociologists, in this case, the possibility of theoretical and empirical progress in the social sciences, the inscription of all scientific activity in a sphere of morality, and its degree of proximity to the lay world.

Despite the relevance of an article of this caliber, it was probably Eliot Freidson who framed, contextualized, and discussed at various levels how tense relations between the HIMC and society, medicine, and sociology are. The topic was explicitly addressed by the author in a speech delivered at St. Thomas Medical School, University of London Special Lecture Series in 1980. His presentation resulted in the article expressively titled "Viewpoint: Sociology and Medicine: A Polemic", published in *Sociology of Health and Illness* in 1983 [9]. We consider it important to take up this article for four reasons. First, although Freidson was not, of course, the only one to see the problem, in this text, Freidson's synthesis of the issues at stake is unique, touching the nerve of the whole. Second, the issues are treated independently of his study of medicalization and largely beyond the analysis of the medical profession for which the author is chiefly remembered, taking a very knowledge-oriented approach. Third, it is an understudied text whose considerations have apparently been left outside the scope of Freidson's so-called 'legacy' in medical sociology and the sociology of professions. Fourth, Freidson focuses on developing several ontological, anthropological, ethical, epistemological, and political grounds specific to both medicine and sociology, or the social sciences in general, that have been subsumed by the methodological constructivism that dominates the discussion.

Freidson's article is a largely speculative text based on the author's one-year experience in the United Kingdom. Margaret Thatcher was then Prime Minister. The more general assertions made by Freidson in this paper are that there is indeed tension between medicine and sociology but that both medicine and sociology face an internal intellectual crisis and a contemporary conjunctural social crisis. These crises, according to the author, could only be overcome through the mutual assistance of medicine and sociology. Let us follow the argumentative structure of the text closely. According to Freidson, the 20th century witnessed political, social, and cultural changes that constituted a source of transformation in medicine. These changes would have weakened the capacity of the medical profession to direct and shape the future in terms comparable to the previous century. This weakening would take place at a time that the author says to be "a time of reckoning which is also a time for reckoning" [9] (p. 208).

The idea of a time of reckoning designates a context of economic crisis characterized by policies of retrenchment or cost reduction of expensive public institutions, mainly affecting the most vulnerable institutions, which are, according to the author, "those that do not produce tangible goods" and "those designed to serve human needs which purely commercial enterprises tend to overlook" [9] (p. 208), namely health institutions, educational institutions, and welfare services. For Freidson, among the effects of this reckoning on the medical institutions is the transformation of medicine's economic position through the attempt to revive the earlier private medical practice and support cheaper physician-substitutes, employing paramedical personnel as practitioners rather than as assistants. These attempts are also followed by an encouragement of lay people to care for themselves.

In Freidson's reading, this transformation was implied, in turn, in a series of exemplary cases of the weakening of the medical profession. On the one hand, the very substance of medical practice undergoes some changes: the rising rationalization and regulation increase the routinization of medical practice, reducing the creativity of physicians and the craftsmanlike character of their activity, and the demarcation boundaries of medical control have been eroded, as have the boundaries of the authority and independence of individual clinical judgment and relations between colleagues in organized clinical practice, which also hinders personal responsibility. At the end of the day, medicine only distinguishes itself, like other specialized professions, for its technical autonomy. On the other hand, while lay and paramedical movements were strengthened, physicians' relations with patients and members of other occupations underwent profound changes.

For Freidson, it is incorrect to interpret these dynamics through the concepts of de-professionalization or proletarianization of medicine. We should instead understand them as representing a

> "movement toward an important reorganization of the profession as a corporate entity, toward greater control of the activities of the practising physician by that corporate entity, and toward a significant redefinition of the profession's relation to other occupations, to its patients, and to agencies of the state" [9] (p. 209).

However, it should be added that, in his text, Freidson makes it very clear that it is not just strictly institutional factors that change. For example, in the same flux, lay cognitive dispositions are also changing. According to Freidson, and in his own formulation, it increased the "public scepticism, if not distrust, of the motives of physicians and of the reliability and value of their expertise", the "fear of medical experiments, and concern about the long-term effects or side-effects of new drugs", "a great deal of interest in self-help and in methods of obtaining care without the need to resort to a doctor" [9] (p. 208). It is not only the medical profession that changes but also the dynamics between the lay reference and the medical reference.

Given the current configuration of medical practice, institutionalized health services, relationships between doctors and other health-related occupations, and their relationships with the lay people and with the state, we may be tempted to classify Freidson's description as excessively prescient, but we should not be rushed into these qualifications. It would perhaps be more accurate and rigorous to assert that it is not a question of prescience per se but of coming across a description that integrates the process of research of the historical process, already studied by several authors and following different frames of reference, of the commodification of nature, knowledge, science, and also health and medicine. Freidson was one of the first to understand the direction and scope that this process was taking with respect to the medical profession and within medical institutions, foreseeing some of its theoretical and practical consequences and prescribing some solutions, also theoretical and practical. In this perception, the foundational tension between medicine and sociology that we have been referring to clearly emerges.

For Freidson, in the context of change analyzed, what is at stake is a macro question of how to establish a health system that guarantees decent and humane care for everyone so that health workers are not reduced to mechanized functionaries and that the economy can support without getting involved in cuts. According to Freidson, once again, in his own clarifying terms, "the critical question for medicine as an organized profession is the role it can play in those changes" [9] (p. 209). Contrary to the conservative attitude that has characterized medicine, its characteristic resistance to and prevention of change, the fundamental question would now be to understand how professionals could participate in it.

As soon as this question is posed, a new web of problems arises because the problems in question are economic, social, and political, with no reasoned answer based on medical knowledge. Medical knowledge is "knowledge of the nature and functioning of the individual organism" [9] (p. 210). To face the problems it faces, medicine needs the "knowledge about the nature and functioning of human institutions" [9] (p. 210). It, therefore, needs knowledge beyond its domain of objects, expertise, and training. In other words: physicians cannot give medicine what medicine needs. Those who can, according to Freidson, would be groups capable of providing knowledge about social processes related to medicine and collecting and evaluating reliable information about medicine, health systems, and health policy. Medicine thus needs knowledge provided by the social sciences, namely sociology. Thanks to these sciences, medicine could understand the institutions in which it participates and the forces in conflict. Ultimately, medicine needs sociology to understand its own social framework. This need is perceived, but is it justified by the effective capacity of the social sciences? Medicine can and should be based on sociological knowledge, but is this concretely possible? Can practiced sociology really support medicine, and medicine support it?

Freidson seems to think that, in fundamental terms, sociology can do it. According to the author, the value of sociology in this respect lies in two aspects. First, sociology more easily questions the settled assumptions and their corresponding political economy and cultural roots of health service and administration because sociology is, to use Freidson's words, "congenitally and deliberately outside" of its routines [9] (p. 219). Second, to use the author's formulation, sociology has a "disciplined character", in the sense that it has methods of data-collection of a systematic and self-conscious character, its analytical methods are theoretically organized, and, thanks to this set of technical and conceptual resources, it allows us to understand the basis for policy-making [9] (p. 219).

Notwithstanding, Freidson finds in real sociology several difficulties that complicate the possibility of responding to the needs of medicine. The first one he mentions is the public hostility towards sociology, which he encountered in English newspapers at the time. The second is the theoretical and practical fragmentation of sociology into three mutually hostile segments. First is the group of practical, empirical, and positivist sociologists, who are not averse to theorizing, although they may ignore its philosophical assumptions, but are mostly oriented to collecting quantifiable data on major institutions to respond to practical problems of the welfare state. Second, the philosophical, phenomenological, and interpretive group, whose members sometimes engage in abstract theorizing and criticism, sometimes carry out empirical studies of a qualitative type, based on direct observation and personal interviews, getting closer to ethnography. Additionally, third, the critical theorists' group, including Marxists, a group that seeks to link theory and practice, rejecting scientific neutrality and seeking through theorizing and history to take an evaluative, critical stand, actively engaging in social and political transformation.

Freidson pays more attention to this second difficulty of sociological fragmentation. According to the author, the contempt between those groups is radical, each having its assumptions, its languages and its own purposes and dealing with mutual hostility. Freidson considers that the focus placed on mutual attacks has made sociology lose intellectual coherence, as, in the name of conflict, it abandons empirical research, which for the author represents a "retreat from the real world" [9] (p. 212). Far from the world, sociology would run the risk of becoming a "scholastic enterprise" or a "technical enterprise", in this case, at the service of its funders [9] (p. 212–213).

Despite the importance of these difficulties, it is necessary to go back and go deeper to discover the central problem as studied by Freidson. For this author, it resides in the self and mutual conceptions of medicine and sociology. Such conceptions are largely fallacious, but they become involved in a tangle that results in a mutual estrangement. In Freidson's terms:

> "Each needs the other, yet each alienates the other by self-serving and essentially dishonest conceptions of itself and the other. Each must face its own self-mystifications, its own myths" [9] (p. 212).

Regarding medicine, the author speaks of three myths especially in need of examination. First, he talks about the myth of experience, that is, the idea that only the physician "can say anything reliable and valid about medical practice and health care" insofar as it is the physician who has experience in these fields [9] (p. 212). This is a myth because it confuses the validity of different forms of knowledge: "the validity of lived experience with the separate validity of systematically gathered data" [9] (p. 213). This myth is reinforced by the belief that physicians' medical training would enable them to make scientific analyses of social processes concerning medical practice and health care. However, physicians' training in this area is minimal, and their particular experience may even bias their understanding of health care systems.

Unlike the first myth, the other two are not just about a certain understanding of medicine but more directly about the relationship between medicine and sociology. This is the myth of simplicity, that is, the idea that the knowledge needed to understand these processes is simple so that learning to study them will also be simple for a physician. In fact, to understand these processes, it is necessary to learn "how to collect data, process it and evaluate it, and how to think about the social world in abstract, conceptual terms" [9] (p. 213).

Like the second one, the third myth Freidson talks about is also directly about the medicine-sociology relationship. However, unlike the first two, this one is not about questions of knowledge but about a practical prejudice. This time it is the myth of technical aid that "if medicine does need sociologists, then they should serve merely as technical aides who study what they are told and merely report the results" [9] (p. 213). This notion leaves sociologists out of the processes of selecting research topics, formulating research questions, and criticizing the considered problems. Freidson thinks that this reduction of sociology to a technical enterprise would have an equivalent in medicine, a doctor whose semiology does not abandon the most superficial symptoms without ever exploring the pathological condition behind them.

In general sociology, that is, outside the narrower scope of the sociological study of health, illness, and medicine, Freidson also finds a number of myths that ultimately take their toll on this particular domain. As was the case in Strong and McPherson's text, the questions that Freidson poses here to think about the relationship between medicine and sociology retrieve fundamental issues left up in the air by the philosophy of science and received by different sociologists in contemporary times. In this case, all the myths referred to by the author cut across traditional problems of epistemology, passing also through fundamental ontological, methodological, and axiological issues, all of which are taken here within the framework of human affairs and social problems. All the myths of which the author speaks in some way "reflect a tendency to confuse the logical constructs and distinctions of theory with practical human activity" [9] (p. 214). It is precisely the myths that arise from this confusion that is, in turn, at the root of the fragmentation that the author had found in the actual exercise of sociology, in its division into mutually hostile groups. In this interpretation, sociology's supposed lack of intellectual coherence seems then to be due less to the underlying theoretical statements than to the putative mythifications they imply or lead to.

It must be said that in pondering these general myths, Freidson reveals much about those who subscribe to them, but he reveals even more about his own theoretical standpoint in the social sciences. Freidson rejects diverse radical ontological, epistemological, methodological, and axiological positions. He does not accept that the structure of reality, the ways of knowing it, and the values that guide the perspective of the one who knows it can be absolutely defined.

Thus, the belief that facts can be known in an absolutely objective way, namely through the use of scientific measurement techniques in empirical research, is referred to by Freidson as the 'myth of objectivity and of positivistic method'. Those who adopt this myth seem to take the world as given, proposing only to describe and analyze it. Against this myth stands the diametrically opposed view that subjectivity is a sufficient guarantor of our knowledge. This view Freidson calls the 'myth of subjectivity'. It would have entailed ignoring or even arguing against the empirical practice, various forms of data collection, formal methods, and analytical techniques.

According to Freidson, this polarization results in itself from the abstract formulation of the theory. However, the author argues that while pure objectivity cannot be guaranteed, neither can we think of the empirical social world from purely logical categories. From the critique of positivism's exaggerations, we cannot derive a denial of all forms of empiricism. The author does not try to pose the question in terms of choice between theory and empirical research. It will be possible for Freidson to take on some values of positivism without being a radical positivist. Freidson declares sociological practice is not faced with epistemological absolutes; it is "a matter of something in between", and what matters is "the question of degree" [9] (pp. 215–216). Theory elevates this practice above technique because it offers insights and guidelines; namely, it allows us to formulate epistemological and methodological criteria. Then, careful empirical research will make it possible to document the characteristics of social units. In this work, qualitative methods should follow the quantitative data, providing them with their social context. This is what medicine needs: "a sociology committed to thinking about theory while testing its mettle in the ambiguous empirical world" [9] (p. 217). We believe that the same can be said about the other social sciences.

Alongside the myth of subjectivity, as a critique of positivism, Freidson finds two other myths. One is the 'myth of commitment', that is, the idea that since there is no axiological neutrality, sociologists should not be interested in research for its own sake; they should choose their values and take them as the ends of their research. The problem here, for Freidson, is the lack of attempt to reduce personal bias.

A correlative myth will be that of criticism, the myth that 'a critical position is truly useful for actually improving the character of human life'. A basis of this myth lies in the idea that there are deep-seated forces that make the world what it is, and in particular, that some of these forces oppress human life. Freidson does not object to this idea. The procedure stemming from this basic idea is that the researcher must actively assess these kinds of forces. However, the author believes that those who adopt a critical position end up being more concerned with the critique than with its substantiation, the actual analysis of the forces in question, and the specification of measures of a social change of an alternative. Ultimately, what ends up happening is that inquiry is replaced by moral judgment and moral commentary, by indignation.

Freidson states that in the context of the study of health, without specifying much further, the Parsonian notion that medicine is a form of social control was reiterated and related in the critique of a capitalist political economy but was largely reduced to a "rhetoric of outrage that medicine is part of a system of social control" [9] (p. 215). Indeed, perhaps we can say that a good deal of this, already with a great deal of forgetting of Parsons' original contribution, is what is going on with current critiques of medicalization in a pandemic context. Freidson tells us that it remains to be seen how medicine can exist without social control, taking what he considers to be the "irreducible elements of social control and authority" arising from medicine's own professional, cognitive, and technological frameworks and seeking to dismantle other oppressive conditions [9] (p. 216). Thanks to the knowledge-based approach, we already have a renewed idea of this relationship, but we cannot stop there.

Freidson ends his text by adding a myth related not to medicine or sociology but to the agencies involved in the process of sponsoring and funding sociological research, which he considers to be the third part of the collaboration between medicine and sociology. It is now the myth of administrative data, that is, the idea that administrative records are transparent, that they speak for themselves. According to Freidson, this is a myth because administrative data are limited by their very nature. They result from participation in a structure or system about which they provide evidence. These data are formed by uniform, standardized activities and operational categories that schematically organize information from official records about certain outcomes of this structure so that they can be compared according to different parameters. To overcome this myth, it is not necessary to abandon administrative data sources but to recognize their limitations and subject them, as in the case of other myths, to the research of the social processes in which they are involved.

We do not have to agree theoretically, or politically, for that matter, with all of Freidson's stances. However, Freidson presents crucial knowledge-based parameters for considering the tense relationships between the HIMC and society and between medicine and the social sciences. These parameters demonstrate that we are not dealing with inert abstractions but with areas of thought that provide theoretical assumptions and practical prejudices about the field of objects that they seek to understand and within whose scope they seek to intervene. The assumptions that Freidson speaks of, the various myths he refers to, are involved in expanding a knowledge-based approach to medicalization. In a way, this expansion corresponds to a theoretical harmonization of the relationship between epistemology and (not only) social ontology, modes of knowledge and conceptions of (not only) social reality.

We are arguing here that what is also at stake is how different forms of knowledge put the relationship between the HIMC and our very conception of society. The two modalities of medicalization that we have been exploring both fit into a somewhat skeptical approach to the possibility of knowledge. The critical attitude, we must recognize, can often, in the case of the medicalization critique movement of which Freidson himself is a part, be reduced to moral judgment and commentary, but this is not necessarily so, provided the substantiation of the oppressing forces which become the object of criticism. At least, in the diverse formulations of medicalization critique, they tend to oppose forms of dogmatism without necessarily falling into radical skepticism. At the very least, there is an evident skepticism in the non-acceptance of the biomedical model, which is widely understood as a set of dogmas originating in the natural sciences. In Freidson's terms, by recognizing the specificity of sociological knowledge in the study of health and medicine, the myths of experience and simplicity are broken. By taking an active stance in the face of the problems in question, one breaks, at least in principle, the myth of technical aid and the myth of administrative data.

However, the conflict between the myths of objectivity and subjectivity seems especially relevant to us, as it is in this that the fundamental field of distinction between the modalities of medicalization and their versions of criticism is inscribed. Seeking to overcome the deficit of reflexivity that we have noticed and dispensing with a merely professional approach, and also understanding that it is not only the role that the concept of social control plays in the critique of medicalization that is at stake, despite its tremendous importance, it is necessary to leave the macroscale of the relationship between social science and medicine to look at the smaller representation of society, or of the social, and social science in this relationship. What our interpretation suggests is, therefore, that the relations between the HIMC and society in general and the critique of medicalization, in particular, are reconstructed from the intersection between the dogmatism–skepticism axis regarding the problem of knowledge and the objectivism–subjectivism axis, concerning the conception of social reality. From what Freidson puts forward, we can observe within the framework of a knowledge-based approach, for example, that, when adopting a realist point of view, the repressive-negative version of medicalization critique does not adopt the subjectivism in which the constructivist version ends up falling. The underlying critical attitude will not allow, in turn, to fall into the contrary myth of objectivity and the positivistic method. We believe that it is in the repressive-negative version of medicalization critique that the degree criterion is met. Nevertheless, it is now essential to underline that this can only be understood consistently following the relevance given to medical knowledge by the constructivist critics of medicalization and the subsequent bio-, cam-, pharma- extensions and the problematization of the notion of social control.

These ideas can be updated in the frame of different contexts. After the scientific and technological transformations that we have witnessed since the 1980s and given the pandemic scenario caused by the global spread of the new coronavirus, a profound reflection on the HIMC and society relationship and the corresponding relation between medicine and social science is imperative. We believe it is within the scope of an enlarged knowledge-based approach that we will be able to lay the foundation for the understanding that the pandemic situation precipitated the emergence of an already agonistic but more latent debate. On the one hand, we have been watching the strengthening of skeptical discourses concerning the regulatory and normalizing status of science and medicine. On the other hand, a certain positivist resurgence of scientific knowledge has also become notorious, namely through the more reiterated and emphatic use of the idea of the consistency of scientific evidence. The disciplinary approaches of these different domains have actually contributed to the escalation of a greater theoretical and epistemological insularity.

11. Concluding Remarks

Contrary to the option adopted by some contemporary authors, the train of thought we sought to develop did not imply the abandonment of the concept of medicalization. As we have seen, the concept of medicalization has integrated various fields, levels, objects, scales, and meanings; it articulated new structures, new agents, and new behaviors; it has been explored by related concepts, such as those of biomedicalization, camization, pharmaceuticalization, or therapeuticalization. The critical reassessments are indicative of the multiple contributions developed, the adaptative nature of the medicalization processes, and the elasticity of this concept itself.

What we sought to do was to scrutinize this long path of theoretical production, with the explicit purpose of showing to what extent some of the foundations that underlie the most widely disseminated trends of social research produce, or reproduce, an analytical narrative whose focus accentuates, in a too generic and totalizing way, ideas that reduce the diversity of forms of knowledge, paying special attention to medicine and the social sciences, integrating and expanding the notion of the transition of the discourse on HIMC.

We hope with this we can also contribute to point out, especially considering the present pandemic conjuncture, the necessity of a broad theoretical clarification in the universe of health, illness, and medicine. From this point of view, we maintain that a certain eagerness to problematize and critically reconstruct the limits of the assumptions of the so-called biomedical model may have a potential effect on the reduction of, on one side, the idea of social science and, on the other, of medicine itself to mere caricatures. For a discussion that seeks to contribute to understanding the implications of these generalizations, it is vital to show to what extent the nature of the social approaches to the HIMC is developed in coherence with some assumptions that, by being constitutive of the most structuring conceptions of some disciplinary fields themselves, can give rise to a potentially sectarian view, assumptions with which we have not ceased to confront throughout our research and from which we have sought to depart.

The first assumption corresponds to a characteristic that is, moreover, at the basis of the very disciplinary identity of sociology of health and concerns its own object of study. It is, basically, about recognizing that there is, since its emergence as a subdiscipline, a well-established division of labor between the social sciences, especially sociology, and medicine. This division is responsible for a segmentation that blocks dialogues and articulations, contributing, in this way, to the emergency of and to feed approaches that are not only distinct from each other but tend to be captive of an insularity that makes common understanding difficult.

A second assumption is often responsible for interpretative generalizations about medical knowledge. This is the use of conceptual categories that shape the historical-sociological analysis of the emergence of the biomedical model and the institutional development of modern medicine in the 19th and 20th centuries. These broad categories allow, in fact, a certain historical tidying up. However, they end up unifying, reifying, and giving a homogenizing coherence to complex realities, subverting the understanding of empirical realities that are not devoid of their theoretical continuities and material contingencies.

Finally, it is also important to consider a third assumption, this one related to the characteristic biophobia of some social scientific approaches, which is prolonged, at least in principle, by the Foucauldian and constructivist conceptualization of the anti-realist-positive modality of medicalization. It is a perspective that neglects the biological and clinical aspects of illness, leading to paradoxically breaking with the very clinical diversity of illness.

What seems to be theoretically more reasonable, analytically more productive, and normatively more responsible is the problematization of the supposedly radical unitary character of medicine, promoting a look that is less totalizing and circumscribed to large generalizing, inadvertently supported on, at the limit, reductive categories. It will not be unimportant to equate an approach that assumes and contemplates the more diverse and fragmented nature of medical vocation. However, not in the sense of presuming them to be erratic or devoid of a specific theoretical or epistemic unity. It is crucial to recognize that medicine, as a practice and field of social action, is not monolithic and, therefore, its empirical reality is not exhausted in the unity and coherence provided by analytical categories, but at the same time, it has ontological, cultural, moral, political, and epistemological frames of reference. In other words, we have to be careful not to fall into the paradox that, between professing the objective of conferring greater neutrality to medicine, or to medicalization processes, or the objective of lending them a strong evaluative charge, we end up neglecting the mosaic of what is understood by health, illness, disease, and medicine. Any effort that entails going beyond the perpetuation of the caricature, whether through unreasonable praise or unlimited criticism, around the biomedical model is in itself a serious and relevant effort with the potential to mitigate mutual misunderstandings and mystifications.

Our reconstruction of the concept of medicalization and of the movement of medicalization critique allows us to defend, against the background driven by the mentioned assumptions, a version of medical skepticism moderated by the recognition of the multi-level conditions of health and illness, namely the constraints of the socio-economic structure produced by the capitalist mode of production. Within the social studies of health, illness, and medicine, this view is contained in, or translated into, an approach to medicalization that is both realist and knowledge-based. This means that it is necessary to collect the results of the development of medicalization studies but also to go back. It is necessary, and in the current pandemic context, this seems to us to be a fundamental task, to take a knowledge-based approach, but to broaden it to include sociological forms of knowledge and thus be able to reevaluate the assumptions that threw us into the very development of the knowledge-based approach. In a context where there is a notorious strengthening of the skeptical problematizations related to the scientific and political status of medicine, a dogmatic response that resurfaces a positivist and imperialist approach to medicine is not acceptable. The necessary re-evaluation needs, in our view, to reorient the knowledge-based approach towards realism, which historically had been parting the way. This is our time for a new reckoning.

Author Contributions: Conceptualization, D.S.d.C. and H.R.; methodology, D.S.d.C. and H.R.; validation, D.S.d.C. and H.R.; investigation, D.S.d.C. and H.R.; resources, D.S.d.C. and H.R.; writing—original draft preparation, D.S.d.C. and H.R.; writing—review and editing, D.S.d.C.; project administration, D.S.d.C. All authors have read and agreed to the published version of the manuscript.

Funding: D.S.C.'s research was financed by Portuguese funds and the European Social Fund through the Doctoral Scholarship awarded by the Foundation for Science and Technology (FCT) with the reference COVID/BD/152011/2021.

Institutional Review Board Statement: Not applicable.

Informed Consent Statement: Not applicable.

Data Availability Statement: Not applicable.

Acknowledgments: We owe deep gratitude to both editors of this special issue, for all the confidence shown in the proposal of this article and throughout the writing process and for all the patience they had negotiating the deadlines. We want to take this opportunity to thank José Luís Garcia, who has supervised several previous works by both authors of the present article. José Luís Garcia was responsible for promoting in Portugal spaces for critical discussion about contemporary techno-scientific transformations, including in the field of biomedicine, a critical point of view followed by classical social theory and a specific modern idea of science. Those spaces served and continue to help us as a source of personal and academic inspiration. Hélder Raposo would also like to thank Noémia Lopes for the opportunity to carry out research, over the last few years, in the field of therapeutic consumptions and for the fact that this context has been conducive to the development of the theoretical debate around concepts such as pharmaceuticalization.

Conflicts of Interest: The authors declare no conflict of interest.

References

1. Fox, R.C. The medicalization and demedicalization of American society. *Daedalus* **1977**, *106*, 9–22.
2. Porter, R. *The Greatest Benefit to Mankind. A Medical History of Humanity*; W. W. Norton & Company: New York, NY, USA, 1997.
3. Le Fanu, J. *The Rise and Fall of Modern Medicine*; Basic Books: New York, NY, USA, 2012.
4. Eisenberg, L.; Kleinman, A. Clinical social science. In *The Relevance of Social Science for Medicine*; Eisenberg, L., Kleinman, A., Eds.; D. Reidel Publishing Company: Dordrecht, The Netherlands, 1981; pp. 1–23.
5. Lupton, D. *Medicine as Culture. Illness, Disease and the Body*; Sage: London, UK, 2012.
6. Marc, B.; Mol, A. (Eds.) *Differences in Medicine: Unraveling Practices, Techniques, and Bodies*; Duke University Press: Durham, NC, USA, 1998.
7. Navarro, V. *Crisis, Health, and Medicine: A Social Critique*; Tavistock: London, UK, 1986.
8. Carapinheiro, G. Do bio-poder ao poder médico. *Rev. Estud. Do Século XX* **2005**, *5*, 383–398.
9. Freidson, E. Viewpoint: Sociology and medicine: A polemic. *Sociol. Health Illn.* **1983**, *5*, 208–219. [CrossRef] [PubMed]
10. Albrecht, G.L.; Fitzpatrick, R.; Scrimshaw, S.C. Introduction. In *Handbook of Social Studies in Health and Medicine*; Albrecht, G.L., Fitzpatrick, R., Scrimshaw, S.C., Eds.; Sage: London, UK, 2000; pp. 1–5.
11. Scrimshaw, S.C.; Lane, S.D.; Rubinstein, R.A.; Fisher, J. Introduction. In *The SAGE Handbook of Social Studies in Health and Medicine*; Scrimshaw, S.C., Lane, S.D., Rubinstein, R.A., Fisher, J., Eds.; Sage: London, UK, 2022; pp. 1–15.
12. Turner, B.S. The history of the changing concepts of health and illness: Outline of a General Model of Illness Categories. In *Handbook of Social Studies in Health and Medicine*; Albrecht, G.L., Fitzpatrick, R., Scrimshaw, S.C., Eds.; Sage: London, UK, 2000; pp. 9–23.
13. Sontag, S. *Illness as Metaphor! AIDS and Its Metaphors*; Anchor: New York, NY, USA, 1989.
14. Scheff, T.J. Elias, Freud and Goffman: Shame as the master emotion. In *The Sociology of Norbert Elias*; Loyal, S., Quilley, S., Eds.; Cambridge University Press: Cambridge, UK, 2004; pp. 229–242.

15. Scheff, T. The Cooley-Elias-Goffman theory. *Hum. Fig.* **2017**, *6*, 1.
16. Turner, B. *Medical Power and Social Knowledge*; Sage: London, UK, 1987.
17. Turner, B. *Regulating Bodies: Essays in Medical Sociology*; Routledge: London, UK, 1992.
18. Raposo, H. A luta contra o cancro em Portugal. Análise do processo de institucionalização do Instituto Português de Oncologia. *Fórum Sociol.* **2004**, *11–12*, 177–203.
19. Kleinman, A. What is specific to Western Medicine? In *Companion Encyclopedia of the History of Medicine*; Bynum, W.F., Porter, R., Eds.; Routledge: London, UK, 1993; Volume 2, pp. 15–23.
20. Vandenberghe, F.; Véran, J.-F. The pandemic as a global social total fact. In *Pandemics, Politics, and Society. Critical Perspectives on the COVID-19 Crisis*; Delanty, G., Ed.; Walter de Gruyter: Berlin, Germany; Boston, MA, USA, 2021; pp. 171–187.
21. Rosen, G. *A History of Public Health*; Johns Hopkins University Press: Baltimore, MD, USA, 1993.
22. Bloom, S.W. *The Word as Scalpel: A History of Medical Sociology*; Oxford University Press: Oxford, UK, 2002.
23. Marx, K. *Capital: A Critique of Political Economy, Book I, the Process of Production of Capital*; Karl Marx & Frederick Engels Collected Works; Lawrence & Wishart: London, UK, 1996; Volume 35.
24. Singer, M.; Erickson, P.I. (Eds.) *A Companion to Medical Anthropology*; Wiley-Blackwell: San Francisco, CA, USA, 2011.
25. Kleinman, A. *Patients and Healers in the Context of Culture*; University of California: Berkeley, CA, USA; Berkeley Press: Berkeley, CA, USA, 1980.
26. Kleinman, A. *Writing at the Margin. Discourse between Anthropology and Medicine*; University of California Press: Berkeley, CA, USA, 1995.
27. Leslie, C. (Ed.) *Asian Medical Systems: A Comparative Study*; University of California Press: Berkeley, CA, USA, 1976.
28. Leslie, C. Medical pluralism in world perspective. *Soc. Sci. Med.* **1980**, *14B*, 191–195. [CrossRef]
29. Canguilhem, G. *The Normal and the Pathological*; Zone Books: New York, NY, USA, 1991.
30. Warner, J.H. The History of Science and the Sciences of Medicine. *Osiris* **1995**, *10*, 164–193. [CrossRef] [PubMed]
31. Sarton, G. The History of Science versus the History of Medicine. *Isis* **1935**, *23*, 315–320. [CrossRef]
32. Sigerist, H.E. The History of Medicine and the History of Science. *Bull. Inst. Hist. Med.* **1936**, *4*, 1–13.
33. Toulmin, S. Knowledge and art in the practice of medicine: Clinical judgment and historical reconstruction. In *Science, Technology, and the Art of Medicine. European-American Dialogues*; Delkeskamp-Hayes, C., Cutter, M.A.G., Eds.; Kluwer Academic Publishers: Alphen aan den Rijn, The Netherlands, 1993; pp. 231–249.
34. Brorson, S. Ludwik Fleck on proto-ideas in medicine. *Med. Health Care Philos.* **2000**, *3*, 147–152. [CrossRef] [PubMed]
35. Carapinheiro, G. *Saberes e Poderes no Hospital. Uma Sociologia dos Serviços Hospitalares*; Afrontamento: Porto, Portugal, 1993.
36. Marques, M.S. *O Espelho Declinado: Natureza e Legitimação do Acto Médico*; Colibri: Lisboa, Portugal, 1999.
37. Gadamer, H. *The Enigma of Health: The Art of Healing in a Scientific Age*; Stanford University Press: Redwood, CA, USA, 1996.
38. Sfez, L. *La Santé Parfaite. Critique D'une Nouvelle Utopie*; Seuil: Paris, France, 1995.
39. Fitzpatrick, M. *The Tyranny of Health*; Routledge: London, UK, 2001.
40. Habermas, J. *The Future of Human Nature*; Polity Press: Cambridge, UK, 2003.
41. Lupton, D. *The Imperative of Health. Public Health and the Regulated Body*; Sage: London, UK, 1995.
42. Martins, M. *Experimentum Humanum. Civilização Tecnológica e Condição Humana*; Relógio D'Água: Lisboa, Portugal, 2011.
43. Garcia, J.L. Engenharia Genética dos Seres Humanos, Mercadorização e Ética. Uma Análise Sociopolítica da Biotecnologia. Ph.D. Thesis, University of Lisbon, Lisbon, Portugal, 2004.
44. Sandel, M. *The Case against Perfection: Ethics in the Age of Genetic Engineering*; Harvard University Press: Cambridge, UK, 2007.
45. Jonas, H. *The Imperative of Responsibility: In Search of Ethics for the Technological Age*; University of Chicago Press: Chicago, IL, USA, 1979.
46. Delkeskamp-Hayes, C.; Cutter, M.A.G. (Eds.) *Science, Technology, and the Art of Medicine. European-American Dialogues*; Kluwer Academic Publishers: Alphen aan den Rijn, The Netherlands, 1993.
47. Gernsheim, E.B. Health and responsability: From social change to technological change and vice versa. In *The Risk Society and Beyond. Critical Issues for Social Theory*; Barbara, A., Beck, U., Loon, J.V., Eds.; Sage: London, UK, 2000; pp. 122–135.
48. Boorse, C. Health as a theoretical concept. *Philos. Sci.* **1977**, *44*, 542–573. [CrossRef]
49. Boorse, C. A rebuttal on health. In *What is Disease?* Humber, J.M., Almeder, R.F., Eds.; Biomedical Ethics Reviews; Humana Press: Totowa, NJ, USA, 1997; pp. 1–134.
50. Nordenfelt, L. *On the Nature of Health: An ActionTheoretic Approach*; Kluwer Academic Publishers: Dordrecht, The Netherlands, 1995.
51. Nordenfelt, L. The concepts of health and illness revisited. *Med. Health Care Philos.* **2007**, *10*, 5–10. [CrossRef] [PubMed]
52. Fulford, K.W.M. Praxis makes perfect: Illness as a bridge between biological concepts of disease and social conceptions of health. *Theor. Med.* **1993**, *14*, 305–320. [CrossRef] [PubMed]
53. Fulford, K.W.M. *Moral Theory and Medical Practice*; Cambridge University Press: Cambridge, UK, 1989.
54. Boorse, C. On the distinction between disease and illness. *Philos. Public Aff.* **1975**, *5*, 49–68.
55. Eisenberg, L. Disease and illness: Distinctions between professional and popular ideas of sickness. *Cult. Med. Psychiatry* **1977**, *1*, 9–23. [CrossRef]
56. Castiglioni, A. *A History of Medicine*; Alfred A. Knopf: New York, NY, USA, 1941.
57. Ackerknecht, E.H. *A Short History of Medicine*; Johns Hopkins University Press: Baltimore, MD, USA, 1968.

58. Ackerknecht, E.H. *Therapeutics from the Primitives to the Twentieth Century*; Hafner: New York, NY, USA, 1973.
59. Roderick, E. (Ed.) *McGrew Encyclopaedia of Medical History*; McGrawHill: New York, NY, USA, 1985.
60. Nutton, V. *From Democedes to Harvey: Studies in the History of Medicine*; Variorum Reprint: London, UK, 1988.
61. Jouanna, J. *Hippocrate*; Librairie Arthème Fayard: Paris, French, 1992.
62. Jouanna, J. *Greek Medicine from Hippocrates to Galen*; Brill: Leiden, The Netherlands; Boston, MA, USA, 2012.
63. Longrigg, J. *Greek Rational Medicine. Philosophy and Medicine from Alcmaeon to the Alexandrians*; Sage: London, UK, 1993.
64. Lloyd, G.; Sivin, N. *The Way and the Word. Science and Medicine in Early China and Greece*; Yale University Press: New Haven, CT, USA; London, UK, 2002.
65. Lloyd, G.E.R. *In the Grip of Disease. Studies in the Greek Imagination*; Oxford University Press: Oxford, UK, 2003.
66. Bynum, W.F.; Porter, R. (Eds.) *Companion Encyclopedia of the History of Medicine*; Routledge: London, UK, 1993; Volume 2.
67. Nutton, V. Murders and miracles: Lay attitudes towards medicine in classical antiquity. In *Patients and Practitioners. Lay Perceptions of Medicine in Pre-Industrial Society*; Porter, R., Ed.; Cambridge University Press: Cambridge, UK, 1985; pp. 24–53.
68. Nutton, V. Healers in the medical market-place: Towards a social history of Graeco Roman medicine. In *Medicine in Society. Historical Essays*; Wear, A., Ed.; Cambridge University Press: Cambridge, UK, 1992; pp. 15–58.
69. Marques, M.S. A Medicina Enquanto Ciência do Indivíduo. Ph.D. Thesis, University of Lisbon, Lisbon, Portugal, 2002.
70. Ackerknecht, E.H. *Medicine at the Paris Hospital 1794–1848*; John Hopkins Press: Baltimore, MD, USA, 1967.
71. Rosen, G. The philosophy of ideology and the emergence of modern medicine in France. *Bull. Hist. Med.* **1946**, *20*, 328–339.
72. Rosen, G. Hospitals, medical care and social policy in the French revolution. *Bull. Hist. Med.* **1956**, *30*, 124–149.
73. Ackerknecht, E.W. Elisha Barlett and the philosophy of the Paris School. *Bull. Hist. Med.* **1950**, *24*, 43–60.
74. Waddington, I. The role of the hospital in the development of modern medicine: A sociological analysis. *Sociology* **1973**, *7*, 221–224. [CrossRef]
75. Foucault, M. *The Birth of the Clinic*; Tavistock Publications: London, UK, 1973.
76. Jewson, N. The disappearence of the sick man from medical cosmology 1770–1870. *Sociology* **1976**, *10*, 225–244. [CrossRef]
77. Armstrong, D. The rise of surveillance medicine. *Sociol. Health Illn.* **1995**, *17*, 393–405. [CrossRef]
78. Vegter, M.W. Towards precision medicine: A new biomedical cosmology. *Med. Health Care Philos.* **2018**, *21*, 443–456. [CrossRef]
79. Nettleton, S. The emergence of e-scaped medicine? *Sociology* **2004**, *38*, 661–679. [CrossRef]
80. Riso, B. A Saúde Armazenada. O Biobanco na Reconfiguração da Saúde na Sociedade Contemporânea. Ph.D. Thesis, Lisbon University Institute, Lisbon, Portugal, 2021.
81. Lloyd, G.E.R. A return to cases and the pluralism of ancient medical traditions. In *Medicines and Markets: Essays on Ancient Medicine in Honour of Vivian Nutton*; Totelin, L.M.V., Flemming, R., Eds.; The Classical Press of Wales: London, UK, 2020; pp. 71–86.
82. Wieland, W. The concept of the art medicine. In *Science, Technology, and the Art of Medicine. European-American Dialogues*; Delkeskamp-Hayes, C., Cutter, M.A.G., Eds.; Kluwer Academic Publishers: Alphen aan den Rijn, The Netherlands, 1993; pp. 165–182.
83. Fischer, E. How to practise philosophy as therapy: Philosophical therapy and therapeutic philosophy. *Metaphilosophy* **2011**, *42*, 49–82. [CrossRef]
84. Carapinheiro, G. Médicos e representações da medicina: Humanismo e tecnicismo nas práticas médicas hospitalares. *Sociol. Probl. E Prát.* **1991**, *9*, 27–41.
85. Stempsey, W.E. Medical humanities: Introduction to the theme. *Med. Health Care Philos.* **2007**, *10*, 359–361. [CrossRef]
86. Antunes, J.L. *A Nova Medicina*; Fundação Francisco Manuel dos Santos: Lisboa, Portugal, 2012.
87. Wiesing, U. From art to science: A new epistemological status for medicine? On expectations regarding personalized medicine. *Med. Health Care Philos.* **2018**, *21*, 457–466. [CrossRef]
88. Gerhardt, U. *Ideas about Illness: An Intellectual and Political History of Medical Sociology*; New York University Press: New York, NY, USA, 1989.
89. Laursen, J.C. Medicine and skepticism: Martin Martinez (1684–1734). In *The Return of Scepticism. From Hobbes and Descartes to Bayle*; Paganini, G., Ed.; Springer: Berlin, Germany, 2000; pp. 305–325.
90. Raynaud, M. Skepticism in medicine: Past and present. *Linacre Q.* **1981**, *48*, 8.
91. Merry, A.; McCall Smith, A. *Errors, Medicine and the Law*; Cambridge University Press: Cambridge, UK, 2001.
92. Kohn, L.; Corrigan, J.; Donaldson, M. (Eds.) *To Err Is Human. Building a Safer Health System*; National Academies Press: Washington, WA, USA, 2000.
93. Harpwood, V. *Medicine, Malpractice and Misapprehensions*; Routledge-Cavendish: Abindon, UK, 2007.
94. Raposo, H. Risco e incerteza no pensamento biomédico: Notas teóricas sobre o advento da quantificação e da prova experimental na medicina moderna. *Anál. Anal. Soc.* **2009**, *44*, 747–765.
95. Stegenga, J. Effectiveness of medical interventions. *Stud. Hist. Philos. Biol. Biomed. Sci.* **2015**, *54*, 34–44. [CrossRef]
96. Stegenga, J. Measuring effectiveness. *Stud. Hist. Philos. Biol. Biomed. Sci.* **2015**, *54*, 62–71. [CrossRef] [PubMed]
97. Stegenga, J. *Medical Nihilism*; Oxford University Press: Oxford, UK, 2018.
98. Cochrane, A.L. *Effectiveness and Efficiency. Random Reflections on Health Services*; The Nuffield Provincial Hospitals Trust: Nuffield, UK, 1972.
99. McKeown, T. *The Modern Rise of Population*; Edward Arnold: London, UK, 1976.

100. McKeown, T. *The Role of Medicine. Dream, Mirage or Nemesis?* Nuffield Provincial Hospitals Trust: London, UK, 1976.
101. McKinlay, J.; McKinlay, S.M. The questionable contribution of medical measures to the decline of mortality in the United States in the twentieth century. *Milbank Meml. Fund Q. Health Soc.* **1977**, *55*, 405–428. [CrossRef]
102. Department of Health and Social Security. *Inequalities in Health: Report of a Research Working Group*; Department of Health and Social Security: London, UK, 1980.
103. Solar, O.; Irwin, A. Discussion Paper 2 (Policy and Practice). In *A Conceptual Framework for Action on the Social Determinants of Health*; World Health Organization: Geneva, Switzerland, 2010.
104. Nunes, J.A. Saúde, direito à saúde e justiça sanitária. *Rev. Crít. Ciênc. Soc.* **2009**, *87*, 143–169. [CrossRef]
105. Hartman, C.E.; González, S.T.; Guzmán, R.G. (Eds.) *Determinación Social o Determinantes Sociales de la Salud?* Universidad Autónoma Metropolitana: Mexico City, México, 2011.
106. Borde, E.; Hernández-Álvarez, M.; Porto, M.F.S. Uma análise crítica da abordagem dos determinantes sociais da saúde a partir da Medicina Social e Saúde Coletiva Latino-americana. *Saúde Debate* **2015**, *39*, 841–854. [CrossRef]
107. Jakovljevic, M.; Fernandes, P.O.; Teixeira, J.P.; Rancic, N.; Timofeyev, Y.; Reshetnikov, V. Underlying differences in health spending within the World Health Organisation Europe Region—Comparing EU15, EU Post-2004, CIS, EU candidate, and CARINFONET countries. *Int. J. Environ. Res. Public Health* **2019**, *16*, 3043. [CrossRef] [PubMed]
108. Jakovljevic, M.; Timofeyev, Y.; Ranabhat, C.L.; Fernandes, P.O.; Teixeira, J.P.; Rancic, N.; Reshetnikov, V. Real GDP growth rates and healthcare spending–comparison between the G7 and the EM7 countries. *Glob. Health* **2020**, *16*, 64. [CrossRef] [PubMed]
109. Jakovljevic, M.; Liu, Y.; Cerda, A.; Simonyan, M.; Correia, T.; Mariita, R.M.; Kumara, A.S.; Garcia, L.; Krstic, K.; Osabohien, R.; et al. The Global South political economy of health financing and spending landscape-history and presence. *J. Med. Econ.* **2021**, *24*, 25–33. [CrossRef]
110. Jakovljevic, M.; Lamnisos, D.; Westerman, R.; Chattu, V.K.; Cerda, A. Future health spending forecast in leading emerging BRICS markets in 2030: Health policy implications. *Health Res. Policy Syst.* **2022**, *20*, 1–4. [CrossRef]
111. Davis, J. How medicalization lost its way. *Society* **2006**, *43*, 51–56. [CrossRef]
112. Zorzanelli, R.T.; Ortega, F.; Bezerra Júnior, B. Um panorama sobre as variações em torno do conceito de medicalização entre 1950–2010. *Ciênc. Saúde Colet.* **2014**, *19*, 1859–1868. [CrossRef]
113. Lupton, D. Foucault and the medicalisation critique. In *Foucault, Health and Medicine*; Petersen, A.R., Bunton, R., Eds.; Routledge: London, UK, 1997; pp. 94–110.
114. Pitts, J. Social control: The concept. In *International Encyclopedia of Social Sciences*; Sills, D., Ed.; McMillan: New York, NY, USA, 1968; Volume 14, pp. 381–396.
115. Strong, P.M. Sociological imperialism and the profession of medicine. A critical examination of the thesis of medical imperialism. *Soc. Sci. Med.* **1979**, *13A*, 199–215. [CrossRef]
116. Wootton, B. Sickness or sin? *20 Century* **1956**, *159*, 433–442.
117. Wootton, B. *Social Science and Social Pathology*; Macmillan Co.: New York, NY, USA, 1959.
118. Szasz, T. The myth of mental illness. *Am. Psychol.* **1960**, *15*, 113–118. [CrossRef]
119. Szasz, T. *The Myth of Mental Illness: Foundations of a Theory of Personal Conduct*; Harper Row: New York, NY, USA, 1974.
120. Szasz, T. *The Manufacture of Madness. A Comparative Study of the Inquisition and the Mental Health Movement*; Syracuse University Press: New York, NY, USA, 1997.
121. Scheff, T.J. *Being Mentally Ill: A Sociological Theory*; Aldine: Chicago, IL, USA, 1966.
122. Lowenberg, J.S.; Davis, F. Beyond medicalisation-demedicalisation: The case of holistic health. *Sociol. Health Illn.* **1994**, *16*, 579–599. [CrossRef]
123. Wolinsky, F.D. The professional dominance perspective, revisited. *Milbank Q.* **1988**, *66*, 33–47. [CrossRef]
124. Freidson, E. *Professional Dominance: The Social Structure of Medical Care*; Atherton Press: New York, NY, USA, 1970.
125. Freidson, E. *Profession of Medicine. A Study of the Sociology of Applied Knowledge*; The University of Chicago Press: Chicago, IL, USA, 1988.
126. Halpern, S.; Anspach, R.R. The study of medical institutions. *Work. Occup.* **1993**, *20*, 279–295. [CrossRef]
127. Bosk, C.L. Avoiding conventional understandings: The enduring legacy of Eliot Freidson. *Sociol. Health Illn.* **2006**, *28*, 637–646. [CrossRef]
128. Conrad, P. Eliot Freidson's revolution in medical sociology. *Health Interdiscip. J. Soc. Study Health Illn. Med.* **2007**, *11*, 141–144. [CrossRef]
129. Illich, I.; McKnight, J.; Zola, I.K.; Caplan, J.; Shaiken, H. *Disabling Professions*; Marion Boyars: London, UK, 1977.
130. Johnson, T. *Professions and Power*; Macmillan Press: London, UK, 1972.
131. Abbott, A. *The System of Professions. An Essay on the Division of Expert Labor*; The University of Chicago Press: Chicago, IL, USA, 1988.
132. Larson, M. *The Rise of Professionalism. Monopolies of Competence and Sheltered Markets*; Transaction Publishers: New Brunswick, NJ, USA, 2013.
133. Starr, P. *The Social Transformation of American Medicine. The Rise of a Sovereign Profession and the Making of a Vast Industry*; Basic Books: New York, NY, USA, 1982.
134. Cockerham, W. Medical Sociology and Sociological Theory. In *The Blackwell Companion to Medical Sociology*; Cockerham, W., Ed.; Blackwell Publishing: Oxford, UK, 2001; pp. 3–22.

135. Cockerham, W. The rise of theory in Medical Sociology. In *Medical Sociology on the Move: New Directions in Theory*; Cockerham, W., Ed.; Springer: New York, NY, USA, 2012; pp. 1–10.
136. Lidler, E. Definitions of health and illness and medical sociology. *Soc. Sci. Med.* **1979**, *13*, 723–731. [CrossRef]
137. Collyer, F. Origins and canons: Medicine and the history of sociology. *Hist. Hum. Sci.* **2010**, *23*, 86–108. [CrossRef]
138. Zola, I.K. Medicine as an institution of social control. *Sociol. Rev.* **1972**, *20*, 487–504. [CrossRef] [PubMed]
139. Waitzkin, H. *The Second Sickness: Contradictions of Capitalist Health Care*; Free Press: New York, NY, USA, 1983.
140. Hedgecoe, A. Geneticization, medicalisation and polemics. *Med. Health Care Philos.* **1998**, *1*, 235–243. [CrossRef]
141. Horrobin, D.F. *Medical Hubris: A Reply to Ivan Illich*; Chuchill Livingstone: Edinburgh, UK, 1978.
142. Eisenberg, L. A Medicina e a ideia de progresso. In *Progresso: Realidade ou Ilusão?* Marx, L., Mazlish, B., Eds.; Bizâncio: Lisboa, Portugal, 2001; pp. 79–109.
143. Illich, I. *Limits to Medicine. Medical Nemesis: The Expropriation of Health*; Boyars: London, UK, 2010.
144. Ferreira, C.A.M. A Medicalização dos Sanatórios Populares: Desafios e Formas de um Processo Social. Ph.D. Thesis, New University of Lisbon, Lisbon, Portugal, 2007.
145. Aïach, P.; Delanoe, D. (Eds.) *L'ère de la Médicalisation. Ecce Homo Sanitas*; Anthropos: Paris, French, 1998.
146. Szasz, T. *The Medicalization of Everyday Life. Selected Essays*; Syracuse University Press: New York, NY, USA, 2007.
147. Hofmann, B. Medicalization and overdiagnosis: Different but alike. *Med. Health Care Philos.* **2016**, *19*, 253–264. [CrossRef] [PubMed]
148. Kaczmarek, E. How to distinguish medicalization from over-medicalization? *Med. Health Care Philos.* **2019**, *22*, 119–128. [CrossRef]
149. Gracia, D. The many faces of autonomy. *Theor. Med. Bioeth.* **2012**, *33*, 57–64. [CrossRef]
150. Turner, B.S. *The Cambridge Dictionary of Sociology*; Cambridge University Press: Cambridge, UK, 2006.
151. Schreier, H.; Berger, L. On medical imperialism. A letter. *Lancet* **1974**, *I*, 1161. [CrossRef]
152. Taylor, R. *Medicine Out of Control. The Anatomy of a Malignant Technology*; Macmillan Education: Victoria, Australia, 1979.
153. Waitzkin, H.; Waterman, B. *The Exploitation of Illness in Capitalist Society*; Bobbs-Merrill: Indianapolis, IN, USA, 1974.
154. Conrad, P.; Schneider, J.W. Looking at levels of medicalization: A comment on Strong's critique of medical imperialism. *Soc. Sci. Med.* **1980**, *14A*, 75–79.
155. Conrad, P.; Schneider, J.W. *Deviance and Medicalization: From Badness to Sickness*; Mosby: St. Louis, MO, USA, 1980.
156. Conrad, P. Medicalization and social control. *Annu. Rev. Sociol.* **1992**, *18*, 209–232. [CrossRef]
157. Wilkinson, D.Y. Sociological imperialism: A brief comment on the field. *Sociol. Q.* **1968**, *9*, 397–400. [CrossRef]
158. Murcott, A. (Ed.) *Sociology and Medicine Selected Essays by P.M. Strong*; Routledge: London, UK, 2018.
159. Foucault, M. *Medicina e Historia. El Pensamiento de Michel Foucault*; Pan American Health Organization: Washington, WA, USA, 1978.
160. Berg, M. Turning a practice into a science: Reconceptualizing postwar medical practice. *Soc. Sci. Med.* **1995**, *25*, 437–476. [CrossRef] [PubMed]
161. Sturdy, S.; Cooter, R. Science, scientific management, and the transformation of medicine in Britain c.1870–1950. *Hist. Sci.* **1998**, *36*, 421–466. [CrossRef] [PubMed]
162. Gordon, D. Clinical science and clinical expertise: Changing boundaries between art and science in medicine. In *Biomedicine Examined*; Lock, M., Gordon, D., Eds.; Kluwer Academic Publishers: Alphen aan den Rijn, The Netherlands, 1988; pp. 257–295.
163. Cunningham, A.; Williams, P. (Eds.) *The Laboratory Revolution in Medicine*; Cambridge University Press: Cambridge, UK, 1992.
164. Burri, R.V.; Dumit, J. (Eds.) *Biomedicine as Culture Instrumental Practices, Technoscientific Knowledge, and New Modes of Life*; Routledge: London, UK, 2007.
165. Clarke, J. Doing the right thing? Managerialism and Social Welfare. In *The Sociology of the Caring Professions*; Abbot, P., Meerabeau, L., Eds.; Falmer Press: London, UK, 1998; pp. 234–254.
166. Carvalho, M.T. *Nova Gestão Pública e Reformas da Saúde. O Profissionalismo Numa Encruzilhada*; Edições Sílabo: Lisboa, Portugal, 2009.
167. Correia, T. New public management in the Portuguese health sector: A comprehensive reading. *Sociol. Line* **2011**, *2*, 573–598.
168. Hunter, D. From tribalism to corporatism: The continuing managerial challenge to medical dominance. In *Challenging Medicine*; Kelleher, D., Gabe, J., Williams, G., Eds.; Routledge: London, UK, 2006; pp. 1–23.
169. Raposo, H. As implicações dos indicadores de desempenho contratualizados na prática clínica da Medicina Geral e Familiar: Um modelo profissional em mutação? *Sociol. Rev. Fac. Let. Univ. Porto* **2018**, *35*, 63–84. [CrossRef]
170. Raposo, H. A padronização em contexto: Uma análise qualitativa sobre a incorporação das Normas de orientação Clínica em Medicina Geral e Familiar. *Anál. Soc.* **2018**, *228*, 702–731. [CrossRef]
171. Raposo, H. Reconfigurações profissionais em contextos de mudança. O papel da medicina geral e familiar. *Sociol. Probl. E Prát.* **2019**, *91*, 77–96.
172. Armstrong, D. *The Political Anatomy of the Body*; Cambridge University Press: Cambridge, UK, 1983.
173. Petersen, A.R.; Bunton, R. (Eds.) *Foucault, Health and Medicine*; Routledge: London, UK, 1997.
174. Jones, C.; Porter, R. (Eds.) *Reassessing Foucault. Power, Medicine and the Body*; Routledge: London, UK, 1994.
175. Rose, N. *Governing the Soul: The Shaping of the Private Self*; Routledge: London, UK, 1990.
176. Fox, N.J. *Postmodernism, Sociology and Health*; Open University Press: Buckingham, UK, 1993.
177. Fox, N.J. *Beyond Health: Postmodernism and Embodiment*; Free Association Books: London, UK, 1999.

178. Bury, M.R. Social constructionism and the development of Medical Sociology. *Sociol. Health Illn.* **1986**, *8*, 137–169. [CrossRef]
179. Hacking, I. *The Social Construction of What?* Harvard University Press: London, UK, 1999.
180. Garcia, J.L.; Martins, H. O *ethos* da ciência e suas transformações contemporâneas, com especial atenção à biotecnologia. *Sci. Stud.* **2009**, *7*, 83–104.
181. Brown, P. Naming and framing: The social construction of diagnosis and illness. *J. Health Soc. Behav.* **1995**, *35*, 34–52. [CrossRef]
182. Barker, K. The social construction of illness. Medicalization and contested illness. In *Handbook of Medical Sociology*; Bird, C., Conrad, P., Fremont, A., Timmermans, S., Eds.; Vanderbilt University Press: Nashville, TN, USA, 2010; pp. 147–162.
183. Stein, H.F. *American Medicine as Culture*; Routledge: London, UK, 2018.
184. Pool, R.; Geissler, W. *Medical Anthropology*; Open University Press: London, UK, 2005.
185. Collyer, F. Max Weber, historiography, medical knowledge, and the formation of medicine. *Electron. J. Sociol.* **2008**, *7*, 1–15.
186. Marques, T.P.; Portugal, S. Medicalização e produção da saúde: Trajetórias de investigação. In *A Saúde Reinventada. Novas Perspectivas Sobre a Medicalização da Vida*; Marques, T.P., Portugal, S., Eds.; CES/Almedina: Coimbra, Portugal, 2021; pp. 11–28.
187. Freese, J.; Li, J.-C.A.; Wade, L. The potential relevances of Biology to social inquiry. *Annu. Rev. Sociol.* **2003**, *29*, 233–256. [CrossRef]
188. Timmermans, S.; Haas, S. Towards a Sociology of Disease. *Sociol. Health Illn.* **2008**, *30*, 659–676. [CrossRef] [PubMed]
189. Williams, S. Sociological imperialism and the profession of medicine revisited: Where are we now? *Sociol. Health Illn.* **2001**, *23*, 135–158. [CrossRef]
190. Halfmann, D. Recognizing medicalization and demedicalization: Discourses, practices and identities. *Health: Interdiscip. J. Soc. Study Health Illn. Med.* **2011**, *16*, 186–207. [CrossRef]
191. Conrad, P. The shifting engines of medicalization. *J. Health Soc. Behav.* **2005**, *46*, 3–14. [CrossRef]
192. Conrad, P. *The Medicalization of Society: On the Transformation of Human Conditions into Treatable Disorders*; Johns Hopkins University Press: Baltimore, MD, USA, 2007.
193. Busfield, J. The concept of medicalisation reassessed. *Sociol. Health Illn.* **2017**, *39*, 759–774. [CrossRef] [PubMed]
194. Light, D. Countervailing powers. A framework for professions in transition. In *Health Professions and the State in Europe*; Johnson, T., Larkin, G., Saks, M., Eds.; Routledge: London, UK, 1995; pp. 25–41.
195. Furedi, F. Medicalisation in a therapy culture. In *A Sociology of Health*; Wainwright, D., Ed.; Sage Publications: London, UK, 2008; pp. 97–114.
196. Arskey, H. Expert and lay participation in the construction of medical knowledge. *Sociol. Health Illn.* **1994**, *16*, 448–468.
197. Torres, J. Medicalizing to demedicalize: Lactation consultants and the (de)medicalization of breastfeeding. *Soc. Sci. Med.* **2014**, *100*, 159–166. [CrossRef] [PubMed]
198. Ballard, K.; Elston, M.A. Medicalisation: A multi-dimensional concept. *Soc. Theory Health* **2005**, *3*, 228–241. [CrossRef]
199. Illich, I. (Ed.) Twelve years after Medical Nemesis: A plea for body history. In *In the Mirror of the Past: Lectures and Addresses, 1978–1990*; Marion Boyars: New York, NY, USA, 1992; pp. 211–217.
200. Clarke, A.E.; Mamo, L.; Fosket, J.R.; Fishman, J.R.; Shim, J.K. *Biomedicalization: Technoscience, Health, and Illness in the U.S.*; Duke University Press: Durham, NC, USA, 2010.
201. Moynihan, R.; Heath, I.; Henry, D. Selling sickness: The pharmaceutical industry and disease mongering. *BMJ* **2002**, *324*, 886–890. [CrossRef] [PubMed]
202. Almeida, J. Towards the Camisation of Health? The Countervailing Power of CAM in Relation to the Portuguese Mainstream Healthcare System. Ph.D. Thesis, University of London, London, UK, 2012.
203. Williams, S.J.; Seale, C.; Boden, S.; Lowe, P.; Steinberg, D.L. Waking up to sleepiness: Modafinil, the media and the pharmaceuticalisation of everyday/night life. *Sociol. Health Illn.* **2008**, *30*, 839–855. [CrossRef]
204. Abraham, J. Pharmaceuticalization of society in context: Theoretical, empirical and health Dimensions. *Sociology* **2010**, *44*, 603–622. [CrossRef]
205. Fox, N.; Ward, K. Pharma in the bedroom . . . and the kitchen . . . The pharmaceuticalisation of daily life. *Sociol. Health Illn.* **2008**, *30*, 856–868. [CrossRef]
206. Lexchin, J. Lifestyle drugs: Issues for debate. *Can. Med. Assoc. J.* **2001**, *164*, 1449–1451.
207. Flower, R. Lifestyle drugs: Pharmacology and the social agenda. *Trends Pharmacol. Sci.* **2004**, *25*, 182–185. [CrossRef]
208. Quintero, G. Rx for a party: A qualitative analysis of recreational pharmaceutical use in collegiate setting. *J. Am. Coll. Health* **2009**, *58*, 64–70. [CrossRef] [PubMed]
209. Vrecko, S. Everyday drug diversions: A qualitative study of the illicit exchange and non-medical use of prescription stimulants on a university campus. *Soc. Sci. Med.* **2015**, *131*, 297–304. [CrossRef]
210. Williams, S.J.; Gabe, J.; Davis, P. The sociology of pharmaceuticals: Progress and prospects. *Sociol. Health Illn.* **2008**, *30*, 813–824. [CrossRef]
211. Pegado, E.; Lopes, N.; Zózimo, J. Pharmaceuticalisation and the social management of sleep in old age. *Aging Soc.* **2017**, *38*, 1645–1666. [CrossRef]
212. Williams, S.; Meadows, R.; Coveney, C. Desynchronised times? Chronobiology, (bio)medicalisation and the rhythms of life itself. *Sociol. Health Illn.* **2021**, *43*, 1501–1517. [CrossRef]
213. Coveney, C.; Gabe, J.; Williams, S. The sociology of cognitive enhancement: Medicalisation and beyond. *Health Sociol. Rev.* **2011**, *20*, 381–393. [CrossRef]

214. Morrison, M. Growth hormone, enhancement and the pharmaceuticalisation of short stature. *Soc. Sci. Med.* **2015**, *131*, 199–206. [CrossRef] [PubMed]
215. Lopes, N.; Clamote, T.; Raposo, H.; Pegado, E.; Rodrigues, C. Medications, youth therapeutic cultures and performance consumptions: A sociological approach. *Health Interdiscip. J. Soc. Study Health Illn. Med.* **2015**, *19*, 430–448. [CrossRef] [PubMed]
216. Lopes, N.; Rodrigues, C. Medicamentos, consumos de performance e culturas terapêuticas em mudança. *Sociol. Probl. E Prát.* **2015**, *78*, 9–28. [CrossRef]
217. Clamote, T.C. Reverberações da medicalização: Paisagens e trajectórias informacionais em consumos de performance. *Sociol. Rev. Fac. Let. Univ. Porto* **2015**, *29*, 35–57.
218. Rodrigues, C.; Lopes, N.; Hardon, A. Beyond health: Medicines, food supplements, energetics and the commodification of self-performance in Maputo. *Sociol. Health Illn.* **2019**, *41*, 1005–1022. [CrossRef] [PubMed]
219. Raposo, H.; Rodrigues, C. Imperativos e investimentos de performance em contextos juvenis: Percepções e formas de gestão do risco e da eficácia. In *Super Humanos. Desafios e Limites da Intervenção no Cérebro*; Barbosa, M., Pussetti, C., Eds.; Edições Colibri: Lisboa, Portugal, 2021; pp. 77–104.
220. Williams, S.J.; Coveney, C.; Gabe, J. The concept of medicalisation reassessed: A response to Joan Busfield. *Sociol. Health Illn.* **2017**, *39*, 775–780. [CrossRef]
221. Correia, T. Revisiting medicalization: A critique of the assumptions of what counts as medical knowledge. *Front. Sociol.* **2017**, *2*, 14. [CrossRef]

MDPI
St. Alban-Anlage 66
4052 Basel
Switzerland
Tel. +41 61 683 77 34
Fax +41 61 302 89 18
www.mdpi.com

Societies Editorial Office
E-mail: societies@mdpi.com
www.mdpi.com/journal/societies

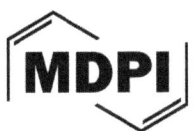

www.ingramcontent.com/pod-product-compliance
Lightning Source LLC
LaVergne TN
LVHW070635100526
838202LV00012B/810